Common Cases in Women's Primary Care Clinics

Massoud Mahmoudi

Editor

Common Cases in Women's Primary Care Clinics

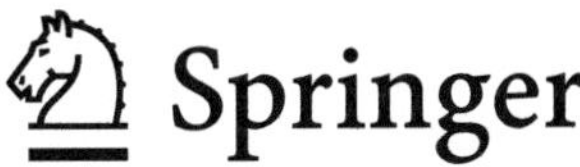 Springer

Editor
Massoud Mahmoudi
Department of Medicine
University of California San Francisco
San Francisco, CA, USA

ISBN 978-3-031-48571-8   ISBN 978-3-031-48569-5   (eBook)
https://doi.org/10.1007/978-3-031-48569-5

This Springer imprint is published by the registered company Springer Nature Switzerland AG
The registered company address is: Gewerbestrasse 11, 6330 Cham, Switzerland

Paper in this product is recyclable

To the memory of my mother, Zohreh, and my father, Mohammad H. Mahmoudi, and to my wife, Lily, and my sons, Sam and Sina, for their continuous support and encouragement.

Preface

I was driven to compile this distinctive collection for two main reasons. First, as I was searching for primary care clinics for women, I surprisingly found only a handful across the United States. Most of the clinics are Ob/gyn clinics or are run by individual providers. Second, when I reviewed clinical interests of primary care medical providers in academic centers, amazingly, there were limited individuals who listed interest for women primary care. Since I joined the UCSF Women's Health Primary Care Clinic as a preceptor, I have been fortunate to be part of a team of enthusiastic, knowledgeable, and interested primary providers of women care. Here in our clinic, a group of faculty members, nurse practitioners, and internal medicine residents work hand-in-hand as a team with the same interest to provide primary care services to women in need.

In addition to my colleagues at UCSF, I have been privileged to extend my hand to my other colleagues, who are very well respected in their fields, to participate and contribute to this collection. This short, yet comprehensive reference presents common cases in women primary care clinics. The book is divided into 19 chapters. Each chapter presents 1–2 common cases followed by discussion. The selected cases are examples of common cases, which are seen in women primary care clinics.

The production of this book would not have been possible without the support of the editorial team at Springer Nature. I am specifically grateful to Michelle Tam, the acquisition editor, and Richard Lansing, Editorial Director of the clinical medicine books team, and the entire production team.

San Francisco, CA, USA

Massoud Mahmoudi

Contents

Part I
Introduction

Chapter 1
Introduction to Women's Primary Care

Amrita Ayer and Massoud Mahmoudi

1.1 Introduction

Primary care comprises the largest interface for health care in the USA today. The field seeks to address acute and chronic health concerns, diagnose the undifferentiated patient, connect patients to appropriate specialty services, and provide data-driven, value-based preventative care. Beyond these diagnostic and therapeutic mandates, primary care providers must also understand and address the social and structural concerns of patients, recognizing that the majority of health outcomes stem from circumstances outside of the clinic. With such a broad scope, the question must be asked: how did primary care become the specialty it is today?

1.1.1 A Brief History of Primary Care

The 1978 International Conference of Primary Health Care and subsequent Declaration of Alma-Alta established primary care as a global priority in achieving "Health for All." This declaration was bookended by the 1961 Millis Report, which underscored the need for general practitioners who would serve as "primary physicians" for their patients, and the Institute of Medicine's creation of a formal definition of primary care in 1996:"the provision of integrated, accessible health care services by clinicians who are accountable for addressing a large majority of personal health care needs, developing a sustained partnership with patients, and practicing in the context of family and community." The past few decades have brought

A. Ayer (✉) · M. Mahmoudi
Women's Health Primary Care Clinic, Department of Medicine, University of California, San Francisco, CA, USA
e-mail: amrita.ayer@ucsf.edu

M. Mahmoudi (ed.), *Common Cases in Women's Primary Care Clinics*,
https://doi.org/10.1007/978-3-031-48569-5_1

3

further revisions to the conceptualization of primary care, as the field has adapted to an evolving landscape of fragmented, costly, inequitable care and, most recently, the COVID-19 pandemic.

The modern-day concept of a primary care physician emerged from World War II. Prior to the twentieth century, the majority of providers served as de facto general physicians, operating alone to provide basic medical care to patients. The growth of subspecialty services leading up to World War II presented an opportunity to reexamine the role of primary care, as physicians increasingly sought to narrow their focus, leaving a vacuum in services. As a result, a number of reports, including the Millis Report above, were published advocating for the establishment of primary care as a specialized field in itself. These efforts led to the creation of Family Medicine as a specialty in the 1960s and the formalization of fields such as generalized internal medicine and pediatrics in academic centers. In the latter half of the twentieth century and moving into the twenty-first century, the model for primary care delivery has changed substantially: moving from the small, private practices of the 1980s to larger, consolidated medical groups with teams of physicians and advanced practitioners. Furthermore, there has been specialization of services within the field, with the rise of sports medicine, geriatric medicine, and sleep medicine among others, reflecting the wide gamut of needs and diversity of patients cared for in primary care settings.

1.1.2   A Primer on Women's Health

Relevant to the main theme of this book, one specific domain for primary care which has gained momentum in the past half century is that of women's health. The women's health movement was born out of the Civil Rights movement in the 1960s, with a predominant focus on inequalities in care of and research surrounding issues related to women's bodies. The initial political and public health context for this movement centered around reproductive rights. As the decades progressed, however, there became increasing recognition of women's needs spanning beyond reproductive health. For example, the 1985 Public Health Service Task Force called for greater attention to non-reproductive, chronic issues affecting women across all ages, due to rising poverty, increasing longevity, and more frequent participation of women in the workforce. Noting that sex and gender were not routinely reported in research studies in the twentieth century and that men were the predominant subjects included in research, the National Institutes of Health pushed for greater involvement in and study of women, establishing an Office of Research on Women's Health. This push resulted in the creation of the Women's Health Initiative, which changed the landscape of post-menopausal hormonal therapy. All in all, the past 50 years have brought tremendous progress to the field of women's health and research.

With increasing data in research and clinical settings which suggest sex-based differences in health concerns and outcomes, the field of women's health has become increasingly important to addressing the health needs of over 50% of the US population. Despite these advances, however, barriers remain. Women's health, on the whole, still remains understudied and underfunded, and there is an urgent need to examine how intersectional identities, such as race, ability, and class, relate to differences in outcomes within women's health. From patients' perspectives, women frequently experience greater difficulty in obtaining health insurance (than men), encounter providers with limited knowledge of women's health and the specific risks they face, and have to seek care from multiple providers to meet their health needs.

Experiences in dedicated women's health clinics find that screening and counseling around some preventative health conditions may be higher in a women's health center compared to a general medicine clinic and that patient satisfaction with providers may similarly be increased . While there is extensive overlap in services provided at a general medicine clinic and a women's health center, there are likely subtle differences in practice due to the majority populations each serves. In a women's health practice, providers may need to more routinely provide reproductive/organ-assessment-based health screening; pay greater attention to trauma-informed care; and develop procedural needs which more frequently include pap smears, long-acting reversible contraception insertion and removal, and advanced procedures such as endometrial biopsies and colposcopies. As such, we write this book with a woman-focused practice in mind, whether in a women's health or general medicine center.

1.1.3 An Overview of this Book

This book will use a case-based format to review a series of common concerns encountered in women's health. Some of these concerns are shared across all aspects of primary care, but may benefit from a woman-centric lens, while others involve concerns more specifically experienced by women and gender minorities. As a note on terminology, in this book, the term "woman/en's health" is largely used to describe health concerns among patients with uteruses, ovaries, and/or breasts who are often assigned female sex at birth. We acknowledge that the term and definition above are socially constructed, do not capture individual gender identities, nor address how identity influences presentation of disease and health needs.

We include some high-yield topics in transgender health care throughout the text, but advocate for further study of the healthcare needs of individuals from gender minorities as part of an essential, integrated approach to primary care. Research suggests that effective care for patients from sexual and gender minorities mandates an understanding of stigmatization; social, legal, and structural barriers to care experienced by sexual and gender minorities; and health risks experienced in greater proportions by some patients with these identities. Social marginalization may influence mental health, substance use, and associated risks to health. A lack of knowledge from healthcare providers may lead to inadequate screening for cancer risks (e.g. cervical, anal, and/or, among individuals who have undergone gender-affirming surgeries, cancers associated with tissue which may be retained following), fewer discussions regarding gender or sexual identity, and inadequate connections to appropriate therapies or care, including hormonal treatments and surgeries. It is imperative that providers receive training on how to address these concerns on an individual and clinic-based level, and that efforts continue in the larger public health and legal sphere to eliminate health disparities disproportionately born by sexual and gender minorities. Our hope is to begin to address the former and stress the importance of the latter in the course of this book.

In the chapters that follow, we will address topics relevant to cardiovascular, immunologic, genitourinary, obstetric, breast, social/psychological, and preventative health. In Chap. 11, we offer a discussion of cardiovascular health, in light of data demonstrating disparities in preventative cardiovascular treatments offered to women, less aggressive treatment goals for hypertension and diabetes, and underappreciated risk factors for CVD. These factors include preterm delivery, hypertensive disorders of pregnancy, gestational diabetes, inflammatory diseases, therapies for breast cancer, depression, and menopause. The understanding and diagnosis of ischemic heart disease similarly continue to lag among women, with a corresponding mortality cost. As such, we aim to orient providers to relevant considerations in triaging cardiovascular concerns and providing primary care cognizant of cardiovascular disease manifestations in women.

Women at are greater overall risk of developing autoimmune conditions when compared to men. Mechanisms for this difference are still under study, but hypotheses include hormonal drivers of autoimmunity, sex chromosome differences, and X-chromosome inactivation. Regardless of the specific molecular cause, the higher preponderance of autoimmune disease among women may influence the women's-health-oriented clinician's differential in assessing a patient with a rash, joint pain, or other common primary care concerns. Furthermore, the natural corollaries of a population's increased risk for autoimmune disease are a greater likelihood of exposure to immunomodulatory agents and closer involvement of specialties such as rheumatology, mandating an understanding of treatment modalities and when to refer. Chapter 10 explores immunity among women and offers guidance on management of related conditions.

In Chap. 4, 5, 6, 8, 17, and 18, we discuss common genitourinary concerns among women: including pelvic and vaginal pain, menstrual disorders, urinary concerns, and sexually transmitted infections (STIs). One in three women will experience a pelvic floor disorder, including urinary continence, fecal incontinence, or pelvic organ prolapse, at some point in her life. Worldwide, prevalence estimates of chronic pelvic pain range from 2.1% to 24%, signaling a high burden on women across the globe. Menstrual concerns are even more common: at least 14–25% of women of childbearing-age report experiencing menstrual irregularity. While these concerns are frequently (appropriately) triaged to obstetric and gynecologic subspecialists, given their high prevalence and a widespread preference among women to receive consolidated care when possible, primary care providers, particularly those working within women's health, must have a knowledge of the relevant history, physical, and diagnostic approach to these concerns. Furthermore, given the stigma which often surrounds discussions of pelvic and sexual health, providers must develop skills in patient-centered communication (with a priority on helping women feel heard and believed) and trauma-informed care.

Reproductive health is another field which has significant overlap in primary medical and obstetric/gynecologic care, with primary care serving as an avenue for expanded access to reproductive health resources and as a point of first contact for many women seeking reproductive planning. Qualitative research findings suggest an expanding role for reproductive health within the primary care clinic, suggesting an emphasis on open-ended questions which do not make assumptions about patients' reproductive preferences. Medically, primary care providers should be prepared to counsel patients on a variety of contraceptive methods and may help pregnancy outcomes by partnering with patients to promote use of prenatal vitamins and reduce substance consumption in pregnancy, for example. Chapters 12 and 13 address elements along the spectrum of reproductive care: with discussions of contraceptives and an approach to pre-conception, early pregnancy, and post-pregnancy care.

Similar to pelvic health, concerns around breast health are frequent among primary care clinic visits. Breast pain, nipple discharge, and breast masses represent three of the most common breast concerns encountered in primary care. Triaging these concerns adequately is a critical skill, in order to accurately provide reassurance and conservative treatment, or, when appropriate, recommend further diagnostics and management. Chapter 7 outlines common breast complaints and their management.

Chapters 9, 13, and 15 offer insight into and tools to address the connection between women's mental and physical health, as both interplay frequently in the primary care domain. The World Health Organization has identified violence against women, including intimate partner violence, as a major global threat, with the National Coalition of Advocacy against Domestic Violence sharing that one in four women and one in nine men experience intimate partner violence in their lifetime. Disordered eating similarly presents disproportionately among women, and mental health concerns are prominent as well. Primary care providers are uniquely situated to address these issues, in part due to their often longitudinal relationships with patients. They must recognize warning signs and act appropriately, given high levels of comorbidity between the three conditions and the significant health risks they each pose.

Lastly, no discussion of women's health and primary care could be complete without guidance on preventative health. In the domain of women's health, this includes preventative cancer screenings, such as for breast and cervical cancers, as well as counseling and management of conditions of aging, such as menopause and osteoporosis. As we have detailed above, the women's health primary care office is an ideal place to address these needs, given a strong opportunity to address preventative measures simultaneously with patient symptom-driven concerns (e.g. breast or pelvic concerns). Chapters 14, 16, and 19 delve into these issues, to provide the primary care provider an armamentarium of tools to preserve and maintain health throughout a woman's lifetime.

In conclusion, women's health represents a field of primary care seeking to address the needs and circumstances of women, recognizing sex- and gender-based differences in disease presentations and health needs. The primary care provider, if able to adopt some of the tools offered here, is uniquely situated to address women and gender and sexual minorities' concerns directly, capitalizing on patient continuity and trust, and expanding access to care. The remainder of this book offers insight into the themes previewed above, with the hope that they guide and inform future practice in primary care and women's health.

Suggested Reading

1. (NICHD), NIH Eunice Kennedy Shriver National Institute of Child Health and Human Development. How many women are affected by menstrual irregularities? 2017. https://www.nichd.nih.gov/health/topics/menstruation/conditioninfo/affected
2. Daniels JP, Khan KS. Chronic pelvic pain in women. BMJ. 2010;341:c4834.
3. Education, Citizens Commission on Graduate Medical. The graduate education of physicians. Chicago: American Medical Association; 1966.
4. Garcia M, Mulvagh SL, Merz CNB, Buring JE, Manson JAE. Cardiovascular disease in women. Circ Res. 2016;118:1273–93.
5. Gharib SD, Manson JA. Women's health care: one size does not fit all. J Gen Intern Med. 2000;15:68–9.
6. Glied S, Jack K, Rachlin J. Women's health insurance coverage 1980-2005. Women's Health Issues. 2008;18:7–16.
7. Institute of Medicine (US) Committee on the Future of Primary Care. In: Donaldson MS, Yordy KD, Lohr KN, et al., editors. *Primary care: America's health in a new era.* Washington, DC: National Academies Press; 1996.
8. Invernizzi P, Pasini S, Carlo Selmi M, Gershwin E, Podda M. Female predominance and X chromosome defects in autoimmune diseases. J Autoimmun. 2009;33:12–6.
9. Klassen CL, Hines SL, Ghosh K. Common benign breast concerns for the primary care physician. Cleve Clin J Med. 2019;86:57–65.
10. Manze MG, Romero DR, Sumberg A, Gagnon M, Roberts L, Jones H. Women's perspectives on reproductive health Services in Primary Care. Fam Med. 2020;52:112–9.
11. Mayer KH, Bradford JB, Makadon HJ, Stall R, Goldhammer H, Landers S. Sexual and gender minority health: what we know and what needs to be done. Am J Public Health. 2008;98:989–95.
12. National Academies of Sciences, Engineering, and Medicine, Health and Medicine Division, Board on Health Care Services, Committee on Implementing High-Quality Primary Care, Robinson SK, Meisnere M, Phillips RL Jr, et al. Implementing high-quality primary care: rebuilding the Foundation of Health Care. Washington, DC: National Academies Press; 2021.
13. NCADV, National Coalition Against Domestic Violence. National statistics domestic violence fact sheet. 2020. https://assets.speakcdn.com/assets/2497/domestic_violence-2020080709350855.pdf?1596828650457
14. NEDA, National Eating Disorders Association. Statistics & research on eating disorders. 2022. https://www.nationaleatingdisorders.org/statistics-research-eating-disorders
15. Nygaard I, Barber MD, Burgio KL, Kenton K, Meikle S, Schaffer J, Spino C, Whitehead WE, Jennifer W, Brody DJ, for the Pelvic Floor Disorders Network. Prevalence of symptomatic Pelvic Floor Disorders in US women. JAMA. 2008;300:1311–6.

16. Organization, World Health. 'Women's mental health: An evidence based review'. 2000.
17. Strobino DM, Grason H, Minkovitz C. Charting a course for the future of women's health in the United States: concepts, findings and recommendations. Soc Sci Med. 2002;54:839–48.
18. Stuenkel CA, Manson JAE. Women's health — traversing medicine and public policy. N Engl J Med. 2021;384:2073–6.
19. White M, Shroff S. A closer look at Women's health centers: historical lessons and future aims. J Women's Health. 2021;31:408–14.
20. Willis J, Antono B, Bazemore A, Jetty A, Petterson S, George J, Rosario BL, Scheufele E, Rajmane A, Dankwa-Mullan I, Rhee K. 2020. The state of primary Care in the United States: a Chartbook of facts and statistics.
21. Women's health. Report of the public health service task force on women's health issues. Public Health Rep. 1985;100:73–106.

Chapter 2
History and Physical Examination of a Woman

Dhuha Alwan and Alexia Markowski

2.1 Short Introduction

Many women, especially those of reproductive age, experience clinical complaints relating to gynecological symptoms, such as pelvic pain, changes to vaginal discharge, and concerns for infection. This is a common presentation within primary care clinics, and many women can experience marked discomfort. In this chapter, we will start with a case of a young female with a common presentation and discuss the important history and physical exam findings that can lead to the correct diagnosis. We will emphasize important points within the history and physical exam of which clinicians should inquire when evaluating women with this chief complaint, including how to best build rapport and trust with patients.

2.2 Case Presentation

A 23-year-old female presented to the clinic due to lower abdominal pain. This patient has no previous medical or surgical history. She has not seen a physician in many years; the last visit she remembers was when she received vaccinations in high school. She was just recently married about 3 months ago. She has had this pain for a few weeks now. The pain is vague and not radiating. She also has some

D. Alwan (✉)
Department of Internal Medicine, The Ohio State University Wexner Medical Center, Columbus, OH, USA
e-mail: dhuha.alwan@osumc.edu

A. Markowski
The Ohio State University College of Medicine, Columbus, OH, USA
e-mail: alexia.markowski@osumc.edu

M. Mahmoudi (ed.), *Common Cases in Women's Primary Care Clinics*,
https://doi.org/10.1007/978-3-031-48569-5_2

vaginal discharge. She has had irregular menstrual periods since menarche. Additionally, this patient is trying to conceive.

2.3　Discussion

2.3.1　*Approach to this Patient: History of Present Illness*

For this patient, it is important to obtain a good history of her current state of illness, and how that compares to her previous state of health. As always, it is important to keep all questions in an open-ended format.

To begin the history, basic questions inquiring about onset and duration are especially important in determining whether this is an acute or chronic problem. A chronic problem could indicate more serious pathology and should be investigated further. Additionally, it would be important to ask the patient whether these symptoms have ever occurred in the past and if so, how often. Recurring episodes of pelvic pain with changes to vaginal discharge may also point to other underlying medical conditions, such as issues with immunity or ability to fight infections. In this case, she has indicated that this pain began a few weeks ago, but the physician should inquire whether the changes to vaginal discharge began at the same time as the onset of pain or if one symptom came before the other. An open-ended question such as "When your symptoms first presented, in what ways had your usual routine changed? Is there anything that has changed recently that you believe may be contributing to your symptoms?"

Next, it is important to clarify the location of her pain, whether it is unilateral, bilateral, pinpoint, generalized, etc. It is best to let the patient describe it in her own words where her symptoms feel at their worst, and then during the physical exam help to confirm that location.

Ask the patient how she would characterize the pain in an open-ended format, and if she has difficulty describing it (such as in this case), give some adjectives to help direct her such as burning, achy, sharp, or dull. Additionally, is the pain constant or waxing and waning? She has already mentioned that the pain is not radiating, but it would be important to ask if the patient is experiencing pain anywhere else, such as back pain or vaginal pain.

Ask the patient what, if anything, makes the pain better or worse. Has the patient tried any medications, herbal remedies, or heating pads to relieve the pain? Is the pain worse with movements, with sexual activity, or in any certain position? Is the pain worse during menstruation? These questions help to determine the underlying cause of the woman's pain and can help with treatment planning as well. In terms of her complaint of increasing vaginal discharge, timing of the onset of symptoms can be extremely important. Changes to hygienic routine or increased sexual activity can both be triggers of vaginitis. Thus, ask questions about any recent changes in soaps, body washes, detergents, deodorants, creams or lotions, and sanitary pads or tampons. These can all contain chemicals or fragrances that can be irritating to the vulva, or change the pH balance of the vagina, which can lead to vaginitis or vulvar dermatitis. Even changes in contraceptive devices like condoms can trigger changes in the vaginal balance. Additionally, the causes of vaginitis can vary with the menstrual cycle (candida infection is more likely to occur before the menstrual period, while Bacterial vaginosis and trichomoniasis tend to occur during or after) so a detailed history about the patient's last period should also be obtained. Additionally, because this patient is trying to conceive, it is very important to know the date of her last menstruation to assess for potential pregnancy. Because of this patient's mention of menstrual irregularities, we will ask more details about her gynecological history later on in the interview. Also, discuss with the patient the timing of her symptoms throughout the day, by asking, "Have you noticed any time of day when your symptoms improve? Likewise, have you noticed any time of day when your symptoms worsen?"

Finally, the quality and quantity of vaginal discharge can vary between women. Questions about this patient's abnormal vaginal discharge should be directed at how this presentation is different from her usual state of health. Examples:

Is the amount of vaginal discharge more or less than the usual amount you have? Can you describe how the odor has changed? Can you describe how the consistency has changed? Can you describe any color changes?

After gathering more details about the patient's present illness, a thorough review of symptoms is important not only for diagnosing her conditions but also looking for underlying pathologies that would be crucial not to miss. Especially for this patient, it would be important to inquire about any vaginal bleeding. If she endorses this, be sure to ask how often and how much bleeding she has experienced. Examples of other general review of systems symptoms to cover include:

- Fever
- Chills
- Unexplained weight loss
- Nausea/vomiting
- Pain or burning with urination
- Blood in the urine or stool
- Urinary or fecal incontinence
- Burning, soreness, swelling in the vulvar area
- Skin changes/rashes
- Pain or discomfort with sexual activity
- Ulcers in the mouth, nose, or genital area
- Changes in mood, such as depression or anxiety

Finally, to finish the history of present illness, ask the patient what concerns she has about her current state of health. This allows the clinician to build rapport with the patient and understand how this is affecting the patient's life. It also helps the clinician counsel the patient and steer the rest of the history and physical exam in a way that will reassure the patient.

Building rapport with the patient is extremely important, especially when she is sharing sensitive details about her health presentation. Studies have shown that female patients have more questions and increased participatory visits compared to male patients, so it is even more vital that clinicians spend adequate time assessing and getting to know the patient and her concerns. Another key question to ask during the history is "What do you believe may be the cause of your symptoms?" Hearing from the patient directly about what she understands about her presentation can build a strong physician–patient relationship. In this way, the clinician listens to what the patient knows and understands about her symptoms and offers the clinician a way to get to know the whole patient. The clinician can empathize with the patient and understand the patient's perspective toward her symptoms. Clinicians should always focus on patient-centered care which includes involving the patient in their own care as much as possible, and responding to the concerns and emotions the patient feels towards his/her presentation or illness. In the primary care setting, patient-centered care resolves around four main principles: the patient's own feelings about being sick, his/her beliefs about what could be causing his/her presentation, how the presentation is impacting his/her daily life and activities, and what he/she expects to be done about the presentation. Vital to the approach of patient-centered care is that the clinician understands the whole of the person and that both the patient and clinician can come together to manage the patient's condition or illness. When clinicians take this patient-centered approach, patients experience better healthcare overall, with improved mental health and less uncomfortability within the overall healthcare process. Patient-centered care was even associated with better efficiency, with less diagnostic tests ordered and decreased referrals to specialists. Thus, these are important questions to emphasize and an imperative approach to adopt during the history so that both the patient and the clinician can achieve a positive outcome from the visit.

When the history has been completed, it may be helpful to summarize what the patient has just told you. This is exceedingly helpful to the creation of a meaningful relationship with the patient. It makes the patient feel comfortable, listened to, and at ease with the fact that her concerns and symptoms are being noted and handled. This gives the patient an opportunity to ensure that all details about the history have been understood correctly and can clear up any confusion or misinterpretations. Once again, this permits the patient to take an active role in her care by confirming the details of her own story, and the clinician can proceed knowing the history is accurate and representative of the patient's presentation.

2.3.2 Approach to this Patient: Past Medical and Surgical History

At this point, it would be appropriate to inquire about past medical and surgical history. In this case, the patient is denying any past history, but a few details are important to clarify, such as any medication history. Inquire about prescription and over-the-counter medications, as well as any vitamins, supplements, or herbal remedies the patient may be using. Also ensure that the patient is not allergic to any foods or medications.

2.3.3 Approach to this Patient: Family History

To be complete, ask the patient about any history of cancers in her family. Multiple first-degree relatives with cancer should be investigated further by the clinician. It is also important to discuss any history of immunodeficiencies or atopy within the family.

2.3.4 Approach to this Patient: Social History

The social history of this patient is very imperative to making a correct diagnosis and for counseling the patient after the diagnosis has been made. Though these questions are more personal, they are vital to understanding the whole patient and the potential triggers of her symptoms.

When beginning the social history, simple and open-ended questions about diet and exercise can start a good conversation. These questions are a good starting point to the social history because they gather more information about the patient's overall health and wellness and begin an open conversation that is inviting and puts the patient at ease.

Next, it is important to inquire about any substance use. This can be done initially with open-ended questions, followed by more specific follow-up questions. Example:

Tell me about any tobacco use.
If the patient uses tobacco products, ask informative follow-up questions such as:
For how many years have you or did you smoke?
How many packs a day do you or did you smoke?

A similar history can be obtained for alcohol use, asking how many drinks consumed per week and what kind of alcohol is consumed (wine, beer, liquor, etc.).

It is also important to ask about any recreational drug use, as use of these can be risk factors for certain infections.

When obtaining a history from any patient, it is always recommended to gather a sexual history, but it is even more imperative for this case or any other gynecological complaint. Because this involves discussing a sensitive topic, it is best to begin by saying, "I would like to ask a few questions about your sexual history, if that is okay with you." This helps the patient feel more at ease with discussing a sensitive subject and creates an environment of comfortability, rather than the patient feeling like she must answer these questions. Once obtaining permission from the patient, begin the sexual history with the following questions:

Are you sexually active? (Though the patient mentioned that she is trying to conceive, details about a patient's history should never be assumed and may be further clarified.)
Do you have sex with men, women, or both?
Within the last 12 months, how many sexual partners have you had?
What, if anything, do you use for protection? (Because this patient is trying to conceive, it is also important to ask about the use of contraception in the past.)
Have you ever been tested for and/or diagnosed with a sexually transmitted infection?
Do you have any sexual concerns at this time?

Once this information has been gathered, thank the patient for answering these questions openly and honestly, for example, by saying, "Thank you for answering these questions and sharing this information with me. Though personal, it is important for us to understand all aspects of your health."

Next, inquire about what the patient does for work or school. This can lead to the discussion of any occupational exposures or hazards that might affect the patient's health. During this time, the clinician can also ask what the patient likes to do for fun or during her free time. Again, questions like this help the clinician and patient build an honest and trusting relationship with one another, which will be a benefit to both parties in the long run.

It is always imperative to ask the patient about homelife and safety at home. It is even more important in this case, because the patient is a young adult female, a demographic that can be associated with an increased risk of domestic violence. In fact, physical and sexual abuse may manifest as different physiologic symptoms, especially gynecological symptoms, such as pelvic pain, menstrual irregularities, and urinary tract infections. Thus, it is important to ensure that patients feel safe in their homes and in their relationships. Here is an example of how to begin the conversation:

First, who lives at home with you? (Acknowledge the patient's response).
The next few questions I would like to ask you are some that we ask all of our patients, and though sometimes difficult to discuss, are important to talk about for your health and well-being.
Do you feel safe at home?
(If the answer is no) Can you tell me more about what makes you feel unsafe at home?

Do you feel safe in your current relationships?
(If the answer is no) Can you tell me more about what makes you feel unsafe in those relationships?
Have you ever felt unsafe in other environments in the past?
(If the answer is no) Can you tell me more about those instances?
Do you feel like you have an adequate support system and others in your life to rely on?

Whenever the patient shares personal stories or sensitive experience, always empathize and acknowledge their feelings by saying, "I'm sorry you had to go through these things, and thank you very much for sharing these experiences with me. This is a safe space to share, and we are willing to help you in any way possible."

This concludes the history, and though very thorough, these are aspects that are not only vital to diagnosing and treating the patient appropriately, but also to establishing a connection between the patient and clinician.

2.3.5 Approach to this Patient: Gynecologic History

For this patient, it is imperative to gather information about her gynecologic history, given her symptom presentation and her mention of menstrual irregularities.

To begin, allow the patient to explain more about her irregularities in her own words: "You mentioned having some menstrual irregularities, can you tell me more about what you have experienced?" This helps the patient feel listened to and involved within her own care, and it also gives her an opportunity to explain her precise issues. After this, more specific and clarifying questions can be asked. These include:

Age of menarche
Approximate between periods
Number of days bleeding
Number of pads or tampons used during bleeding
Pain or other symptoms experienced during periods
Bleeding between periods
Changes in mood during periods
If the patient endorses any of these, also ask if she has tried anything to improve those symptoms.

This patient also mentioned that she is trying to conceive. It is important to obtain an obstetric history well, which includes:

History of prior pregnancies
History of miscarriages, ectopic pregnancies, abortions, or preterm births

If the patient has been pregnant and delivered a child, more history can be obtained, including:

Issues conceiving or using reproductive assistance
Gestational age at the time of delivery
Mode of delivery
Delivery complications (such as use of vacuum or forceps, or shoulder dystocia)
Maternal complications during pregnancy and delivery
Fetal complications during pregnancy and delivery
Neonatal complications
Other aspects of the gynecological history include inquiring about contraceptive use (now and in the past), history of abnormal pap test (because this patient has not seen a physician in many years, it is unlikely she has ever had a pap test), and any gynecologic diagnoses such as ovarian cysts or fibroids.
Lastly, ask the patient if she has received any or all of the human papilloma virus vaccinations, as this is an important aspect of preventable medicine and could be offered to the patient if she so wishes.

2.3.6 Approach to this Patient: Physical Exam

Now that the historical information has been obtained, it is next appropriate to ask if the clinician can perform a physical exam on the patient.

The exam starts by simply looking at the patient and deciding whether she is ill- or well-appearing. Next, auscultate the heart for rate, rhythm, and murmurs, and then the lungs for good air movement and any focal findings.

Because of this patient's complaint of abdominal pain, it is important to complete a thorough abdominal exam. Ideally, the patient is in a gown already, but it can also be completed by asking the patient if the examiner can lift the patient's shirt to get a closer look at her abdomen. The first step in the abdominal exam is assessing for any skin changes, rashes, marks, or atrophy. Next, listen for bowel sounds in multiple quadrants and also auscultate the abdominal aorta for any bruits.

When palpating the abdomen, begin with light palpation in all four quadrants using one hand. As you palpate, watch the patient's reaction, as this can show you if they are experiencing pain within any of the quadrants. After light palpation, the clinician can also ask if the patient felt any pain and where it was located. Next, perform deep palpation using two hands and again watch for the patient's reaction to any pain she may be experiencing. When palpating the liver and the spleen, ask the patient to take a deep breath in and as she breathes out, assess for the presence of hepatomegaly or splenomegaly.

After palpation, perform percussion in each of the four quadrants. Lastly assess for costovertebral tenderness by palpating each flank.

When performing the pelvic exam, begin by asking the patient if it is okay to proceed with the examination. It is also important to ask if the patient would like another individual in the room during the exam to serve as a chaperone. First, inspect all areas of the vulva for any bruising, rashes, excoriations, skin changes, scarring, or atrophy. Always tell the patient when she will feel any touch, and ask if there is any pain or discomfort associated with where she is being touched. Ask the patient to characterize the discomfort she is feeling. In some cases, the vaginal discharge may be assessed at this point, but it can also be assessed during the speculum exam. During this time, a q-tip test can also be performed, which is where the clinician probes various areas of the vulva and vaginal introitus with a q-tip to look for areas of pain or discomfort. Again, the clinician should always inform the patient about what this next part of the exam entails so the patient is prepared and more at ease. When subjected to a gynecological exam, women have felt more comfortable and less pain when the clinician explains what he/she is doing during each aspect of the exam, and more importantly, why he/she is doing it. When inspecting the vulva, the clinician can also look for any genital lesions or warts, as well as looking for any foreign bodies near the introitus.

The next part of the physical exam is the speculum examination to further inspect the vagina, vaginal wall, and cervix. Assess the vaginal wall for lesions, retained foreign bodies, warts, scar tissue, or inflammatory changes like swelling or erythema. Assess the cervix for changes in appearance or for any discharge from the cervix. To detect for friability of the cervix, use a cotton swab to detect for any bleeding or irritation.

The quality and quantity of the vaginal discharge can also be assessed at this time. While normal vaginal discharge can vary, it is typically transparent, white or yellow in color and typically odorless or with some malodor. The quantity can range between one and four milliliters within a 24 hour timespan.

During the bimanual examination, assess for normal anatomy of the uterus and ovaries, evaluate for any masses, and look for any cervical motion tenderness.

During the physical exam, pH testing can be performed and swabs of the vaginal discharge can be obtained for other diagnostic tests.

2.4 Conclusion

Gynecological complaints are extremely common among women, especially those of reproductive age like the patient presented in this case. This chapter serves as a guide to obtain a thorough and accurate history and physical exam. Performing a detailed history and physical exam such as this one can not only help to diagnose the patient but it can also build a strong relationship between the clinician and the patient. When taking an approach rooted in patient-centered care, the clinician and patient can come together to evaluate and manage the patient holistically. Though gynecological complaints are common (especially within a setting of primary care), they can involve a comprehensive history and physical exam that should take into account the patient's physical, mental, and emotional health. Above all, the trust and respect between the clinician and the patient can lead to better outcomes and a more rewarding healthcare visit for all persons involved.

Suggested Reading

1. Sobel JD. Vaginal discharge (vaginitis): Initial evaluation. UpToDate. 2022, October 14. Accessed 23 Dec 2022.
2. Hainer BL, Gibson MV. Vaginitis. Am Fam Physician. 2011;8b(7):807–15.
3. Bertakis KD, Azari R. Patient-centered care is associated with decreased health care utilization. J Am Board Family Med. 2011;24(3):229–39.
4. Stewart M, Brown JB, Donner A, Mcwhinney IR, Oates J, Weston WW, Jordan J. The impact of patient-centered care on outcomes. J Fam Pract. 2000;49(9):796.
5. Mark H, Bitzker K, Klapp BF, Rauchfuss M. Gynecological symptoms associated with physical and sexual violence. J Psychosom Obstet Gynecol. 2008;29(3):167–75.
6. Petravage JB, Reynolds LJ, Gardner HJ, Reading JC. Attitudes of women toward the gynecologic examination. J Fam Pract. 1979;9(6):1039–45.

Chapter 3
Procedures in Women's Primary Care Clinic

Sondos Al Sad

3.1   Case Study

JF is a 48-year-old female coming in for an annual check-up for the first time since the COVID pandemic started. She reports weight gain and irregular periods with heavy flow. She can't leave home without being anxious about the bleeding. She is not interested in having more children. She doesn't have a gynecologist. She is wondering if she needs to see a gynecologist regarding her periods separate from her annual physical today. She reports a distant history of an abnormal pap test with no treatment needed. No history of HPV and she is not HPV vaccinated. She is a former light smoker and has been smoke-free for 18 years. She is currently monogamous with one partner and is G3P0030. Her pap test was 5 years ago, and her mammogram was benign 2 years ago. She takes multivitamins inconsistently with no other daily medications. She reports that she was on oral contraceptives in college and did not like how they made her feel.

3.2   Introduction

Expanded services with attention to women's needs are more likely to be utilized and make a difference in providing effective and timely care. Primary care providers with procedural skills and well-rounded expertise have become a pillar for access to universal care. Moreover, primary care settings with a women's health focus are a

S. Al Sad (✉)
Family and Community Medicine Department, Women's Health Primary Care Center,
University of California San Francisco, San Francisco, CA, USA
e-mail: Sondos.Alsad@ucsf.edu

M. Mahmoudi (ed.), *Common Cases in Women's Primary Care Clinics*,
https://doi.org/10.1007/978-3-031-48569-5_3

sign of growth in the right direction. It reduces health disparities and builds on longitudinal care with established rapport. Patients would benefit from understanding that women's health primary care provides comprehensive interdisciplinary care in the context of community medicine. The patient's question may indicate inadequate marketing of the primary care role in fulfilling the service gap in all regions: both metropolitan and underserved areas, inconsistent training of primary care residents, and under utilization of internal referrals within the one practice.

Our patient will need a detailed medical history intake, physical examination, a basic workup for abnormal uterine bleeding with irregular cycles, diagnostic procedures, and likely a therapeutic intervention. All of this can be ordered and done by her primary care provider. Refer to history and physical examination (Chap. 2), and menstrual disorders (Chap. 6) for more details.

Table 3.1 refers to common procedures done in primary care settings depending on location, population served within the practice, and demand for these procedures. Rural and underserved areas may invest in even more procedures in their primary care residency training such as obstetrics and loop electrosurgical excision procedure (LEEP). In this chapter, I will focus on pelvic procedures provided in women's health primary care settings for adult females (Figs. 3.1, 3.2 and 3.3).

Table 3.1 Common in-office primary care procedures

Procedure	Uses	Equipment	Logistics
Pelvic examination	Diagnostic Therapeutic Preventive	Sterile speculum Lubricant Reliable lighting source	Minimal for clinic/no insurance involvement
Intrauterine device (IUD) insertion and removal	Therapeutic	Pelvic examination tools Betadine Ring forceps[a] Tenaculum Paracervical block[b] Uterine sounding tool IUD of choice Scissors	Average cost depending on the volume/coverage depends on insurance, regional reproductive health politics, and type of IUD
Implant insertion and removal	Therapeutic	Sterile marker Measurement meter Alcohol prep Local anesthetics (Lidocaine/ Epinephrine) Betadine Implant Kerlix wrap/gauze (Blade 11 for removal)	It is a reasonable cost for the practice Often covered by insurance Removal is more operator-dependent than insertion

Table 3.1 (continued)

Procedure	Uses	Equipment	Logistics
Bartholin cyst I&D	Therapeutic	Betadine Local anesthetic Small forceps Blade 11 or 15	Available in most outpatient settings Covered by insurance Recurrence may warrant referral
Endometrial biopsy	Diagnostic	Pelvic examination tools Betadine Ring forceps[a] Tenaculum Paracervical block[b] Sterile cervical dilators Uterine sounding tool Endometrial Pipelle Formalin container	Available in clinics with high volume and demand Covered by insurance Needs volume for credentialing
Colposcopy	Diagnostic	Pelvic examination tools Colposcope Acetoacetic acid Cotton swabs Cervical punch biopsy Endocervical curette Toothpicks Formalin container Hemostatic agent Endocervical speculum (optional)	Available in clinics with high volume and demand Cost of colposcope and maintenance Covered by insurance Needs volume for credentialing
Ultrasound (PoCUS)	Diagnostic Therapeutic	Ultrasound machine Sterile gel	The device and its maintenance are of high cost Needs special documentation Certification and credentialing are needed
Pessary placement	Therapeutic	Pelvic examination tools Pessaries	Providers need training Low cost in clinic
Cervical polyp removal	Therapeutic Diagnostic	Pelvic examination tool Ring forceps Paracervical block Endocervical curettage Hemostatic agent (silver nitrate sticks or Monsel's solution) Formalin container	Low cost for clinic operations Minimal training needed Credentialing dependent on practice policies

(continued)

Table 3.1 (continued)

Procedure	Uses	Equipment	Logistics
Skin biopsy (vulvar or non-gyn)	Diagnostic Therapeutic	Reliable lighting source Local or topical anesthetic Desired punch biopsy 2–6 mm Formalin container Needle holder Suture 4.0 or 5.0 nylon Iris scissor Hemostatic agent	Depends on volume and the provider's comfort Billing differs based on pathology report findings
Joint aspiration/ injection	Therapeutic Diagnostic	Antiseptic solution Local anesthetic 3 syringes and needles Therapeutic medication solution Hemostat Culture and lab supplies Band-aids +/– Ultrasound	Availability of local anesthetics and injectable therapeutic medications is expensive if there is no volume of patients Ultrasound-guided procedure has more cost and different billing. Needs credentialing and volume Sterility can be a challenge
Neoplastic ablation (Cryotherapy)	Therapeutic	Liquid nitrogen (pressed or in a cryotherapy gun)	Simple and low cost

[a]Ring forceps are used to hold Betadine swabs for sterilization unless you use your Betadine in a cup with long and large cotton swabs, it is used for IUD removal as well
[b]Paracervical block is an intradermal injection of an anesthetic into the cervix (lidocaine; buffered or plain)

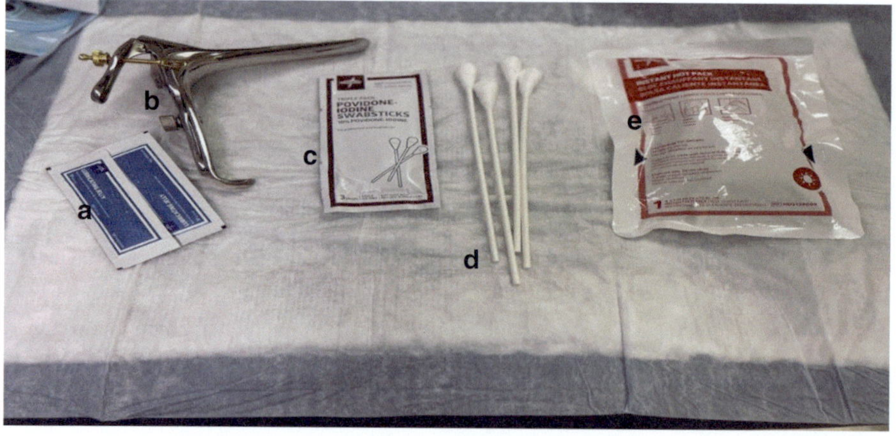

Fig. 3.1 (**a**) Lubricant, (**b**) Vaginal Speculum, (**c**) Betadine, (**d**) Large cotton swabs, (**e**) Heat Pack

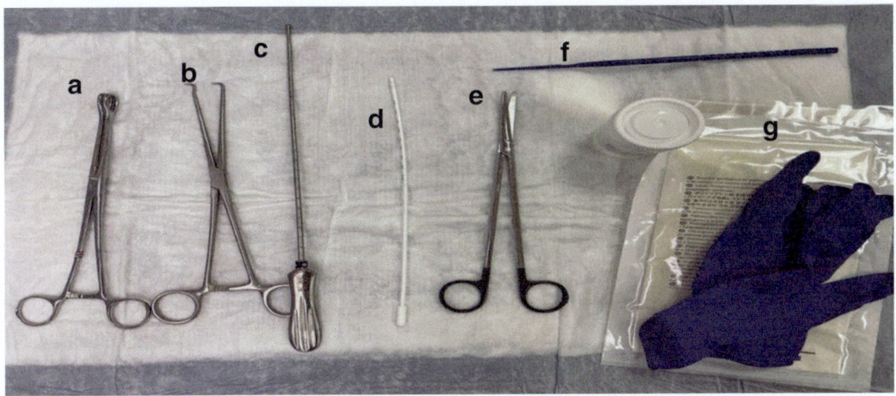

Fig. 3.2 (**a**) Ring forceps, (**b**) Tenaculum, (**c**) Uterine Sound, (**d**) Pipelle, (**e**) Scissors, (**f**) Cervical dilator, (**g**) Sterile gloves

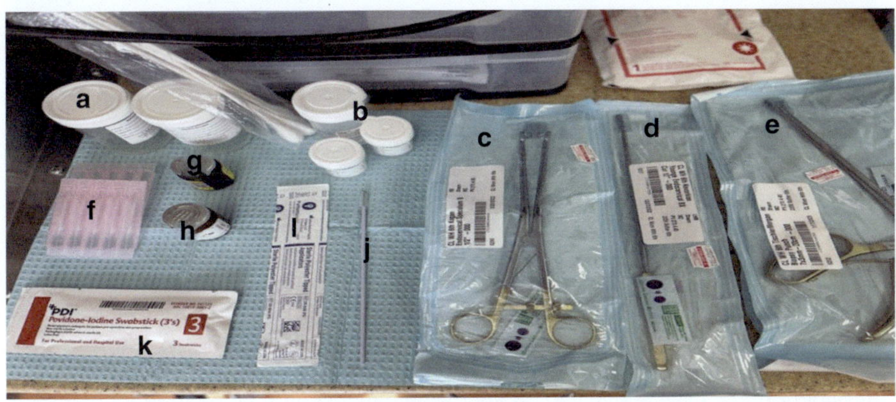

Fig. 3.3 (**a**) Container with Acetoacetic acid, (**b**) Formalin container for specimen collection, (**c**) endocervical speculum, (**d**) Endocervical curette, (**e**) Cervical biopsy punch, (**f**) Normal saline vials, (**g**) Monsel's solution (for homeostasis), (**h**) Lugol's solution, (**I**) cotton swabs, (**j**) Cytobrush, (**k**) Iodine swabsticks

3.3 Women's Health Primary Care Clinic Model

The women's health primary care (WHPC) model is evolving and has the potential to grow with adequate funding. It refines clinical skills for providers, reduces health disparities, provides primary care practitioners with career satisfaction, nourishes a focused women's health research, optimizes utilization of social services, and fosters to interdisciplinary education and training. WHPC is a woman-centered approach to health provision and provides a one-stop shop for most health needs encountered by women throughout their lifespans.

Providing in-office procedures minimizes referrals to specialists, reduces the utilization of high-cost radio-imaging, and offers a longitudinal approach to management planning. Procedural training for primary care providers can increase retention, provide professional growth in healthcare administrative tasks, and offers better insight into the billing and coding of these services, hence improving compensation rates.

In-office procedures may be challenged by limited resources, cost, maintenance of needed equipment, low volume, inadequate staffing to assist during procedures, inconsistent certification criteria, the burden of training primary care providers during residency or after graduation, and the variability of credentialing process in healthcare systems.

Building in-office procedure skills and practices within a WHPC setting would require involved practice leadership, interested providers, and adequate patient volume in training to be credentialed. It is important for residents and junior providers to explore the culture of practices they are joining to cater to their interest in providing procedural services for female patients.

Primary care providers are expected to be well-versed in counseling patients for informed consent, providing educational material to prepare patients for procedures, and arranging a follow-up plan with patients. Comprehensiveness is a time-honored value in primary care, and recent evidence shows that it lowers Medicare costs.

3.4 Primary Care Outpatient Procedures

3.4.1 Gynecological Procedures

Our Case

Our patient in the case above had an abnormal pap test with atypical glandular cells and negative HPV. Her blood work was inconclusive of her irregular bleeding, however, showed mildly elevated triglycerides, and mild iron deficiency anemia. She was scheduled to follow for a colposcopy and endometrial biopsy per American Society for Colposcopy and Cervical Pathology (ASCCP) guidelines. The patient was concerned and had many questions about the procedure and the prognosis of her results. She was relieved that she could get her procedures done with her primary care provider and not have to wait a long time for answers.

Patient Comfort and Procedural Preparation

All pelvic procedures need a reliable light source and satisfactory visualization of the vulva and cervix with minimal discomfort to patients. In pelvic procedures, pain is impacted by multiple factors(parity, history of dysmenorrhea, provider's skill and expertise, history of vaginal delivery, estrogen state of the pelvis, operative duration, anxiety, and anticipated pain). Here are some tips to achieve patient comfort:

- Prior to the procedure consider sharing resources with your patients either via electronic chart messaging or in pre-procedural counseling while the patient is dressed.
- Alternatives for the procedure and its steps should be thoroughly discussed prior to signing a consent.
- Identify any history of trauma and provide trauma-informed care by empowering your patients and providing them with all options for management and details of the procedure, showing them the equipment to be used in the procedure, and identifying how they prefer to be addressed during the procedure. You may use "table" instead of "bed" and "footrest" instead of "stirrups."
- Attend to patient's privacy and modesty preferences. A paper or cloth drape may be used to avoid unnecessary exposure, and a pad available for use after the procedure for patient comfort.
- Make sure you have all the instruments you need prior to the procedure, huddle with your medical assistant for any potential needs such as chaperoning, and check the date on your local anesthetics (e.g., lidocaine with or without epinephrine).
- Consider checking the examination table and availability of the electric outlets for your light or colposcope prior to rooming patients. It is not uncommon for examination tables to be too high or not adjustable. Tables often vary across exam rooms within one practice.
- Use adequate lubrication and latex-free gloves to reduce irritation.
- Bimanual examination for trained providers can be helpful in identifying the direction of the uterine fundus and mobility of the cervix. You can reposition a mobile cervix into mid-position from an anteverted or retroverted direction by gently pushing on the uterine fundus on the abdominal side, this tactic can reduce the traction needed by a tenaculum for endometrial biopsy or IUD insertion. Generally, the uterus is considered anteverted if both of your fingers were to come above the cervix on bimanual examination, and retroverted when your fingers come underneath the cervix. If the uterus is anteflexed or retroflexed you may have difficulty estimating fundal height.
- Avoid blind entry to the introitus and allow the speculum to slide into the vagina without force or pushing.
- Use the smallest vaginal speculum needed to fully visualize the cervix. Bear in mind that choosing a big speculum may be more comfortable if it provides satisfactory visualization of the cervix than choosing a smaller one with frequent adjustments.
- Watch for perineal skin when locking your speculum in place, it is not uncommon to pinch that area. Consider holding the speculum as shown in Fig. 3.4.

- If you have a medical assistant, you may suggest the McRoberts maneuver or have the patient cross their arms across their chest to reduce the occurrence of vasovagal response.
- For pain management and patient's comfort, you may use pharmacotherapy (NSAIDs and anxiolytics prior to the procedure, applying topical lidocaine gel

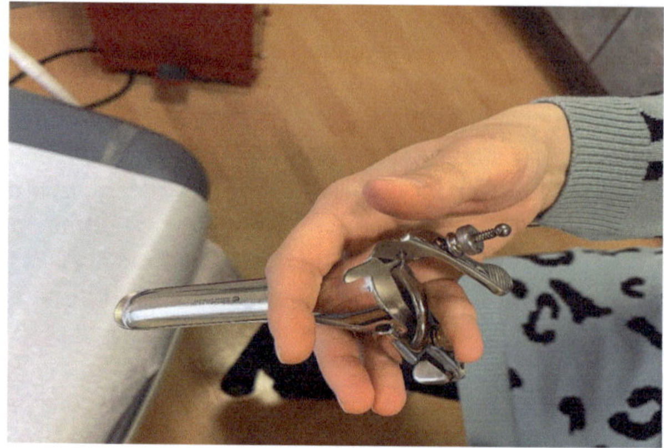

Fig. 3.4 Holding the speculum where the locking part is shielded from the patient's skin and allows spontaneous sliding into the vaginal vault without active pushing

10–15 minutes to the vaginal vault prior to the procedure, paracervical block – intradermal lidocaine 1%-, or endometrial lidocaine 2% infusion using Pipelle) or nonpharmacological (heating pack, support individual, use their phone for music, or distracting conversation).

– Paracervical block: pain scores are reduced by using the paracervical block into the cervical stroma prior to placing a tenaculum. You can do it by either injecting a local anesthetic into the cervicovaginal junction in either a four-point (at 2, 4, 8, and 10 o'clock) or two-point (at 4 and 8 o'clock only) fashion. A total dose of 5–20 mL of anesthetic agent (e.g.,1% lidocaine) is found to be adequate in 3 minutes to achieve satisfactory pain management.

• For cervical stenosis, consider using the cytobrush, rubber dilators, and endometrial Pipelle to sound before reaching out to metal sounds or dilators. Misoprostol is effective in women with no history of vaginal delivery but is not favorable for cervical dilation due to its side effects. Discuss topical estrogen for women with a recurring need for endometrial biopsy or colposcopy to reduce pain and trauma.
• Keep notes of each patient's needs for a successful and uneventful visualization in future appointments.

Sterility and Disinfection

Procedures in outpatient settings do not require an operating room's level of sterility. Using sterile gloves is not a guarantee to a sterile procedure, as it is possible to contaminate equipment, it is acceptable to use a "no touch technique" whereby no equipment that enters the uterus is touched.

While there is some evidence on cervical cleaning in improving pap smear quality, there is not much evidence to support the need for cervical cleaning with an antiseptic solution to reduce infection. Both povidone-iodine and chlorhexidine were reportedly used as antiseptic agents. There is no requirement to wear protective gear for any of the procedures discussed in this chapter.

All sharps should be installed in a biohazard container. Secure a box to place your reusable tools in for sterilization. Each practice addresses waste differently, not all waste goes to biohazard containers, review your practice policy and identify labels on the receptacles in your exam room for proper discarding.

Aftercare Instructions and Follow-Up

Longitudinal follow-up is a priceless virtue of primary care compared to specialty interaction. It is important to go over aftercare instructions with patients and discuss preferences for follow-up on results or postprocedural symptoms for optimally shared decision-making. Provide a printout or refer them to an electronic after-visit summary and consider providing those in the patient's preferred language if feasible.

It is important for patients to know that they may get two different bills: one for the procedure and one for pathology results if applicable.

Inform patients of potential next steps for management with diagnostic procedures and the need for follow-up with therapeutic ones.

Billing and Coding

It is important to keep up to date with billing and coding for in-office procedures, especially in primary care settings. Compliant and proper documentation of physician-led steps such as paracervical block, cervical dilation, and procedural complications secures a better appreciation of the complexity of the encounter and proper compensation.

Diagnostic(screening) Procedures

- *Endometrial biopsy*

    An endometrial biopsy (EMB) is a procedure during which a sample of the endometrial tissue is obtained using a small suction device that is inserted into the uterus to sample cells of the uterine body. The tissue obtained is examined by a pathologist and used to guide treatment or additional diagnostic workup.

    - Indications

        It is clinically indicated when there is abnormal uterine bleeding with an unopposed estrogen in a female's health profile. It is indicated for abnormal pap test findings as well. (See Table 3.2). The risk of malignancy is directly proportionate to the patient's age.

        Patients who are younger than 49 years of age are less likely to have a malignancy, it is left to the provider's discretion and the patient's preferences to wait and monitor symptoms if the patient is at low risk for endometrial cancer.

    - Contraindications

        EMB is contraindicated in cases of pregnancy, acute vaginitis, cervicitis, pelvic inflammatory disease, cervical cancer, and relatively in coagulopathy.

Table 3.2 Clinical indications for endometrial biopsy

AUB	Abnormal cervical cytology	Other
• <= 45 years old: • Unopposed estrogen: chronic ovulatory dysfunction, BMI >30, estrogen therapy without progesterone • Failed medical treatment for AUB • High risk of endometrial cancer (e.g., Lynch syndrome) • > 45 years old: any postmenopausal bleeding, metrorrhagia, menorrhagia, prolonged amenorrhea > 6 months	• Presence of AGC-endometrial. • Presence of AGC-all subcategories other than endometrial – If ≥35 years of age **or** at risk for endometrial cancer (risk factors or symptoms). • Presence of benign-appearing endometrial cells in patients ≥40 years of age who also have abnormal uterine bleeding or risk factors for endometrial cancer.	• Monitoring of patients with endometrial pathology (e.g., endometrial hyperplasia). • Screening in patients at high risk of endometrial cancer (e.g., Lynch syndrome).

AUB Abnormal uterine bleeding, *BMI* Body mass index, *AGC* Atypical glandular cells

- Risks and complications

  Inadequate sampling is the most disappointing complication long term. Other risks can be intolerance to the procedure, pelvic infection, pain, cramping, bleeding, and very rarely uterine perforation. Diagnostic errors are unlikely; EMB is 90% sensitive to endometrial malignancy and 82% to atypical hyperplasia and 100% specific in postmenopausal and premenopausal patients.

- Procedure steps

  1. Make sure an informed consent is signed and confirm the patient's name and date of birth.
  2. Prepare the patient for pelvic examination in the lithotomy position and ensure their comfort and yours by adjusting the examination table.
  3. Perform a bimanual examination to identify the cervical position and uterine fundal height if possible.
  4. Visualize the cervix using a reliable light source and proper vaginal speculum and lock your speculum once the cervix is satisfactorily visualized.
  5. Apply antiseptic agent using long oversized cotton swabs or hold pre-packaged betadine with a ring forceps.
  6. A paracervical block may be used or topical lidocaine to the cervix to reduce cramping when placing the tenaculum. We recommend injecting each quadrant of the cervix in case you had to change the tenaculum's position.
  7. Position your tenaculum on the cervix and apply gentle traction to stabilize and straighten the uterus. A heating pad may be of use to reduce cramping if the patient is able to hold it on their suprapubic area.
  8. See above for cervical dilation if cervical stenosis is noted.

9. Insert the Pipelle (suction sampler) in the uterus, pull the suction catheter, and twirl the Pipelle inside the uterus with an intentional scraping of the endometrial lining. If cervical stenosis is noted, refer to the tips above to dilate.
10. Make sure your formalin container is within reach to push the sample inside it without touching any other surface.
11. You can use multiple passes to get an adequate sample if the Pipelle doesn't touch any other surface in between passes.
12. Make sure your container has a patient label on it with the biopsy type written on it.
13. Remove the tenaculum and the speculum, check hemostasis of the cervix, and notify the patient of the procedure's conclusion. Praise them for their patience and cooperation.
14. Relieve your patient from the lithotomy position, allow the supine position for a few minutes for the patient to recover, and leave them a pad to use while getting dressed privately afterward. Hand your patient their user card and document the details of your procedure including the information about the device inserted.

– Procedural findings.

   You may notice a pale vulva indicative of low estrogen and a scanty endometrial sample. Consider suggesting a topical lubricant or hormonal therapy empirically to address the genitourinary syndrome of menopause.

– Moderate to copious samples can be indicative of a thick endometrial lining or phase of the cycle at the time of the biopsy and must be correlated with the clinical scenario. For premenopausal women, knowing their last menstrual period (LMP) can predict pathology findings of a proliferative or secretory phase of the cycle.

- *Colposcopy*

   Colposcopy is a diagnostic procedure in which a colposcope (a dissecting microscope with different magnifying lenses) is used to provide a magnified and illuminated view of the cervix to identify vulvar, vaginal, cervical, or anal dysplasia. For purposes of this chapter, we will focus on cervical colposcopy following an abnormal cervical screening test.

   Primary care providers are perfectly suited to counsel patients presenting for colposcopy about human papilloma virus (HPV) vaccine, and modifiable risk factors such as tobacco use, as well as educate them on updated cervical cancer screening guidelines (Fig. 3.5).

– Indications

   Providers can use the smartphone application of the American Society for Colposcopy and Cervical Pathology (ASCCP) for prompt and efficient clini-

Fig. 3.5 Colposcope

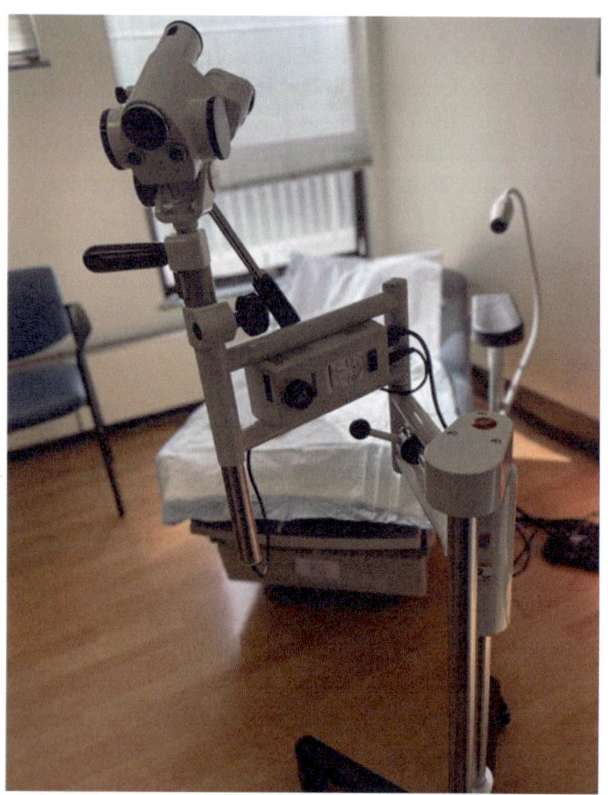

cal decision-making. ASCCP 2019 guidelines are updated to manage based on the patient's risk profile than merely on pathology results. Refer to Chap. 19 for more details on indications for colposcopy evaluation. The persistence of HPV infection for more than 12 months on a pap test is a major indication for a colposcopy examination. Dysplastic squamous changes of low grade or higher and any glandular atypia are other pathological indications for colposcopy regardless of HPV status.

– Contraindications

There are no absolute contraindications for colposcopy, however, either refer or reconsider the timing of the procedure if your patient is pregnant, has acute cervicitis, coagulopathy, or is immunocompromised. If in doubt, refer your patient to a cervical dysplasia clinic unless you are in a low-resource area.

Risks and complications

Unlikely to have any complications if there was no cervical biopsy collection. Potential complications are discomfort with the exam, cramping, inadequate sampling, and inability to fully visualize squamocolumnar junction

Table 3.3 Tips to overcome common challenges to colposcopy

Challenge	Tip (s)
Blood obscuring field during biopsy	Biopsy posterior cervical lip first
Limited visualization to SCJ (cervical stenosis or distorted due to history of previous treatment or large multiparous cervix)	Use a tenaculum with counter traction, graduated metal dilators, or even a small incision with a scalpel to open the os for adequate tissue sampling; consider a paracervical block for the treatment of discomfort. Endocervical speculum or use of sterile cotton swabs to manipulate external os
IUD strings with cervical mucus	Large-tip swabs with a generous acetic acid application will act as a mucolytic Use a cytobrush and twirl it inside the os to collect the cervical mucous Bozeman forceps or a small cotton swab to push the IUD strings up inside the cervix until the biopsy is completed, then gently bring them back down through the external os
Low estrogen (GSM)	Use a small lubricated (either tap water or gel) speculum or consider two to four weeks of topical estrogen cream, then repeat the examination, and minimal redirection of the speculum
Patient's habitus and mobility	A longer speculum needed to adequately visualize the cervix and complete the examination Traditional large metal Graves speculum is more durable and adjustable Reposition the patient low on the examination table and elevate legs for positional advantage; padded leg rests or surgical stirrups to assist with leg support Adjustable procedure room tables often start lower to the ground
Patient with intellectual disability	Always have a chaperone

(SCJ). To minimize complications: use tactics for optimal visualization and pain management described earlier in the chapter. Consider targeted sampling, especially with positive HPV type 16 and 18 to minimize missing dysplastic changes, and use cervical speculum for full SCJ visualization. Our colposcopy procedure is considered satisfactory when the SCJ is fully visualized.

There are minimal risks with performing colposcopy, however, we could have some challenges. See Table 3.3.

– Procedure steps

1. Review your patient's record thoroughly (LMP, tobacco use, immune status, parity, allergies) and document previous abnormal results and any past treatments.
2. Make sure an informed consent is signed and confirm the patient's name and date of birth.
3. Master your colposcopy skills

   a. Check your colposcope and adjust the intraocular distance between eyepieces to ensure binocular vision.

   b. Most colposcopes have a focal length of 30 cm between the lens and target tissue to allow enough room for instrument navigation.

   c. Fine focusing can be done by turning a knob, and coarse focusing is performed by moving the instrument toward or away from the patient.

   d. Low power (2× to 10×) is useful to obtain an overall impression of surface architecture. Medium (10× to 20×) and high (20× to 25×) powers are utilized to evaluate the vagina and cervix, with high power being particularly useful for close inspection of vascular patterns, which can signify high-grade or invasive disease. A consistent plan for magnification (usually starting at 15×) is important so that examinations are comparable and reproducible.

   e. A green filter switch is present to toggle between the two light settings. Green filter light may help identify vascular changes.

4. Prepare the patient for pelvic examination in the lithotomy position and ensure their comfort and yours by adjusting the examination table.

5. Visualize the cervix using a reliable light source and proper vaginal speculum and lock your speculum once the cervix is satisfactorily visualized.

6. Generously apply acetoacetic acid (AA) using long oversized cotton swabs. In 30–60 seconds, the acidic solution dehydrates cells so that squamous cells with relatively large or dense nuclei (e.g., metaplastic cells, dysplastic cells, and cells infected with HPV) reflect light and thus appear white. This is referred to as "acetowhite change." Blood vessels and columnar cells are not affected but they become easier to visualize against the white background. Fading of acetowhite changes usually occurs after three minutes, and therefore, acetic acid should be reapplied, as needed, after this time. If excessive acetic acid pools in the vagina, it should be removed with dry swabs as it can cause irritation. The squamous cells of the ectocervix have a smooth gray-pink appearance, and the glandular cells of the endocervix have a pink-red cobblestone appearance.

7. If no lesions are seen after AA is applied, a dilute **Lugol** solution may be applied to the cervix. Lugol's iodine consists of 5 g of iodine and 10 g of potassium iodide in 100 mL of distilled water. Uniform uptake of stain would confirm the colposcopist's impression that no lesion is present. Glycogen-containing cells will take up iodine and become dark brown (Chocolate color). Non-glycogenated cells, such as normal columnar or glandular cells, high-grade lesions, and many low-grade lesions, will not take up iodine and remain light yellow (mustard color). We would only

recommend this step if there were a high suspicion of neoplasia as it can interfere with the pathology's examination.

8. If any abnormal findings are noted, obtain a targeted cervical biopsy (1–2 mm) using a cervical punch biopsy instrument. Multiple targeted biopsies increased the detection of CIN 2 or worse compared with single ones. The sensitivity of two (82%) or three or more (83.3%) biopsies was superior to one biopsy (68%).

9. To minimize the impact of bleeding after a biopsy, start with the posterior cervical lip first, take smaller biopsies, specifically for cancerous-looking lesions, apply pressure with cotton swabs, and use silver nitrate for small bleeds and Monel's solution for prominent ones.

10. Endocervical curettage (ECC) is performed by inserting a long straight curette into the endocervical canal and scraping the four quadrants of the canal. An endocervical brush is then inserted and rotated to remove any exfoliated tissue. These specimens should be collected and labeled separately. A drop of mucus and blood is often seen at the os after ECC, and this should be included in the specimen.

    a. Per ASCCP 2019 guidelines ECC is not indicated in pregnant patients and is not recommended for all colposcopies. Of note, some data suggest that ECC increases the sensitivity of the examination, particularly in older patients, as it can sample skin lesions -noncontiguous- seen in glandular neoplasia.

    b. Indications for ECC include atypical squamous cells that cannot exclude HSIL (ASC-H), high-grade squamous in situ lesion (HSIL), atypical glandular cells (AGC); adenocarcinoma in situ, inadequate colposcopy, no lesion visualized in ASCUS or LSIL exam in a high-risk patient, or ablative treatment is contemplated.

11. Make sure your formalin container is within reach to push the sample inside it, you may use toothpicks to push the sample into the container.

12. Make sure your container(s) has a patient label, biopsy type, and location written on it (them). Confirm the date of birth and name with the patient prior to sending specimens to pathology.

13. Remove the speculum and notify the patient of the procedure's conclusion. Praise them for their patience and cooperation.

14. Relieve your patient from the lithotomy position, allow the supine position for a few minutes for the patient to recover, and leave them a pad to use while getting dressed privately afterward.

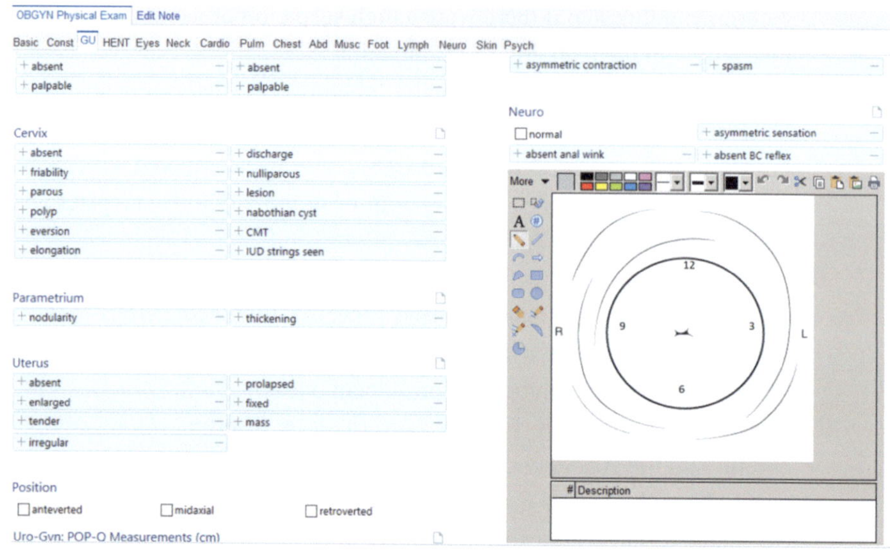

Fig. 3.6 Electronic record documentation of colposcopy findings

Table 3.4 Pathological Findings on colposcopy warranting biopsy

Colposcopic sign	Normal	Abnormal
Transformation zone (TZ)	Nabothian cysts Gland openings Glycogenated epithelium Faint acetowhite epithelium (squamous metaplasia)	Acetowhite epithelia after AA application Vascular abnormalities (punctation, mosaicism, atypical vessels) Ulcerations
Rubin and Barbo's assessment Color Vessels Borders Surface	Pink/Translucent Fine/lacy/Normal branching Normal TZ Flat	White/red/yellow/gray Punctation/mosaic/irregular/bizarre Diffuse/geographic/peeling/rolled edges Papillary/raised/nodular/ ulcerated/necrotic/exophytic
Reid's Colposcopic Index Margin Color Vessels Iodine staining	Indistinct margins No acetowhite epithelia Unform vessel patterns with no dilation No iodine uptake (chocolate brown color)	Sharp peripheral margins or internal borders between areas of different appearances Shiny gray-white or dull gray Definite punctuation or dilated vessels in well-defined patterns. (Suspicious yet organized behavior) Partial or large iodine intake with yellow staining (mustard-yellow appearance)

15. Your findings must be documented in detail; visualization of SCJ, size, and location of biopsies and abnormalities, and evaluation of vulva and vaginal orifices. The locations of abnormalities are noted in numbers as on the face of the clock (e.g., 1 o'clock location). (See Fig. 3.6).

– Procedure findings

To biopsy or not to biopsy is the decision every colposcopist must make. There are few systems to differentiate abnormal findings from normal, hence deciding on taking a biopsy. In general, any acetowhite or vascular abnormalities would warrant a biopsy and the ability to detect a dysplastic lesion improves significantly when two or more biopsies are taken.

The transformation zone is the area bordered laterally by the original squamocolumnar junction (SCJ) and medially by the new SCJ. In between both, the squamous metaplasia is characterized by high cellular activity and is at risk of neoplastic transformation. So, visualizing the SCJ is crucial for satisfactory evaluation and sampling process. The normal transformation zone contains mature squamous epithelium, squamous metaplasia, Nabothian cysts, gland openings, and fine reticular blood vessels.

Rubin and Barbo's colposcopic assessment system and Reid's Colposcopic index (RCI) can be used to identify pathological findings. (See Table 3.4) RCI gives a score to each colposcopic sign from 0–2 depending on tissue changes noted on colposcopy, a sum score higher than 5 is considered a high-grade disease.

Primary care providers are likely to refer high-grade dysplasia to a dysplasia clinic or gynecology when found on colposcopy unless in low resource area and they are trained to provide LEEP and cryotherapy.

- *Vulvar biopsy*

  – Indications

  Any lesions suspicious for malignancy following the ABCD for skin changes (Asymmetry, Border irregularity, Color variation, Diameter change), bleeding, non-healing ulcers, or firm to the touch. If a diagnosis is inconclusive by visual inspection or a lesion is not responsive to standard treatments.

  – Contraindications

  Pregnancy, bleeding disorders, and current infection. We recommend referring blistering or ulcerating lesions to a specialty clinic unless primary care clinicians have advanced training for dysplastic vulvar lesions.

  – Risks and complications

  Bleeding, infection, inadequate biopsy, scarring, and pain.

  – Procedure steps

    1. Place the patient properly on an examination table in a lithotomy position, and inspect the vulva for skin changes. If the lesion is in the clitoris, urethra, or anal opening refer to a specialist.

2. Prepare the selected with a cleansing solution then apply a topical anesthetic as early as possible for it to be effective. Topical lidocaine-prilocaine cream is found to significantly reduce pain scale prior to the injectable anesthetic. A topical anesthetic may take up to 15 minutes on mucous membranes and more on keratinized tissue. Thereafter, inject 1–2 ml of 1 to 2% lidocaine with or without epinephrine into the biopsy site. Ensure effective analgesia with the patient using the needle before taking the biopsy.

3. For shave biopsy a sterile surgical Dermablade is fine to use. Shave biopsies can be adequate for epidermal lesions with no depth suspected. They are not recommended when melanoma is suspected. A punch biopsy is warranted if dermal and subcutaneous involvement is suspected. A cervical punch biopsy forceps can be used if low suspicion for cancer and a punch biopsy (2–6 mm) for full-thickness biopsy if the cancer diagnosis is most likely on your differential.

4. Hemostasis can be achieved by either pressure or a chemical agent. If bleeding persists a suture of the wound may be warranted. Your office setting should have 4–0 absorbable sutures available to reduce discomfort and infection rate.

5. Send tissue to pathology and prepare your patient for your result wait time and future management.

6. For wound care counsel your patient to keep the site dry and clean with no dressing needed. Sitz bath with lukewarm water to reduce swelling or pain if any and may apply plain petrolatum to it.

Therapeutic (prevention)

- LARC

  Long-acting reversible contraceptives (LARC) indications and contraindications are discussed in Chap. 12.

  – Risks and complications of the procedure:

    IUD insertion: infection, bleeding, cramping, menstrual irregularities, secondary amenorrhea, lost IUD strings, and very rarely perforation of the uterus.

    IUD removal: most IUD removals are uneventful. Visibility of the IUD strings and removing the IUD device intact are the optimal outcome. IUD strings may be missed due to retraction into the cervical canal, misplacement, migration, perforation, or expulsion. Lost IUD strings are reported in up to 18% of IUDs.

Implant insertion: *local effects*: bruise to the arm, misplacement of the implant, swelling, pain, hematoma, and erythema. *Systemic side effects*: irregular menstrual bleeding, weight changes, emotional lability, headaches, and acne.

Implant removal: difficult removal due to deeply located rod or broken rod, bleeding, hematoma, bruising of the skin, and skin scarring from incision to remove the implant.

– Procedure steps

IUD insertion

1. Same steps (1–8) in endometrial biopsy procedure.
2. Proper sounding using either a metal sound or a Pipelle reduces the risk of misplacement. Most IUDs can be reliably placed into uterine cavities of a depth between 6 and 10 cm, small or larger cavities are more likely to experience expulsion or misplacement.
3. Remove the tenaculum ensure hemostasis, then remove the speculum and notify the patient of the procedure's conclusion. Praise them for their patience and cooperation.
4. Relieve your patient from the lithotomy position, allow the supine position for a few minutes for the patient to recover, and leave them a pad to use while getting dressed privately afterward.
5. Hand your patient their user card and document the details of your procedure including the information about the device inserted.

IUD removal

1. Place the patient on the examination table in a lithotomy position.
2. Use ring forceps to grasp the IUD strings and gently pull the IUD strings out.
3. For lost strings, consider using a cytobrush, forceps alligator (blind or ultrasound-guided), or refer to gynecology for further evaluation and removal in an operating room.
4. Confirm that the IUD is intact, show it to the patient, remove the speculum, and relieve them from the lithotomy position.
5. Document alternative plans for bleeding, contraception, or conception counseling.

Implant insertion.

1. Place your patient supine on an examination table
2. You may position the patient's nondominant arm extended at a full length or the upper inner aspect of it in a bending position by flexing the

patient's elbow 90 degrees and rotating the arm upward and outward so that the patient's hand is next to their head.

3. Identify the planned insertion site 8–10 cm (3–4 inches) from the medial epicondyle of the humerus and 3–5 cm (1.25–2 inches) posterior to (below) the sulcus (groove) between the biceps and triceps muscles" (i.e., overlying the triceps muscle and not the sulcus itself). Some new insertion sites have been identified in the literature, but outside the scope of primary care settings (e.g., the Scapular region, supraumbilical region, and medial side of the thigh). A sterile drape may be placed under the patient's arm.

4. Warn your patient of a burning sensation from the injectable lidocaine Use a 25-gauge, 1.5-inch needle on a 2–5 ml syringe to inject a local anesthetic(1 to 2 mL of 1% lidocaine) into the dermis to raise a small wheal along the planned track of the rod insertion needle.

5. You better be seated and view the insertion site from the side, not from above the device to ensure a subdermal insertion that avoids the sulcus.

6. The sharp, beveled trocar easily penetrates the skin; a separate incision is not needed. Grasp the applicator above the needle cap on its textured surface between the thumb and forefinger, remove the clear plastic needle cover, and place the needle against the insertion site holding the applicator at an angle of 30 degrees to the skin. While applying counter traction to the skin around the insertion site, puncture the skin with the needle tip. Lower the applicator so that it is parallel to the skin and advance the needle in the subdermal connective tissue while lifting the skin with the tip of the needle without forcing the tip into the skin above. You must advance the needle to its full length. If the needle is not fully advanced under the skin, the implant will not be correctly inserted. Lastly, unlock the slider with downward finger pressure on the lever, and then, move the slider fully backward (distally) and remove the applicator.

7. Immediately after insertion, palpate the skin to verify the correct placement of the rod; both ends should be palpable. Ask the patient to feel the implant, then place an adhesive closure (e.g., "Steri strip") on the insertion puncture and wrap the site with a pressure bandage. Check the applicator to make sure the implant is no longer in the cannula.

8. Hand your patient their user card and document the details of your procedure including the information about the device inserted.

Implant removal.

1. Position your patient with their arm bent as described for the implant insertion. It is crucial to palpate the implant, if the implant is not palpable, we recommend radio imaging and referral to gynecology for removal.

2. Use your sterile gloves to cleanse the site where the incision will be made with an antiseptic. Drape above and below the implant.

3. Identify your incision site by pushing down on the proximal end of the rod (the end closest to the axilla) and inject no more than 0.5 mL of lidocaine with epinephrine subdermal under the elevated distal tip of the rod, raising a small wheal (<5 mm). Massage this area to disperse the anesthetic. We recommend using epinephrine to reduce the bleeding.

4. Make a 2–3 mm longitudinal incision with a #11 scalpel through the skin over the end of the rod. Deepen the incision until you feel a rubbery sensation against the point of the scalpel blade; this is the rod encased in a fibrous sheath. Nick the fibrous sheath covering the end of the rod with the tip of the scalpel blade. It may take several nicks in different directions to fully open the sheath.

5. Use your fingers to apply pressure on the proximal (axillary) end of the implant so that the distal (elbow) end pushes up against the skin. Pushing the rod against the incision with finger pressure is critical for success with this "Pop Out" technique. If pressure is released, the rod will slip back into the fibrous sheath in the subdermal tissue. That is where most of the bruising may occur.

6. The end of the rod will come into view as the sheath is opened. Continue to exert finger pressure on the proximal (axillary) end of the rod to push the distal (elbow) end through the incision until it can be grasped with mosquito forceps or fingers and pulled out. Confirm that all 40 mm of the rod has been removed.

7. Close the incision with a Steri strip and cover it with a pressure bandage to minimize bruising.

- Polyps' removal.

  – Indications
    Symptomatic polyps (e.g., abnormal uterine bleeding, postcoital bleeding,
  – Contraindications
  – Pregnancy, infection, or bleeding disorder.
  – Risks and complications

- Recurrence, pain, bleeding, and infection.
- Procedure steps

1. Place patient properly for pelvic examination.
2. Visualize the polyp.
3. You may use a paracervical block to reduce pain and cramping.
4. Place long Kelly or ring forceps as close to the base of the polyp as possible and clamp.
5. Twist the polyp in one direction until it easily breaks off. Place the polyp and tissue collected in a formalin container.
6. Use an EC curette to scrape the base of the endocervical canal to remove any polyp remnants. An endocervical brush can also be used.
7. Use Silver nitrate or Monsel's solution for hemostasis.
8. Send the specimen to pathology for review.

3.5 Our Case

JF results came back benign for the EMB and CIN1 from the colposcopy. She was scheduled for co-testing in 12 months since her last three pap tests charted were normal and HPV negative. She was interested in a hormonal IUD placement to stop her bleeding and was agreeable to lifestyle modifications for her weight gain.

3.6 Summary

Procedures in primary care outpatient settings are cost-effective, improve patient access, reduce specialty clinics' burden, and provide professional growth to primary care clinicians. Training primary care residents and clinicians to provide merits emphasis in graduate medical education.

Suggested Reading

1. Ravindran TS. Universal access: making health systems work for women. BMC Public Health. 2012;12(Suppl 1):S4. https://doi.org/10.1186/1471-2458-12-S1-S4.
2. Pace LE, Dolan BM, Tishler LW, Gooding HC, Bartz D. Incorporating long-acting reversible contraception into primary care: a training and practice innovation. Womens Health Issues. 2016;26(2):131–4.

3. Striepe MI, Coons HL. Women's health in primary care: Interdisciplinary interventions. Fam Syst Health. 2002;20(3):237–51. https://doi.org/10.1037/h0089578.

4. Loveys AJ. "A family doctor can do that!" Is there a role for a formalized referral network for office procedures in family practices of Newfoundland and Labrador? In: Electronic thesis and dissertation repository; 2015. p. 3408.

5. Arnold MJ, Jonas CE, Carter RE. Point-of-care ultrasonography. Am Fam Physician. 2020;101(5):275–85.

6. Shen-Wagner J, Deutchman M. Point-of-care ultrasound: a practical guide for primary care. Fam Pract Manag. 2020;27(6):33–40.

7. Cattoni E, Sorice P, Leidi-Bulla L. Pessary: A rediscovered tool. In: Management of pelvic organ prolapse. Cham: Springer; 2018. p. 81–94.

8. Planer R. Cervical polyp removal. In: Primary care procedures in women's health. Cham: Springer; 2020. p. 93–100.

9. Picone ML. Vulvar Skin Biopsy. In: Primary Care Procedures in Women's Health. New York: Springer; 2010. p. 265–74.

10. Williams LK, Weber JM, Pieper C, Lorenzo A, Moss H, Havrilesky LJ. Lidocaine–Prilocaine cream compared with injected lidocaine for vulvar biopsy: a randomized controlled trial. Obstet Gynecol. 2020;135(2):311–8.

11. Rifat SF, Moeller JL. Basics of joint injection: general techniques and tips for safe, effective use. Postgrad Med. 2001;109(1):157–66.

12. Poulin EA, Swartz AW, O'Grady JS, Kersten MP, Angstman KB. Essential office procedures for medicare patients in primary care: comparison with family medicine residency training. Fam Med. 2019;51(7):574–7. https://doi.org/10.22454/FamMed.2019.659478.

13. Ireland LD, Allen RH. Pain management for gynecologic procedures in the office. Obstet Gynecol Surv. 2016;71(2):89–98.

14. Trolice FC, McGrady S. Anesthetic efficacy of intrauterine lidocaine for endometrial biopsy: a randomized double-masked trial. Obstetrics and Gynecology (New York. 1953). 2000;95(3):345–7. https://doi.org/10.1016/S0029-7844(99)00557-8.

15. Hashem AT, Mahmoud M, Aly Islam B, Ibrahem Eid M, Ahmed N, Mohamed Mamdouh A, et al. Comparative efficacy of lidocaine–prilocaine cream and vaginal misoprostol in reducing pain during levonorgestrel intrauterine device insertion in women delivered only by cesarean delivery: A randomized controlled trial. Int J Gynecol Obstet. 2022.

16. Hellekson K. AAP issues recommendations on infection control in physicians' offices. Am Fam Physician. 2001;63(4):787–9.

17. Kotaska AJ, Matisic JP. Cervical cleaning improves Pap smear quality. CMAJ. 2003;169(7):666–9.

18. Cartier S, Mayrand MH, Gougeon F, Simard-Émond L. Endometrial biopsy in low-risk women: Are we over-investigating? J Obstet Gynaecol Can. 2022;44(10):1097–101.

19. Long S. Endometrial biopsy: indications and technique. Prim Care. 2021;48(4):555–67.

20. Burness JV, Schroeder JM, Warren JB. Cervical colposcopy: Indications and risk assessment. Am Fam Physician. 2020;102(1):39–48.

21. Wentzensen N, Walker JL, Gold MA, et al. Multiple biopsies, and detection of cervical cancer precursors at colposcopy. J Clin Oncol. 2015;33(1):83–9.

22. Gage JC, Hanson VW, Abbey K, et al. ASCUS LSIL Triage Study (ALTS) group. Number of cervical biopsies and sensitivity of colposcopy. Obstet Gynecol. 2006;108(2):264–72.

23. Buscema, Woodruff JD. Significance of neoplastic a typicalities in endocervical epithelium. Gynecol Oncol. 1984;17(3):356–62. https://doi.org/10.1016/0090-8258(84)90221-X.
24. Verma U, Astudillo-Dávalos FE, Gerkowicz SA. Safe and cost-effective ultrasound-guided removal of retained intrauterine device: our experience. Contraception. 2015;92(1):77–80.
25. Reed S, Heinemann K. Events associated with Nexplanon insertion and removal: interim results from the Nexplanon observational risk assessment study (NORA). Contraception. 2016;94(4):409.
26. Prabhakaran, Chuang A. In-office retrieval of intrauterine contraceptive devices with missing strings. Contraception (Stoneham). 2011;83(2):102–6. https://doi.org/10.1016/j.contraception.2010.07.004.
27. Stabile G, Foti C, Mordeglia D, De Santo D, Mangino FP, Laganà AS, Ricci G. Alternative insertion site of nexplanon: description of a case report and systematic review of the literature. J Clin Med. 2022;11(11):3226.

Part II
Non Infection Medical Condition in Women

Chapter 4
Pelvic Pain

Molly Heublein

4.1 Case

Amy is a 27 year old woman who presents to establish care and get help with pelvic pain. She reports since she was a teen she had intermittent pelvic pain, now happening more frequently and getting to the point that sometimes it is so uncomfortable she misses work and she avoids sexual intercourse. She has a history of migraine headaches, but is otherwise healthy. She takes ibuprofen and acetaminophen for the pain but no other medications. We find some information in her past charts—she has had some prior workup with her last PCP including negative screening for sexual transmitted infections, a normal urinalysis, and an unremarkable pelvic ultrasound.

4.2 Introduction

Clinic visits for chronic pelvic pain are a common scenario that we need to feel comfortable managing in primary care. An estimated one-quarter of women struggle with chronic pelvic pain, and in 80% the cause may not be gynecologic. We in primary care are in the perfect position to identify all organ systems that may be involved and initiate treatment to help our patients improve their quality of life.

Chronic pelvic pain is defined by the American College of Obstetrics and Gynecology as pain perceived by clinician or patient to come from anywhere in the pelvis (below umbilicus including lower back, vagina, and vulva) persistent for typically at least 6 months, although when associated with disability, may qualify if

M. Heublein (✉)
Department of General Internal Medicine, Women's Health Primary Care, UCSF,
San Francisco, CA, USA
e-mail: molly.heublein@ucsf.edu

M. Mahmoudi (ed.), *Common Cases in Women's Primary Care Clinics*,
https://doi.org/10.1007/978-3-031-48569-5_4

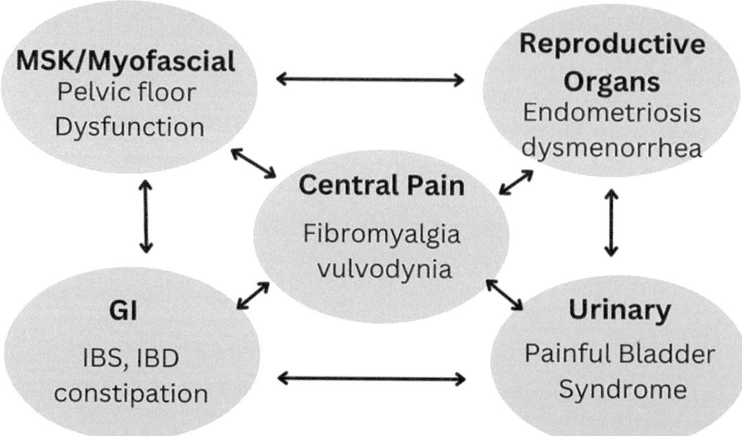

Fig. 4.1 Organ system approach to pelvic pain

persistent for a shorter period of time (i.e. 3 months). Chronic pelvic pain now includes recurrent cyclic pelvic pain or dysmenorrhea as well as more persistent pain conditions.

Because the pelvis is so complex, it can be helpful to use an organ system approach to addressing chronic pelvic pain focusing on the 5 organ systems: (1) Reproductive organs (endometriosis, ovarian cysts, etc.) (2) Musculoskeletal or myofascial (pelvic floor dysfunction, referred back/hip pain); (3) GI (IBS, IBD, etc.); (4) Urinary (painful bladder syndrome); (5) Central pain (fibromyalgia/neuropathic pain, vulvodynia). Considering each of these should allow the clinician to tailor evaluation and treatment (Fig. 4.1).

4.3 Differential Diagnosis

In patients with chronic pelvic pain, 20–40% will have more than one cause. Thinking through each organ system can help identify areas that require more evaluation and then help direct treatment.

Viscero-visceral cross-sensitization or convergence is an important concept for understanding pelvic pain syndromes. The nerve pathways in the pelvis are physically closely linked, and stimulation of one pathway can trigger nerve responses in neighboring organs. For example, when the uterus contracts during menstruation or childbirth, this frequently triggers colon contraction which can lead to bowel changes or bladder spasm which can cause urinary symptoms. This can make determining a set of symptoms or single underlying pathology challenging, but being aware of this can help patients understand their symptoms more fully.

4.3.1 Reproductive Organs

Reproductive organs are immediately thought of as a primary cause for pelvic pain in women, but in reality, they are only etiology in the minority of chronic pelvic pain patients. Most urgent causes of pelvic pain of course need to be considered and ruled out, but these are rarely chronic. Patients with chronic pelvic pain should be screened for pelvic inflammatory disease with sexually transmitted infection (STI) screening, gynecologic cancers with pap smears and pelvic ultrasound, and structural causes such as fibroids and ovarian cysts with pelvic ultrasound. In reality, most patients with chronic pelvic pain will have a non-structural or functional cause and will thus have normal pelvic imaging and negative STI screening. Aspects of history that suggest a gynecologic cause of pelvic pain is dysmenorrhea or pelvic pain that is now chronic but has progressed from pain that originally was cyclic with menses. Chronic pelvic pain associated with heavy menstrual bleeding also can suggest a gynecologic cause (Fig. 4.2).

Primary dysmenorrhea is a condition where patients present with painful menses without another identifiable cause. Research suggests this may be due to increased prostaglandin production which triggers uterine contraction, leading to reductions in blood flow which can trigger anaerobic metabolites that trigger nerve pain transmission. Patients complain of cramping pain which may be severe during their cycle and can also be associated with bowel changes and nausea.

Endometriosis does need to be considered as imaging is insensitive and diagnosis is frequently delayed. Endometriosis is a condition in which the endometrium, the cells which shed with menses every month which is usually contained within the uterus, is found freely in the pelvis. This tissue can implant on the ovaries, the lining of the abdominal cavity (peritoneum), and the bowel. It can cause chronic pelvic pain, pain with sex, and infertility. When bowel or bladder is involved, patients can present with tenesmus, hematuria, dysuria, or bowel changes. Prevalence rates are challenging to determine, but an estimated 5–10% of reproductive age women may experience symptoms or morbidity related to endometriosis in their lifetime. The

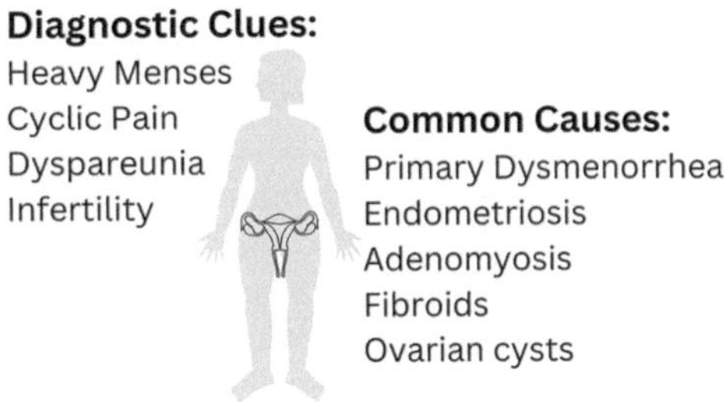

Fig. 4.2 Reproductive organ causes of chronic pelvic pain

numbers vary widely, another study found endometriosis in 82% of symptomatic women and 24% of asymptomatic women.

There are several proposed mechanisms for the etiology of endometriosis, but actually research has not conclusively shown a cause. Retrograde menstruation is posited as the origin; however, this seems to be a common/physiologic occurrence and why some women develop endometriosis and others do not is unclear. Fascinatingly, endometriosis can be found in distant sites almost anywhere in the body—higher in the abdominal cavity on liver/kidneys, at prior surgical sites, or in the lungs. A few case studies have even found endometriosis in men. Another possible cause for endometriosis that may explain this diversity of location is that progenitor cells in the peritoneum give rise to endometrial cells spontaneously or due to local/systemic influences.

Regardless of the underlying etiology, once endometrial cells are present outside the endometrium, there is a complex interplay between immune response to these endometrial deposits (either clearing them or causing chronic inflammation and scarring) may affect the development of endometriosis. Another important factor in the symptomatic development of pain from endometriosis seems to be nerve transmission thresholds and the way pain is processed in the central nervous system which varies between different people. Some women with severe endometriosis seen on laparoscopy done for other causes may experience no pain. Others with small deposits may have debilitating symptoms.

The most difficult thing about diagnosing this condition is that imaging is insensitive, and endometriosis may require laparoscopy to identify. Understandably, women with milder symptoms, and clinicians treating, may be hesitant to pursue an invasive procedure. Unfortunately MRI and ultrasound can only see large lesions, so have a low sensitivity. It is important to keep endometriosis on the differential for patients with painful periods or cyclic pelvic pain.

Adenomyosis is a condition in which the endometrium invades the myometrium and can be linked with heavy menses and pelvic pain. This was initially considered a rare condition, more common as women near menopause since it was diagnosed on hysterectomy. Lately, adenomyosis is becoming increasingly recognized as ultrasound and MRI imaging techniques of the pelvis improve, visualizing this condition in younger women. The etiology of adenomyosis is still being determined, but seems to involve an interplay of hormone receptor alterations, inflammation/fibrosis, and growth factors/neuroangiogenic factors. An estimated 10–35% of women have evidence of adenomyosis, but not all will have symptoms.

Another common structural cause of pelvic pain due to a gynecologic etiology includes *fibroids or uterine myomas* (benign growths of the uterus muscle). These are common and when small may be asymptomatic, but when large can cause bulk symptoms of painful periods, progressing to persistent pressure or pain, or pain with sex. Symptoms usually progress gradually as the fibroid slowly enlarges. Fibroids are very estrogen sensitive and so tend to increase in size during reproductive years and then shrink after menopause. Fibroids are readily imaged on ultrasound.

Adnexal masses or cysts when large or ruptured may cause pelvic pain and these are generally easily visualized on pelvic imaging. Small adnexal cysts are physiologic with menstruation and typically do not cause pelvic pain, cyst rupture may cause acute pain but they are rarely implicated in chronic pelvic pain. Full evaluation of adnexal masses is beyond the scope of this chapter, but if there is concern for pelvic malignancy, consultation with a gynecologist is suggested.

4.3.2 Musculoskeletal or Myofascial Pain

Musculoskeletal or myofascial pain is a common cause of pelvic pain and is often overlooked (Fig. 4.3).

Pelvic floor dysfunction is becoming an increasingly recognized cause of pelvic pain. This can occur when there is either weakness or spasm of the muscles in the base of the pelvis that support the bladder, uterus, and colon. Clues on history can be associated dyspareunia, overactive bladder symptoms, chronic constipation, or pelvic organ prolapse. Examination with a bimanual examination can be very helpful to evaluate resting tone of the pelvic floor, identify focal muscle tenderness or spasm on palpation, and examine for prolapse.

Referred pain from the low back or hips can manifest as pelvic pain. Performing a careful history which elicits symptoms related to movement or positional changes and an examination of the patient's adjacent joints can help suggest these pathologies. A full scope of evaluation of orthopedic complaints is outside the scope of this chapter, but clinicians should not ignore their orthopedic training when the complaint is female pelvic pain.

4.3.3 Gastrointestinal

Gastrointestinal causes of pelvic pain are not uncommon, and we as primary care providers are in an excellent position to help determine this etiology. A careful history of bowel patterns looking for constipation, diarrhea, tenesmus, or

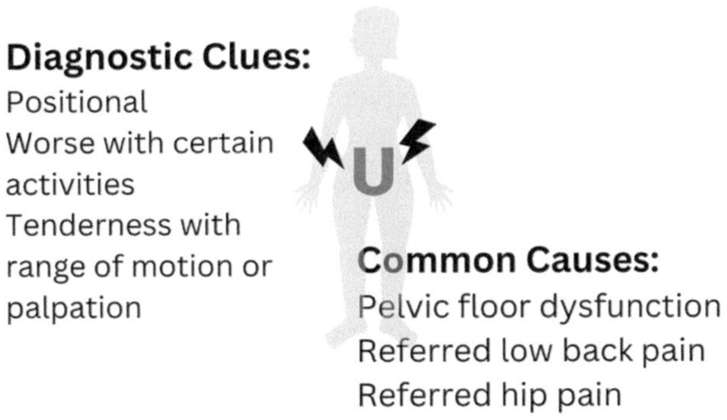

Fig. 4.3 Musculoskeletal causes of chronic pelvic pain

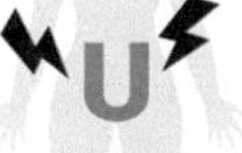

hematochezia should be elicited. It is beyond the scope of this chapter to fully discuss colonic causes of pelvic pain, but appropriate to rule out serious pathology such as colon cancer or inflammatory bowel disease in appropriate patients, and important to be aware that irritable bowel syndrome (IBS) can be a common cause of pelvic pain that seems to fluctuate with bowel function.

4.3.4 Urinary

Urinary causes of pelvic pain are common. Ruling out more acute or serious causes such as urinary tract infection, nephrolithiasis, and/or bladder tumors may be appropriate in select patients. In patients with a normal urinalysis and no other risk factors (younger age, no hematuria, etc.), bladder pain syndrome is an important entity to not miss. Patients with *bladder pain syndrome* (previously termed interstitial cystitis) may complain of pelvic pain and urinary urgency or frequency. The typical patient would be one who reports recurrent sensations of a bladder infection with repeatedly negative urinalysis and culture and definitely should be considered in a patient who fails to respond to antibiotics for UTI symptoms and has negative cultures. This condition is still an area of active research, but the current understanding is that it is a central pain condition leading to heightened pain transmission from the bladder. It may include aspects of overactive bladder symptoms and pelvic floor dysfunction. These patients often struggle with other overlapping central pain conditions (see below). Helping patients receive this diagnosis can help limit the exposure to unhelpful and unnecessary antibiotics for dysuria symptoms. In a low risk patient with appropriate symptoms and normal urinalysis, recurrent episodes or symptoms of dysuria, frequency, and pelvic pain are sufficient to make the diagnosis without advanced urologic testing (no need for urodynamic studies).

4.3.5 Central Pain Disorders

Central pain disorders such as fibromyalgia or central sensitization should be explored. A growing body of research reliably shows a variety of differences in how pain processing occurs across the population. Pain transmission is complex and begins with peripheral nerves obtaining enough input to cross a threshold for passing signals. The density of pain sensing c-fibers varies between individuals. The signals are then summed and passed to the spinal cord where they are processed in the dorsal root ganglion. Some signals here may be downregulated or upregulated. Pro-nociceptive (pain upregulating) including substance p and glutamate and anti-nociceptive (pain downregulating) molecules like endogenous opioids, cannabinoids, and norepinephrine present in the spinal fluid can increase or decrease transmission. Neural impulses that do continue on are passed on to the brain, where differences in brain interconnectivity and pain processing have been seen on functional MRIs. Together this variety can cause a significant difference between people in how pain, temperature, and vibration signals are experienced. These differences can be genetic—differences in genes important in catecholamine metabolism have been prospectively linked to the development of chronic painful conditions. Environmental and psychosocial factors impact pain transmission as well. Prior trauma, depression, lack of sleep as well as beliefs around pain and health can contribute to an increased pain sensitivity (Fig. 4.4).

In *fibromyalgia*, this upregulation of pain transmission is diffuse and patients experience widespread pain across multiple regions of the body, typically also associated with central symptoms of fatigue, lack of restful sleep, cognitive dysfunction, or depression. Fibromyalgia can be diagnosed using the American College of Rheumatology 2010 criteria, with a Widespread Pain Index (WPI) and Symptom Severity Score above thresholds. There is no specific laboratory or imaging finding that diagnoses fibromyalgia. Fibromyalgia prevalence is estimated around 2–3% of the population, with a significant female predominance. Understanding the patient's other underlying medical conditions and symptoms rather than focusing just on pelvic pain can help a clinician identify these patients. While a patient may present specifically for pelvic pain, if on questioning you also learn that she is experiencing headaches, neck pain, nausea, dizziness, fatigue, paresthesias, and exercise intolerance, it is appropriate to consider a broader cause beyond pelvic specific pathology, such as fibromyalgia.

Vulvodynia is an important diagnosis to be aware of in the central sensitization disorders that can contribute to chronic pelvic pain. Vulvodynia is diagnosed when there is significant vulvar pain, often described as burning and associated with dyspareunia, without a clear visible or structural cause (so excludes conditions like postherpetic neuralgia or genitourinary syndrome of menopause). Vulvodynia is estimated to effect 8–10% of reproductive age women and can lead to significant

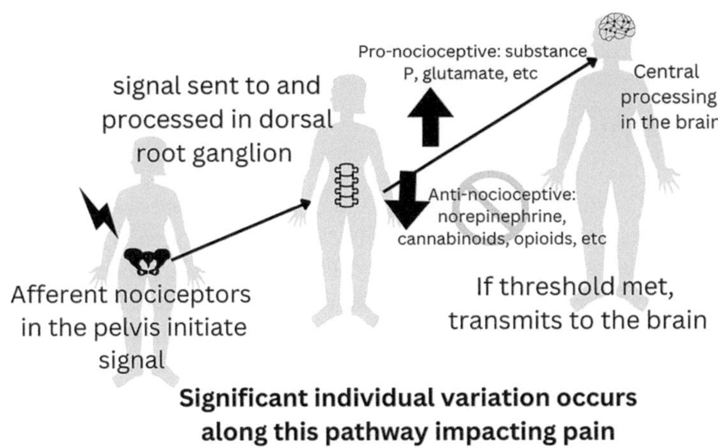

Fig. 4.4 Pain transmission

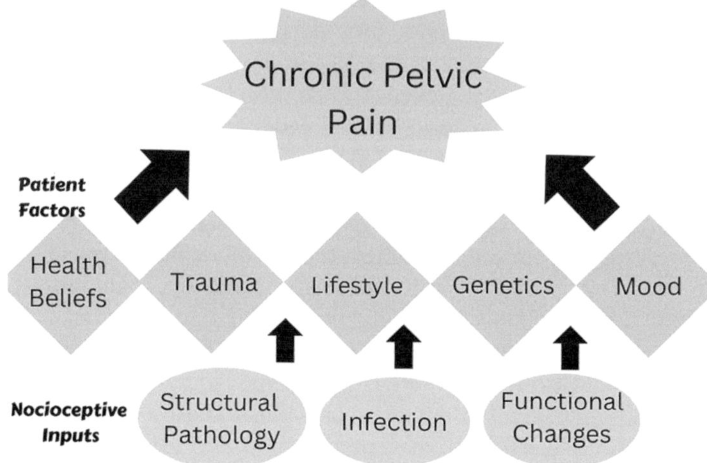

Fig. 4.5 Central sensitization

morbidity due to its effect on sexual intimacy, psychological wellbeing, and daily activities. It is understood to be caused by dysfunctional pain signaling that is giving the patient the feeling of pain without structural damage (Fig. 4.5).

Patients without an overt diagnosis of fibromyalgia may still have central sensitization and upregulation of pain transmission. This can lead to small changes in structural pathology (for example, small endometrial deposits on the adnexa) causing severe pain in one patient and no symptoms in another. Chronic pain conditions frequently overlap; patients with chronic pelvic pain have significantly higher rates of headache disorders, temporomandibular dysfunction, and irritable bowel syndrome. Understanding the patients broader medical history can help point toward this diagnosis.

4.4 Evaluation

The first step in evaluation is ruling out acute pathology or conditions which may need more emergent treatment to prevent further tissue damage such as pelvic inflammatory disease, urinary infections, or pelvic masses concerning for malignancy. Most patients with chronic pelvic pain will have already had a basic evaluation, but if they have not already been checked, testing for sexually transmitted infections, obtaining a urinalysis, and getting a pelvic ultrasound are important. If these tests have already been run and were normal, repeating them for ongoing, unchanged symptoms is low yield and should be discouraged as it does not improve patients functionality or increase diagnostic yield.

When a patient presents with chronic pelvic pain, they have often had painful or traumatic examinations in past medical visits and may not be ready or willing to undergo a pelvic examination at the first visit. Respecting patient autonomy and building a relationship is important; only perform an internal pelvic exam if and when the patient is ready. With the patient's consent, a pelvic exam can be helpful in evaluating causes of pain. Evaluating for external hyperesthesia is valuable. Checking for pain on light touch of the external genitalia can suggest vulvodynia. On the internal exam, start with just a gloved finger—speculum exam is of limited value in chronic pelvic pain and is often intolerable for patients. Evaluate for resting pelvic muscle tone, masses or prolapse, and focal muscle tenderness with a digital exam which can suggest pelvic floor dysfunction. Cervical motion tenderness is rare in chronic pelvic pain, but could suggest pelvic inflammatory disease. Bimanual exam is of limited value, as it is insensitive for pelvic masses, and patients with chronic pelvic pain should undergo pelvic imaging (typically a pelvic ultrasound) which is significantly more sensitive. Examining adjacent joints (back and hips) can be helpful to evaluate if other musculoskeletal conditions are contributing.

For most patients, a pelvic ultrasound is sufficient imaging to evaluate structural causes. In patients who may not be able to tolerate the intravaginal probe, a pelvic MRI can be helpful. Pelvic MRI has similar sensitivity to ultrasound for conditions such as endometriosis or cysts, so does not add significant value for primary care providers as secondary imaging.

If a patient presents with warning features that suggest more serious pathology such as weight loss, hematochezia, hematuria, or fevers or have a significant family or personal history that may suggest more worrisome pathology such as a strong family history of colon cancer or inflammatory bowel disease appropriate referral to specialists or more targeted testing like a colonoscopy is appropriate.

4.5 Case

In the case of Amy, we elicit more history and learn that Amy has regular menstrual periods that last 7 days with 4 days of heavy bleeding and it is on these days that she has the worst of her pain. She intermittently experiences constipation, but denies hematochezia or weight loss. She has had a single urinary tract infection that responded promptly to antibiotics last year. When her pain flairs, she feels worse with prolonged standing or at the end of a busy day. The pain often radiates to her back. She has become increasingly discouraged that no one can tell her why she has the pain, and she is concerned it is a sign of an undiagnosed cancer or infection. She is not seeking pregnancy.

We identify that her pain seems to have begun as primary dysmenorrhea with now possible contributions of constipation and myofascial pain. We affirm the impact her pelvic pain is having on Amy and recognize that it is quite distressing for her. We spend time building a relationship with Amy and help her understand that her testing has been appropriate and no further testing is valuable at this time, and we can feel confident that we have ruled out pathology that would progress to tissue damage like cancer. We partner with her to trial therapeutics, including a referral to pelvic physical therapy, constipation treatment, and NSAIDs during her menses. Her pain is somewhat improved, but still quite uncomfortable. We start continuous combined oral contraceptive pills and her menstrual cramps and bleeding decrease significantly. She is happy with the results.

4.6 Treatment

Education is key when addressing a patient with chronic pelvic pain. When a patient is given information around a more specific diagnosis, it can help reduce ongoing testing which has little value. Many patients with chronic pelvic pain will see multiple providers and have the same testing repeated with the same negative results in the effort to explain their pain. Many may feel discouraged and unheard by their medical providers. Being told that testing is normal when you are in pain is not always helpful, as it can make patients feel that providers do not believe the pain is real. Approaching these patients with sympathy and reassurance is extremely valuable. Explaining the limits of our testing, the fact that most patients with chronic pelvic pain have normal imaging or tests, and that does not negate their experience can help build a therapeutic relationship.

The reality is that most cases of chronic pelvic pain do not progress to pathologic damage or morbidity. Helping patients understand the differences between acute pain which may suggest pathologic damage, and chronic pain which is a dysregulation of pain transmission pathways that typically is not explained by actual tissue damage can be helpful in reframing thoughts around the pain experience. The fear-avoidance behaviors that often develop in patients with chronic pain can contribute to perpetuation of pain, and helping patients reengage in activities, understanding that pain does not equate with physical damage, can help break these cycles.

Lifestyle measures are helpful for most patients. Because rest is a common reaction to being in pain, and physical inactivity is linked with muscle spasm, reduced bowel function, and negative psychological effects, helping patients establish a tolerated exercise routine is important. The impact of lack of sleep on pain should be discussed, focusing on helping patients improve sleep hygiene. Pain and depression interact significantly being in chronic pain and loss of enjoyment in activities can often cause depression and worsening depression can heighten pain experience. Working with a psychologist, especially one trained in chronic pain can be valuable for most patients.

The overall goals of treatment should be to improve function, restore the patient's ability to engage in activities they enjoy, and reduce pain to a tolerable level. Setting expectations that complete resolution of the pain may not be possible is important, while also partnering with the patient that this will be an ongoing relationship to continue to work with them to manage symptoms.

Fig. 4.6 Chronic pelvic pain treatment

First line for all:
Education
Lifestyle Measures
Physical Therapy
Pain Psychology

For Cyclic or MSK:
NSAIDS
other pain relievers

For Central Pain:
TCAs, gabapentinoids, SNRIs

For Cyclic Pain:
oral contraceptives, IUS or implant

Refer to Specialist:
injections, refractory cases, surgery

When addressing specific diagnoses, primary care providers are in an excellent position to initiate *pharmacologic treatment* (Fig. 4.6).

For conditions arising from *reproductive organs* such as endometriosis, adenomyosis, or primary dysmenorrhea, nonsteroidal anti-inflammatories (NSAIDs) are appropriate first line treatment. Scheduling high dose NSAIDs like ibuprofen 600–800 mg three times daily or naproxen 500 mg twice daily during menses can help the patient use adequate doses. If NSAIDs are insufficient or not tolerated, hormonal treatments are often successful. In patients who prefer oral treatments, using continuous cycle oral contraceptive pills (OCPS) (either combined estrogen-progesterone OCPS or progesterone only OCPS in patients who have contraindications to estrogens) is usually preferred over cyclic dosing. Skipping placebo weeks and starting new pill packs immediately can reduce menstrual bleeding and cramping. Long acting reversible contraceptives such as the levonorgestrel intrauterine system or the etonogestrel implant can be a convenient and low side effect option. In cases where these are insufficient to manage symptoms, referral to gynecologic specialists is appropriate to review more advanced hormonal treatments like gonadotropin releasing hormone agonists or for surgical treatments such as endometriosis resection or hysterectomy. Referral to a specialist can be helpful in cases where the patient is also actively seeking fertility.

Primary care providers often address *musculoskeletal complaints* and should feel confident addressing low back pain associated with pelvic pain or pelvic floor dysfunction causing pain. Focused physical therapy, especially pelvic floor physical therapy from a trained professional can be very helpful. NSAIDS and other pain relievers are appropriate treatments. Referral to a specialist for spinal or myofascial lidocaine or steroid injections or pelvic floor injections with onabotulinum toxin is sometimes helpful in refractory cases.

Helping patients have regular and nonpainful bowel movements can help reduce *gastroenterologic sources* of pelvic pain in cases of IBS or chronic constipation. Discussing dietary interventions, recommending fiber supplementation, and prescribing constipation treatment can relieve symptoms. Referral to a nutritionist or gastroenterologist is appropriate in refractory cases.

Urinary symptoms of painful bladder syndrome can be challenging to address, but pelvic physical therapy is often helpful as many patients may have overlapping pelvic floor muscle dysfunction. Medications for overactive bladder such as anticholinergics (i.e. oxybutynin) or beta-3 agonists (i.e. mirabegron) or muscle relaxants such as baclofen have value for some patients. Using centrally acting medications such as tricyclic antidepressants TCAs (i.e. amitriptyline) may help relieve symptoms in some patients. In refractory cases, referral to urogynecology to consider intravaginal suppositories or bladder instillations is appropriate.

In *central sensitization* causes, centrally acting medications such as TCAs, gabapentinoids (i.e. pregabalin) and serotonin-norepinephrine reuptake inhibitors SNRIS (i.e. duloxetine or milnacipran) have evidence for benefit in pain reduction. Centrally acting muscle relaxants like cyclobenzaprine which has a very similar chemical structure to TCAs may be valuable.

4.7 Summary

Chronic pelvic pain can have a serious negative impact on a patient's life. A carefully detailed history and basic physical exam with testing can help rule out more worrisome causes of pelvic pain and allow clinicians to narrow down a diagnosis. By considering reproductive organs, GI pathology, musculoskeletal causes, urinary etiologies, and central pain disorders, a clinician can systematically evaluate possible contributing causes. Providing diagnoses and education is the first step in treatment, as it allows patients to understand the nature of their condition and reduce ongoing medical evaluation which is low yield. Primary care providers can feel comfortable prescribing common pharmacologic treatments as first and second line therapies for these painful conditions and should know when to refer to specialists for refractory patients.

Suggested Reading

1. Lamvu G, Carrillo J, Ouyang C, Rapkin A. Chronic pelvic pain in women: a review. JAMA. 2021;325(23):2381–91. https://doi.org/10.1001/jama.2021.2631.
2. Chronic pelvic pain: ACOG practice bulletin, number 218. Obstet Gynecol. 2020;135(3):e98–e109. https://doi.org/10.1097/AOG.0000000000003716.
3. Ferries-Rowe E, Corey E, Archer JS. Primary dysmenorrhea: diagnosis and therapy. Obstet Gynecol. 2020;136(5):1047–58. https://doi.org/10.1097/AOG.0000000000004096.
4. Klemmt PAB, Starzinski-Powitz A. Molecular and cellular pathogenesis of endometriosis. Curr Womens Health Rev. 2018;14(2):106–16. https://doi.org/10.2174/1573404813666170306163448. PMID: 29861704; PMCID: PMC5925869
5. Kho KA, Chen JS, Halvorson LM. Diagnosis, evaluation, and treatment of adenomyosis. JAMA. 2021;326(2):177–8. https://doi.org/10.1001/jama.2020.26436.

6. Vannuccini S, Petraglia F. Recent advances in understanding and managing adenomyosis. F1000Res. 2019;8:F1000 Faculty Rev-283. https://doi.org/10.12688/f1000research.17242.1. PMID: 30918629; PMCID: PMC6419978

7. Torres-Cueco R, Nohales-Alfonso F. Vulvodynia-it is time to accept a new understanding from a neurobiological perspective. Int J Environ Res Public Health. 2021;18(12):6639. https://doi.org/10.3390/ijerph18126639. PMID: 34205495; PMCID: PMC8296499

8. Bresler L, Westbay LC, Fitzgerald CM. Bladder pain syndrome in women. JAMA. 2019;322(24):2435–6. https://doi.org/10.1001/jama.2019.16927.

9. Schwartz ES, Gebhart GF. Visceral pain. Curr Top Behav Neurosci. 2014;20:171–97. https://doi.org/10.1007/7854_2014_315.

10. As-Sanie S, Harris RE, Harte SE, Tu FF, Neshewat G, Clauw DJ. Increased pressure pain sensitivity in women with chronic pelvic pain. Obstet Gynecol. 2013;122(5):1047–55. https://doi.org/10.1097/AOG.0b013e3182a7e1f5. PMID: 24104772; PMCID: PMC3897295

Chapter 5
Vaginitis

Anne W. Chang

5.1 Introduction

Vaginitis is the most common gynecologic diagnosis made in primary care. Bacterial vaginosis accounts for up to 50% vaginitis cases when a cause is identified. This is followed by vulvovaginitis candidiasis which accounts for up to 25% of the cases, and trichomoniasis which accounts for up to 20% of the cases. Non-infectious vaginitis is less common and may account for up to 10% of cases. Patients usually present with one or more of the following: change in vaginal discharge, irritation, burning, itching, dyspareunia, spotting, odor, and dysuria. A history should be taken, noting the presenting symptoms as well as the last LMP, sexual activity, recent antibiotic use, and use of contraceptives, tampons, or douches. The physical examination should include examination of the vulva, vagina, cervix, and pelvis. A cervical, vaginal, and urine specimen should be obtained, and sexually active patients should be tested for gonorrhea, chlamydia, and trichomoniasis. HIV testing should be performed if warranted. Vaginal pH should be checked if thinking about bacterial vaginosis or trichomoniasis is suspected as the pH would be higher than 4.5. Microscopic examination of the vaginal discharge is done with adding a drop of 10% KOH or 0.9% normal saline to the vaginal secretion. The amine test is performed by smelling the slide after applying KOH to detect the fishy odor of BV. Microscopic slides are examined for Candida hyphae and/or buds, clue cells, motile trichomonas, and increased PMNs. Laboratory testing may include NAAT to diagnose BV, candidiasis, trichomoniasis, gonorrhea, and chlamydia. Vaginal discharge may also be sent for culture to diagnose Candida nonalbicans infections. Treatment for diagnosed bacterial vaginosis includes oral metronidazole and intravaginal metronidazole or clindamycin. Treatment for vulvovaginal candidiasis

A. W. Chang (✉)
University of California, San Francisco, San Francisco, CA, USA
e-mail: anne.chang@ucsf.edu

M. Mahmoudi (ed.), *Common Cases in Women's Primary Care Clinics*,
https://doi.org/10.1007/978-3-031-48569-5_5

infections consists of oral fluconazole or topical azoles. For pregnant women with candida infection only topical azoles are recommended. Trichomonas infection is treated with oral metronidazole or tinidazole and the sexual partners need to be treated. Non-infectious vaginitis can be treated when the underlying cause is determined which includes hormones, steroids, and antibiotics.

5.2 Case Presentation

39 y/o Carol with a history of depression, obesity (BMI 31), tobacco use, and hypothyroidism presents today with complaints of 2–3 months of abnormal vaginal discharge and occasional odor. The vaginal discharge may be white to grayish and thin. Sometimes the patient notices a distinct odor, other times it is less. Patient is sexually active with one partner and her menses is regular. She uses an IUD for contraception and denies recent antibiotic use, or douching. Physical examination reveals normal vulva, vagina, and cervix. Vaginal secretions have been obtained for microscopy and NAAT to rule out STD gonorrhea, chlamydia, and trichomoniasis. Also, the pH of the vaginal secretion was >4.5 and amine whiff test was done and did not give any odor. Microscopy showed more than 20% clue cells.

5.3 Discussion of Case

Bacterial vaginosis (BV) is the most common vaginitis accounting for 40–50% of cases when the cause is identified. This patient is sexually active, and lack of condom use fits the demographics of BV. Also, the history of smoking is associated with higher risk of BV as smoking has antiestrogenic effects and benzo[a]pyrene diol epoxide (BPDE) is found in the vaginal secretions of smokers. BPDE increases bacteriophage induction in Lactobacillus spp. The thin vaginal secretion which can be grayish in color and odor also fits the diagnosis of BV with a pH greater than 4.5. Finally, microscopy showed more than 20% clue cells, so the patient meets 3–4 Amsel criteria (Table 5.1).

First-line treatment for BV includes metronidazole or clindamycin either orally or intravaginally. Adverse effects should be discussed with the patient and patient

Table 5.1 Amsel diagnostic criteria for bacterial vaginosis

• **Thin homogenous vaginal discharge**
• **Vaginal pH > 4.5**
• **Positive whiff test (produced when a drop of KOH is added to the vaginal sample – amine odor)**
• **20% Clue cells present on microscopy**
3 out of 4 criteria must be met to diagnose bacterial vaginosis

Source of information: Paladine and Desai 2018; Eckler et al. 2022 preference should be considered. For oral metronidazole common side effects include a metallic taste, nausea, transient neutropenia prolongation of INR and peripheral neuropathy. Although the manufacturer's labeling advises against alcohol consumption during treatment with oral metronidazole the data supporting this are rare, so we do not advise people to stop drinking. However, patients taking disulfiram should not use metronidazole because it can cause psychosis. Oral clindamycin is usually less preferred because of the potential risk of Clostridioides difficile-associated diarrhea.

Our Carol was treated with intravaginal 0.75% metronidazole gel which is inserted into the vagina once a day for 5 days. After completing the treatment her vaginal secretions cleared to a white discharge and the vaginal odor has resolved. And her STD tests came back normal. However, after 1 month she again had the same grayish vaginal discharge with odor and was treated again for BV this time with clindamycin cream 2% intravaginally, 5 grams of cream for 7 days. After the second episode the patient had not had no more BV. Our Carol had another episode of BV after the first treatment which was also treated. She does not meet the criteria for recurrent BV which is defined as 3 or more confirmed episodes within 1 year.

5.3.1 Bacterial Vaginosis

Approximately 7.4 million cases of bacterial vaginosis occur each year in the USA. It is a disease of women of childbearing age with a prevalence of up to 15% in pregnant women, 20–25% in young women seen at student health centers and up to 30–40% in women seen at sexually transmitted disease clinics. Bacterial vaginosis is a clinical diagnosis in which there is a change in the vaginal microbiome from Lactobacillus species to a mixed flora including Gardnerella vaginalis, Mycoplasma hominis, Ureaplasma urealyticum, Fannyhessea vaginae. Species of Porphyromonas, Bacteroides, Peptostreptococcus, Mobiluncus, Megasphaera, Sneathia, Clostridiales, and Fusobacterium are also common in BV. With the loss of lactobacilli, the pH rises and there is an increase in anaerobic gram-negative rods. These anaerobes produce enzymes that break down vaginal peptides into amines which are volatile and malodorous.

BV is associated with reproductive age sexual activity, having sex with women, lack of condom use, tobacco use, and douching. BV can be symptomatic or asymptomatic and may not require treatment. Before doing a PAP smear ask about abnormal vaginal discharge and odor; if there are no symptoms and the PAP cytology comes back with possible BV, then no treatment is needed.

In patients with symptoms, BV can be diagnosed when 3 out of 4 Amsel criteria are met or the NAAT result is positive for BV. The Amsel criteria include thin vaginal discharge, pH >4.5, a positive whiff test in which the vaginal sample is mixed with the 10% KOH and an amine odor is detected, and 20% or more clue cells seen by microscopy. The sensitivity using the Amsel criteria is 79% to 97% and the specificity is 90% to 94% compared to the Gram stain, which is the standard and

Table 5.2 Recommended treatment for bacterial vaginosis

Medication	Treatment directions
Recommended Meds	
Metronidazole	500 mg orally twice a day for 7 days
Metronidazole 0.75% gel	One applicator (5 gm) intravaginally once a day for 5 days
Clindamycin 2% cream	One applicator (5 gm) intravaginally at bedtime for 7 days
Alternative Meds	
Clindamycin	300 mg orally twice a day for 7 days
Clindamycin ovules	100 mg intravaginally at bedtime for 3 days
Tinidazole	2 gm orally once a day for 2 days
Tinidazole	1 gm orally once a day for 5 days

Source of information: https://www.cdc.gov/std/treatment-guidelines/bv.htm

most commonly used for research purposes. The DNA probe for detection of Gardnerella vaginalis or detection of vaginal fluid sialidase activity has a sensitivity of 92% to 100% and specificity of 92% to 98% compared to Gram stain. If BV is diagnosed then other STD tests should be performed including chlamydia, gonorrhea, HIV, and syphilis.

Treatment of BV is for symptomatic patients and patients undergoing gynecologic procedures involving the vagina regardless of symptoms. The most common treatment is oral or topical metronidazole or intravaginal clindamycin (Table 5.2). Both metronidazole and clindamycin are safe during pregnancy and have similar cure rates of 75% to 86%. Other drugs to consider if metronidazole or clindamycin are intolerable are oral tinidazole or secnidazole. At this time, probiotics are not recommended for treatment because larger studies are needed before their efficacy is known.

Recurrent BV is defined as 3 or more confirmed episodes in 1 year. Patients with confirmed BV who are asymptomatic are not treated. However, asymptomatic BV patients who undergo gynecologic procedures involving the vagina are treated, as this reduces the rate of post gynecologic infections. Many reasons may contribute to recurrent BV, including inadequate treatment, reinfection, antimicrobial resistance, recurrent infection, or possible genetics. Treatment considerations include cost and availability of medications, previous medications used, and patient preference. If possible, consider using medications that were not used in previous treatments or use medication that produced the best response.

5.3.2 *Vulvovaginal Candidiasis*

This is the second most common type of vaginitis. And it is the most common cause of vulvovaginal itching and discharge. Vulvar erythema is also a common complaint. This vaginal discharge is curd like and white with no odor. The diagnosis is made with vulvovaginal symptoms and the presence of Candida species. The Candida species alone is not considered a disease, as it is considered normal flora in 25% of women. Also, vulvovaginal candidiasis (VVC) is not considered a sexually transmitted disease. Risk factors for VVC include pregnancy, diabetes, antibiotic use, immunosuppression, and glucocorticoid use. Heat, moisture, and occlusive clothing are likely to contribute to VVC.

Vaginal pH and microscopy (wet mount) are the preferred method of diagnosis because they provide immediate results. Typically, the pH is <4.5 and microscopic examination with 10% KOH shows hyphae, budding yeast and/or spores. The sensitivity of the wet mount is 40% and the specificity of 100%. Diagnosis can also be made by DNA probe testing with sensitivity of 77% to 97% and specificity of 77% to 99%.

VVC is usually treated with topical vaginal antifungals or a single dose of 150 mg fluconazole, with comparable cure rates of 80% to 90% (Table 5.3). Topical

Table 5.3 Recommended treatment for vulvovaginal candidiasis

Medication	Treatment directions
Over the Counter Intravaginal Meds	
Clotrimazole 1% cream	One applicator 5 gm intravaginally once a day for 7 to 14 days
Clotrimazole 2% cream	One applicator 5 gm intravaginally once a day for 3 days
Miconazole 2% cream	One applicator 5 gm intravaginally once a day for 7 days
Miconazole 4% cream	One applicator 5 gm intravaginally once a day for 3 days
Miconazole 100 mg vaginal suppository	One suppository intravaginally once a day for 7 days
Miconazole 200 mg vaginal suppository	One suppository intravaginally once a day for 3 days
Miconazole 1,200 mg vaginal suppository	One suppository intravaginally once
Tioconazole 6.5 % ointment	One applicator 5 gm intravaginally once
Prescription Intravaginal Meds	
Butoconazole 2% cream	One applicator 5 gm intravaginally once
Terconazole 0.4% cream	One applicator 5 gm intravaginally once a day for 7 days
Terconazole 0.8% cream	One applicator 5 gm intravaginally once a day for 3 days
Terconazole 80 mg vaginal suppository	One suppository intravaginally once a day for 3 days
Prescription Oral Meds	
Fluconazole 150 mg tablet	One tablet orally once
Ibrexafungerp 150 mg tablet	Two tablet orally twice a day for 1 day

Source of information: Eckler et al. 2023

treatments include miconazole, clotrimazole, tioconazole, butoconazole and terconazole creams, ointments, or vaginal suppositories. Usual topical treatments are for 3–7 days; however, one-day topical treatments are available. Studies show that patients prefer to take oral medications for cure due to the ease. However, topical medications have fewer side effects and are faster at relieving symptoms than oral medications. Along with antifungal meds use of topical corticosteroid can give more relief to vulvovaginitis symptoms.

Patients have complicated VVC when there are severe signs/symptoms, have Candida species other than C. albicans, particularly C. glabrata, pregnancy, poorly controlled diabetes, immunosuppression, debilitation, or history of recurrent culture verified VVS. If so, treatment may vary, and oral fluconazole may be given for 2 or 3 doses at least 72 hours apart. The number of doses depends on the severity of the disease. An alternative to fluconazole is ibrexafungerp 150 mg tabs taken twice daily. The optimal duration of therapy is not known. Recurrent VVC is defined as 3 or more episodes of symptomatic infection within one year and this may be treated with long-term fluconazole treatment taken for weeks to months.

5.3.3 Trichomoniasis

The most common non-viral sexually transmitted disease in the world is caused by Trichomonas vaginalis, a protozoan. Many people have the STD for months or years before diagnosis because the infection is often asymptomatic. However, women may present with malodorous frothy thin greenish-yellow vaginal discharge, vulvar irritation, abdominal pain, or dyspareunia. Physical findings include vulvar and vaginal erythema. Punctate hemorrhages may be seen on the cervix (strawberry cervix) and/or vaginal mucosa.

Diagnosis is made by testing vaginal discharge for pH and microscopy or nucleic acid amplification test (NAAT). Vaginal pH is >4.5 and motile trichomonads on wet mount are diagnostic of infection. However, the sensitivity of microscopy is 44% to 68% compared to NAAT. Therefore, the CDC recommendation is to use NAATs since sensitivity and specificity are close to 100%. Before NAAT, culture was the gold standard. However, it is now only used when neither NAAT nor microscopy are

Table 5.4 Recommended treatment for trichomoniasis[a]

Medication for Women[b]	Treatment directions
Metronidazole	500 mg orally twice a day for 7 days
Tinidazole	2 gm orally once
Recurrent Trichomoniasis in Women	
Metronidazole	2 gm orally once a day for 7 days
Tinidazole	2 gm orally once a day for 7 days

[a]Need to treat partners
[b]Because of high rate of reinfection, retest in 3 months
Source of information: https://www.cdc.gov/std/trichomonas/treatment.htm

available. Patients with trichomoniasis identified by PAP should be evaluated by NAAT, wet mount microscopy or culture. And if trichomoniasis is diagnosed other STDs will need to be tested including chlamydia, gonorrhea, HIV, and syphilis.

Treatment of trichomoniasis infection is available for both symptomatic and asymptomatic individuals and their sexual partners. Metronidazole, tinidazole, and secnidazole are the only classes of drugs that can cure trichomoniasis (Table 5.4). The cure rate is reported to be 90–95%. The preferred treatment is metronidazole 500 mg taken orally twice daily for 7 days for both pregnant and non-pregnant women. There are single-dose options that may provide greater compliance but are less effective. And metronidazole vaginal preparations should not be used to treat trichomoniasis. Patients and partners should be counseled to abstain from sex until all parties have completed antibiotic treatment and are asymptomatic. All female partners should be retested for trichomoniasis since reinfection rates of up to 17% have been reported. Females should be tested by NAAT 3 weeks to 3 months after completion of antibiotic treatment. If infection persists despite treatment, then the trichomonas must be evaluated for resistance or be referred to an infectious disease specialist.

5.3.4 Non-infectious Vaginitis

The two most common types of non-infectious vaginitis are vulvovaginal atrophy or atrophic vaginitis and desquamative inflammatory vaginitis (DIV). Vulvovaginal atrophy and the associated genitourinary symptoms are the result of low estrogen levels, usually due to menopause. However, other less common causes include hyperprolactinemia, hypothalamic amenorrhea, lactation, and use of antiestrogenic medications. Sometimes symptoms can be seen with the use of extra low-dose contraceptive pills and cancer therapy. The etiology of desquamative inflammatory vaginitis is unknown. It was first described in 1956, but few studies have been published in the last 50 years. A major reason is that it was uncommon to be diagnosed with DIV in the past however in the last 5 years more studies have been published on DIV leading to more diagnosis.

Genitourinary symptoms of atrophic vaginitis include vulvovaginal dryness, dyspareunia, vaginal bleeding, decreased libido or orgasm, vulvovaginal burning or itching, vaginal discharge, dysuria, urinary frequency, recurrent urinary tract infections and urethral prolapse. Physical findings in atrophic vaginitis include loss of connective tissue substance resulting in the shrinkage of the labia majora. The labia minora may be completely atrophied and the introitus may be reduced in size. The vagina is pale and dry with the walls being smooth and unrugated. The entire vagina may be shortened and the fornices may have disappeared so that the cervix is flush with the vault. Submucosal petechial hemorrhages may also be seen in the vaginal wall. The diagnosis of atrophic vaginitis is made by changes on physical examination, increase in vaginal pH of >5 and presence of parabasal cells on saline

Table 5.5 Recommended treatment for atrophic vaginitis

Medication	Treatment directions
Over the Counter Intravaginal Meds- Moisturizers	
RepHresh Vaginal gel	Prefilled applicators use intravaginally every 3 days
Replens	Prefilled applicators use intravaginally every 3 days
Luvena	Prefilled applicators use intravaginally every 3 days
Canesintima Intimate Moisturizer	Pump onto finger and apply to vaginal area
Ah! Yes	Prefilled applicators use intravaginally every 3 days
Sylk Natural Intimate Moisturizer	Squeeze drops onto finger and apply to vaginal area
HyaloGyn	Prefilled applicators use intravaginally every 3 days
Revaree	Prefilled applicators use intravaginally every 3 days
K-Y Liquibeads	Insert one ovule intravaginally everyday
Intravaginal Lubricants	
K-Y Jelly Water Based Lubricant	Apply with fingers
Astroglide Gel	Apply with fingers
ID Glide	Apply with fingers
Wet Original Gel	Apply with fingers
Durex Play Feel Pleasure Gel	Apply with fingers
Good Clean Love Almost Naked	Apply with fingers
H2O Sliquid Naturals	Apply with fingers
Pjur Women Nude	Apply with fingers
Ritex Senstiv Gel	Apply with fingers
Simply Slick	Apply with fingers
Ah! Yes	Apply with fingers
Swiss Navy	Apply with fingers
K-Y True Feel	Apply with fingers
Prescription Meds	
Estring – 7.5 mcg estradiol daily	One ring inserted into vagina every 3 months
Imvexxy – 4 mcg estradiol tablet	One tablet intravaginally daily for 2 weeks, followed by twice weekly
Imvexxy – 10 mcg estradiol tablet	One tablet intravaginally daily for 2 weeks, followed by twice weekly
Vagifem – 10 mcg estradiol tablet	One tablet intravaginally daily for 2 weeks, followed by twice weekly
Yuvafem – 10 mcg estradiol tablet	One tablet intravaginally daily for 2 weeks, followed by twice weekly
Premarin Vaginal Cream – 0.625 mg conjugated estrogen/gm cream	0.5 gm intravaginally daily for 2 weeks, followed by twice weekly; maybe dose adjusted to patient's response
Estrace Vaginal Cream – 100 mcg estradiol/gm cream	0.5 gm intravaginally daily for 2 weeks, followed by twice weekly; maybe dose adjusted to patient's response

Source of information: Bachmann et al. 2023

microscopy. The degree of atrophic changes does not correlate with symptoms. Therefore, symptoms alone dictate the need for treatment.

Treatment of atrophic vaginitis is symptom relief. Many patients with symptoms do not seek medical attention because of cultural, religious, or social beliefs, embarrassment, or lack of awareness of effective treatments. And many clinicians do not ask about symptoms of atrophic vaginitis. The first-line treatment for symptomatic atrophic vaginitis is nonhormonal vaginal moisturizers and lubricants and sexual activity (Table 5.5). Atrophy can be prevented with regular sexual activity. These treatments work well for mild vaginal symptoms. Vaginal moisturizers are used regularly 2–3 times a week, while lubricants are used only during sexual activity. However, if vaginal moisturizers or lubricants are not enough to treat symptoms, oral or topical estrogen treatment is more effective.

Vaginal estrogen is the treatment for moderate to severe symptoms of atrophic vaginitis when moisturizers and lubricants are ineffective. Low-dose estrogen therapy can restore the vaginal acidic pH and microflora, thicken the epithelium, and increase vaginal secretions. Vaginal estrogen is usually preferred to oral estrogen because of lower blood levels of estrogen. Since vaginal estrogen preparations can be detected in the blood, be sure there are no contraindications for its use. Vaginal estrogen is available in cream, tablet, capsule, and ring formulations (Table 5.5). All the different formulations are equally effective in relieving symptoms and the lowest systemic absorption is from the tablet, capsule, or ring. Oral estrogen can also be used to treat the symptoms of atrophic vaginitis when more systemic estrogen is needed for other purposes other than treating genitourinary symptoms.

Desquamative inflammatory vaginitis (DIV) is diagnosed by the symptoms of diffuse exudative inflammation of the vagina, profuse purulent discharge, and dyspareunia. Recently, DIV has become more widely recognized and diagnosed. The average age of women to be diagnosed is 41.8 years old and 37% were menopausal. The etiology of DIV is not known however these women tend to have low estrogen levels and gram stain of the vagina show lack of lactobacilli. Usually, the microflora in DIV includes Escherichia coli, Staphylococcus aureus, Group B Streptococcus or Enterococcus faecalis. In the absence of lactobacilli, the vaginal pH is elevated. The preferred method of diagnosis is wet mount microscopy which shows increased leukocytes and parabasal epithelial cells. Treatment of DIV is usually with antibiotics or corticosteroids. Differential diagnosis includes infectious vaginitis such as trichomoniasis or group A streptococcus, erosive lichen planus, mucous membrane pemphigoid and vulvo-gingival syndrome.

5.4 Conclusion

Vaginitis affects women of all ages. It is one of the top 25 reasons women seek medical care, resulting in 5 to 10 million office visits annually. Inflammation and infection of the vagina is caused by many pathogens, allergic reaction to condoms or other products, lack of estrogen and friction during coitus. Most of the diagnoses are made with careful history, physical examination, pH of vaginal secretions, microscopy, and NAAT. Since diagnosis of some vaginitis is associated with increased likelihood of having STDs, sexually active individuals are tested for STDs. Many types of vaginitis can be treated with antibiotics, corticosteroids, and estrogen therapy. There are many prescriptions and over-the-counter medications to treat vaginitis and understanding of the cause of vaginitis will help in determining the most effective treatment.

Suggested Reading

1. Leclair C, Stenson A. Common causes of vaginitis. JAMA. 2022;327(22):2238–9.
2. Paladine HL, Desai UA. Vaginitis: diagnosis and treatment. Am Fam Physician. 2018;97(5):321–9.
3. Eckler K, Barbieri RL, Marrazzo J, Sobel JD. Vaginal discharge (vaginitis): initial evaluation. Up To Date. 2022; Retrieved February 24, 2023 from https://www.uptodate.com/contents/vaginal-discharge-vaginitis-initial-evaluation
4. Paavonen J, Brunham RC. Bacterial vaginosis and desquamative inflammatory vaginitis. NEJM. 2018;379(23):2246–54.
5. Lev-Sagie A, Nyirjesy P. Noninfectious vaginitis. In: Goldstein AT, Pukall CF, Goldstein I, editors. Female sexual pain disorders. Blackwell Publishing Limited; 2008.
6. Papadakis MA, McPhee SJ, Rabow MW. editors. Lange current medical diagnosis & treatment 2022. In: Vaginitis. McGraw Hill; 2022. p. 789–90.
7. Eckler K, Barbieri RL, Marrazzo J, Sobel JD. Candida vulvovaginitis. Up to Date. 2022; Retrieved February 27, 2023 from https://www.uptodate.com/contents/candida-vulvovaginitis-treatment
8. Eckler K, Barbieri RL, Marrazzo J, Sobel JD. Trichomonas: treatment. Up to Date. 2022; Retrieved February 27, 2023 from https://www.uptodate.com/contents/trichomoniasis-treatment
9. Eckler K, Barbieri RL, Marrazzo J, Sobel JD, Mitchell C. Trichomonas: clinical manifestations and diagnosis. Up to Date. 2022; Retrieved February 27, 2023 from https://www.uptodate.com/contents/trichomoniasis-clinical-manifestations-and-diagnosis
10. Bachmann G, Pinkerton JAV, Barbieri RL, Burstein HJ, Chakrabarti A. Genitourinary syndrome of menopause (vulvovaginal atrophy): treatment. Up to Date. 2023; Retrieved February 28, 2023 from https://www.uptodate.com/contents/genitourinary-syndrome-of-menopause-vulvovaginal-atrophy-treatment
11. https://www.cdc.gov/std/treatment-guidelines/bv.htm
12. https://www.cdc.gov/std/trichomonas/treatment.htm

Chapter 6
Menstrual Bleeding Disorders

Katherine Sherif

6.1 Introduction

PCOS is not only a reproductive disorder with oligomenorrhea and infertility but it is primarily a metabolic disorder that is accompanied by insulin resistance, risk for type 2 diabetes, and fatty liver. PCOS is underdiagnosed primarily due to a lack of familiarity with diagnostic criteria. Early detection and prompt attention to metabolic issues will prevent the high morbidity associated with PCOS.

6.2 Normal Menstrual Cycle

Worldwide, the mediation age of menarche is 12 years, and the range is 12–14 years.

The follicular (proliferative) phase of the menstrual cycle begins at the onset of menses and is characterized by low serum hormone concentrations of estradiol (E_2) and progesterone (P). In response to low sex hormones, the hypothalamus secretes gonadotropin releasing hormone (GnRH), which increases follicular stimulating hormone (FSH) secretion by the pituitary. FSH, in turn, triggers folliculogenesis. Primordial follicles develop into antral (fluid-filled) tertiary follicles and secrete E_2. E_2 in turn inhibits FSH and LH. GnRH pulse frequency increases over the follicular phase, culminating in an abrupt LH surge. As a dominant follicle emerges, other follicles undergo atresia. The mid-cycle LH surge signals the onset of the luteal (secretory) phase of the menstrual cycle. The oocyte is released from the follicle

K. Sherif (✉)
Department of Medicine, Sidney Kimmel College of Medicine, Thomas Jefferson University, Philadelphia, USA
e-mail: Katherine.sherif@jefferson.edu

M. Mahmoudi (ed.), *Common Cases in Women's Primary Care Clinics*,
https://doi.org/10.1007/978-3-031-48569-5_6

(ovulation). The granulosa cells of the follicle produce P, which in turn reduces LH secretions. In the absence of fertilization, E_2 and P decrease and menstrual bleeding ensues. This marks the first day of the follicular phase. Median menstrual intervals are 28 days (range 25–32 days) with duration ranging from 2 to 9 days. Menstrual patterns are most variable in adolescence and perimenopause. Blood volume loss is difficult to estimate in any one individual but is estimated to be approximately 30 mL on average. Oligomenorrhea is defined as cycle intervals >35 days. Blood volume loss exceeding 80 mL is considered menorrhagia.

In the PCOS menstrual cycle in PCOS, GnRH pulse frequency and amplitude are exaggerated, driving an increase in LH and inhibiting folliculogenesis. No dominant follicle emerges and immature antral follicles become the peripheral ovarian "cysts" visualized on ultrasound. The absence of ovulation results in oligomenorrhea.

6.3 Case

A healthy 32-year-old woman was prescribed the oral contraceptive pill (OCP) at age 15 years for dysmenorrhea. She lost her health insurance 8 months ago and has not refilled the OCP, which is the first time she has been off the OCP in 17 years. Since she has been off the OCP, she has had only one menstrual period (3 months ago). She has had sexual intercourse during this time and has not conceived. She has gained about 8# in the last 6 months. Her hair seems to be thinner, but she is not sure. She has no acne. Her vital signs and physical exam are normal. Labs show a negative pregnancy test, normal TSH and free T4, normal prolactin and elevation in serum free testosterone, total testosterone and DHEAS (DHEA sulfate), pelvic ultrasound shows polycystic ovary morphology.

The Rotterdam Criteria are the most widely used criteria by PCOS experts, are simple and require 2 out of 3 criteria:

- A history of irregular menstrual periods (oligo-anovulation)
- Hyperandrogenism:

  - Signs of hyperandrogenism (hirsutism, alopecia, cystic acne) OR.
  - elevated serum androgens.

- Polycystic ovary morphology on transvaginal ultrasound ($\geq$ 12 follicles measuring 2–9 mm in diameter and/or an ovarian volume > 10 mL in at least one ovary).

The patient meets the Rotterdam Criteria for the diagnosis of PCOS with irregular menstrual intervals and elevated serum androgens. As many as 50% of women have not been diagnosed with PCOS due to the erroneous belief that they need to have an elevated body mass index (BMI) or hirsutism in order to meet criteria. As many as 25% of women with PCOS have a normal body mass index (BMI Factors such as hirsutism, alopecia and overweight are phenotypic traits that depend on receptor status in various ethnic groups and their absence should not be used to exclude the diagnosis. For example, a woman of Chinese descent may have an elevated serum testosterone of 90 mg/dL but no hirsutism due to an absence of cutaneous androgen receptors.

One of the most common reasons that women are not diagnosed with PCOS is that like the patient in this case, they are prescribed OCPs before establishing a diagnosis of PCOS. Young women will often report "regular" periods but without further questioning, the clinician may miss the fact that they have oligomenorrhea. The most common reasons to prescribe OCPs, besides contraception, include dysmenorrhea, oligomenorrhea or menorrhagia, or some combination. When women discontinue the OCP in their 20 s or 30 s, PCOS may be unmasked. They develop oligomenorrhea and may be told that this is due to the fact that they were on the OCP "for a long time." They may develop hyperandrogenemic symptoms such as alopecia, hirsutism, and cystic acne. They may develop insulin resistance and rapidly gain weight, e.g., 30# in 6–12 months. When they finally do receive a diagnosis of PCOS, many women are informed that they will be infertile but the rates of fertility are excellent.

Another source of failing to establish the diagnosis of PCOS includes blood testing for androgens. Any contraceptive with sex hormones will suppress endogenous hormone levels, including the levonorgestrel-containing IUD, oral contraceptive pills, contraceptive patches and rings, and the subcutaneous implant. Accurate sex hormones should be obtained when the patient has discontinued hormonal contraception for at least 6–8 weeks. If the patient has been cycling every 28–32 days, obtain sex hormones on day #21 of the menstrual cycle.

The initial workup for oligomenorrhea includes a urine HCG, TSH, and a serum prolactin. Women with oligomenorrhea who are taking a low-dose ethinyl estradiol-containing OCP may have oligomenorrhea due to the low level of estrogen and should be reassured. An elevated serum prolactin due to a pituitary adenoma is not common, but should not be missed. Elevated prolactin does not necessarily cause galactorrhea or visual field cuts. In PCOS, serum prolactin levels are frequently slightly elevated in the 30 mg/dL range (normal <20 mg/dL). Clinically significant prolactin adenomas serum concentrations are usually greater than 150 mg/dL.

If oligomenorrhea is not due to pregnancy, hypothyroidism or elevated prolactin, test for sex hormones if the patient is not taking hormonal contraception.

- Serum total and free testosterone.
- LH and FSH.
- DHEA sulfate (not DHEA, and not "DHEA serum").
- 17-alpha-hydroxyprogesterone
- Anti-müllerian hormone (AMH).

A caveat to serum testosterone concentrations is that there is inconsistency in assays for both total and free testosterone resulting in underestimate of serum sex hormones. An elevated DHEAS above 500 mg/dL or 17-alpha hydroxyprogesterone above 200 mg/dL should prompt a search for an adrenal source of hyperandrogenism, i.e., congenital adrenal hyperplasia (most likely non-classical). Patients with Cushingoid features should undergo a 24-h urinary cortisol with referral if >100 mg/dL. Although as many as 75% of women with PCOS are insulin resistant [5], measuring insulin levels is not helpful in management. Anti-müllerian hormone is a reflection of ovarian reserve. AMH levels are generally higher in PCOS compared with age-matched women and measurements are not affected by exogenous sex steroids.

The comorbidities of PCOS include both metabolic issues as well as pregnancy complications. PCOS confers increased risk for insulin resistance, impaired glucose tolerance, gestational diabetes, and type 2 diabetes. Other pregnancy comorbidities include a higher prevalence of first trimester miscarriage, pre-eclampsia and NICU admissions. Additionally, women with PCOS have dyslipidemia, characterized as high triglycerides and low high-density lipoprotein (HDL) cholesterol, elevated blood pressures and fatty liver disease. The latter is particularly significant due to the fact that the primary indication for liver transplant is now non-alcoholic steatohepatitis. Finally, women with PCOS also are more likely to have sleep apnea than weight-matched controls and hidradenitis suppurativa, depression, and anxiety.

The pathophysiology of PCOS is not entirely understood. Increased GnRH pulsatility increases LH production which inhibits folliculogenesis. Insulin resistance and resultant hyperinsulinemia modulates GnRH pulsatility, directly stimulates theca cells and decreases sex hormone binding globulin (SHBG) which increases unbound testosterone. In the last several years, research findings demonstrate the role of the intestinal microbiome in the genesis of PCOS. PCOS women have a less diverse microbiome, a factor that favors inflammation. PCOS mice who receive a fecal microbial transplant (FMT) show improvement in PCOS symptoms.

Treatment for PCOS should treat both anovulation and underlying insulin resistance. Anovulation can be treated with hormonal contraception if the patient desires contraception or with an insulin sensitizer, such as metformin. Metformin and other measures to improve insulin resistance act by decreasing serum insulin and preventing insulin-mediated androgen increase by the ovaries. Ways to improve insulin resistance include

- Exercise that increases muscle mass.
- Consistent sleep 7–9 h per night.

  - screen for sleep apnea.

- Dietary changes:

  - Decrease simple carbohydrates and processed foods.
  - Consuming more probiotics (supplements and fermented foods).
  - Consuming more prebiotics (approximately 25–30 g fiber daily).

- Medications such as metformin, thiazolidinediones and GLP1-receptor antagonists.
- Supplements.

  - inositol (myo-inositol and d-chiro inositol),

- N-acetyl cysteine (NAC).
- Vitamin D3.

6.4   Conclusion

PCOS is a highly prevalent condition with both reproductive and metabolic comorbidities. Up to 50% of women and girls are undiagnosed. Lack of recognition of the diagnosis prevents early intervention to prevent or attenuate gestational diabetes, pre-eclampsia, type 2 diabetes and fatty liver, among other comorbidities. Clinicians need to become more familiar with the Rotterdam diagnostic criteria and aggressively intervene (Fig. 6.1).

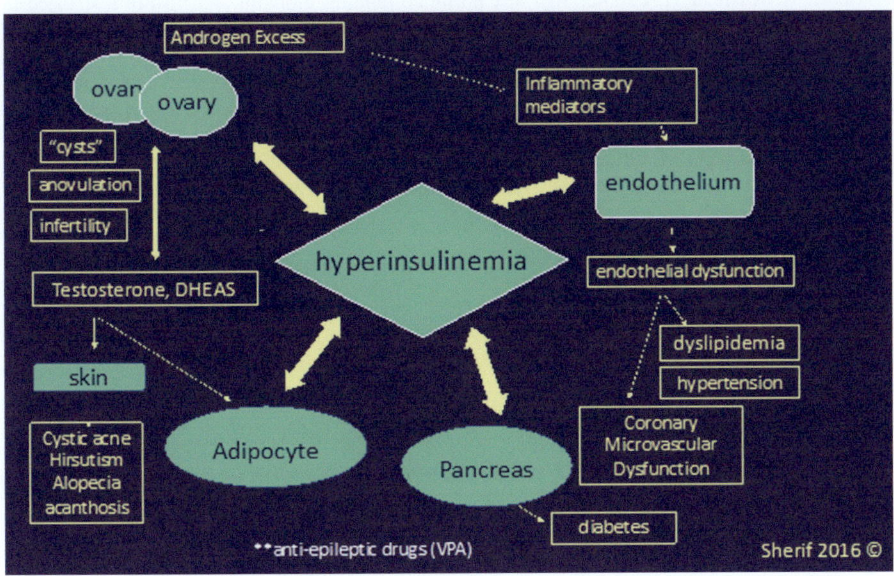

Fig. 6.1 The central role of insulin resistance in the pathophysiology of PCOS

Suggested Reading

1. Richards JS. Chapter one – the ovarian cycle. In: Litwack G, editor. Vitamins and hormones, vol. 107. New York: Academic Press; 2018. p. 1–25. https://doi.org/10.1016/bs.vh.2018.01.009.
2. Rotterdam ESHRE/ASRM-Sponsored PCOS consensus workshop group. Revised 2003 consensus on diagnostic criteria and long-term health risks related to polycystic ovary syndrome (PCOS). Hum Reprod. 2004;19(1):41–7. https://doi.org/10.1093/humrep/deh098.
3. Smet ME, McLennan A. Rotterdam criteria, the end. Australas J Ultrasound Med. 2018;21(2):59–60. https://doi.org/10.1002/ajum.12096.
4. Sherif K, Coborn J, Hoovler A, Gill L. Medical journey of patients with polycystic ovary syndrome and obesity: a cross-sectional survey of patients and primary care physicians. Postgrad Med. 2023;135(3):312–20. https://doi.org/10.1080/00325481.2022.2140511.
5. Cassar S, Misso ML, Hopkins WG, Shaw CS, Teede HJ, Stepto NK. Insulin resistance in polycystic ovary syndrome: a systematic review and meta-analysis of euglycaemic-hyperinsulinaemic clamp studies. Hum Reprod. 2016;31(11):2619–31. https://doi.org/10.1093/humrep/dew243.
6. Yang S-W, Yoon S-H, Kim M, Seo Y-S, Yuk J-S. Risk of gestational diabetes and pregnancy-induced hypertension with a history of polycystic ovary syndrome: a Nationwide population-based cohort study. J Clin Med. 2023;12(5):1738. https://doi.org/10.3390/jcm12051738.
7. Sherif K, Kushner H, Falkner BE. Sex hormone binding globulin and insulin resistance in African-American women. Metab Clin Exp. 1998;47(1):70–4. https://doi.org/10.1016/S0026-0495(98)90195-0.
8. Torres PJ, Ho BS, Arroyo P, et al. Exposure to a healthy gut microbiome protects against reproductive and metabolic dysregulation in a PCOS mouse model. Endocrinol. 2019;160(5):1193–204. https://doi.org/10.1210/en.2019-00050.
9. Sherif K, Heublein M, Grant K, Okamoto E, Watto MF. "#198 PCOS: polycystic ovary syndrome with Katherine Sherif MD". *The Curbsiders Internal Medicine Podcast* http://thecurbsiderscom/episode-list March 9, 2020.

Chapter 7
Breast Complaints

Audrey Tran and Massoud Mahmoudi

7.1 Introduction

Breast lumps are a hallmark concern for patients in women's primary care clinics. While most breast concerns are benign, and often cystic in nature, it is essential to discern the high risk features of breast masses so there can be timely workup and early referral to specialists if malignancy is confirmed. Of all breast concerns, breast cancer is the most feared and most comorbid. Primary care providers are also tasked with guiding asymptomatic patients in discussion about appropriate intervals of breast cancer screening, based on their personal risk factors, and appropriate assessment of the associated risks and harms of screening. Therefore, primary care clinicians must be adept at addressing both benefits and harms of our screening interventions to engage in full shared decision-making.

7.2 Epidemiology for Breast Cancer

Breast cancer remains a leading cause of morbidity and premature mortality for women in the USA. According to the American Cancer Society Facts and Figs. 2023, breast cancer is the most common cancer diagnosis annually for women worldwide, accounting for 31% of new cancer cases in women patients in a year. Extrapolated to the US population, invasive breast cancer is estimated to impact more than 297,790 women annually, compared to 2,800 men. Breast cancer is also the second leading cause of cancer-related death for women and accounts for more than 43,170

A. Tran · M. Mahmoudi (✉)
University of California, San Francisco, San Francisco, CA, USA
e-mail: audrey.tran2@ucsf.edu

M. Mahmoudi (ed.), *Common Cases in Women's Primary Care Clinics*,
https://doi.org/10.1007/978-3-031-48569-5_7

deaths annually. It also can impact women at a relatively younger age than most cancers.

Based on estimations from current incidence rates, about 12.9% of Americans will develop breast cancer in their lifetime. This means roughly 1 in 8 women are at risk of develop breast cancer at some point in their life, compared to men, who have a 1 in 800 chance. Amount of estrogen exposure is one of the most important risk factors for developing breast cancer. Risk also increases with age, exposure to radiation, genetic predisposition, diet and sedentary lifestyle, and tobacco/alcohol use.

The mainstay of managing this massive health condition is through screening and diagnostic mammograms. We recommend an urgent referral to Breast Oncology when clinical suspicion for malignant or premalignant disease is confirmed, and counseling and education when suspicion is low. Despite dramatic improvements in screening and earlier detection for both men and women since the 1980s, reduction in annual breast cancer morbidity and mortality has only slowly decreased for women over the past decade since 2010.

In this chapter, we will discuss workup of a symptomatic case of an abnormal breast mass from the primary care perspective, and an asymptomatic screening case to compare the various diagnostic vs. screening tools available for providers. We will also discuss how to assess an individual patient's risk factors for breast cancer, how to utilize appropriately breast cancer risk prediction tools to guide screening frequency recommendations. Lastly, we will explore strategies to modify behaviors that put patients at higher risk for the development of breast cancer.

7.3 Case 1:Guidance and Management of Clinically Suspicious Breast Lump

7.3.1 Patient Case

Mrs. Houston is a 47-year-old nulliparous woman with obesity, hypertension, and hyperlipidemia who presents with 5–6 months of a right-sided breast lump. It is hard, painless, and immobile. It does not change in size with her menses. She has a strong family history of breast cancer, including maternal grandmother diagnosed in her late 40s, maternal aunt diagnosed in her late 50s, and mother diagnosed in early 60s, though *BRCA* status is unknown. Two weeks ago, she received an indeterminate reading on a screening mammogram. Given that her great grandmother was diagnosed with breast cancer at age 48, Mrs. Houston wishes to discuss additional imaging needed to definitively characterize this breast mass.

She takes no medications and uses a levonorgestrel-containing intrauterine device for contraception. Her vital signs are notable for a blood pressure of 130/72, heart rate of 79, and body mass index of 33.0 kg/m². She is well appearing, well nourished, with a normal cardiopulmonary, abdominal, and neurological exam. Her breast exam is notable for a firm, immobile breast mass, measuring 3 cm roughly

2 cm at the 4 o'clock position at the right nipple. It is nontender to palpation. There are no signs of skin puckering, rashes, erythema, or fluctuance on either breast.

Question: How would you work up this patient's complaint, and what factors of her case are most concerning to you?

7.3.2   Workup of a Breast Mass

In the case above, the patient has multiple features concerning for a potentially malignant breast lump. These risk factors include a painless mass or lesion that is fixed, immobile, does not fluctuate in size or tenderness with her hormonal cycles, and a strong family history of breast cancer. The patient's age, BMI, and nulliparous history are additional risk factors, given her uninterrupted exposure to estrogen and estrone in adipose tissue. During the history, context of patient's hormonal cycle is important. It is also important to elicit if the lump is associated with a rash, if afore-mentioned rash is steroid responsive, if the lump has grown, if the patient is breast-feeding, and when patient last had her menses or if she is still menstruating.

The clinical breast exam can be an important part of the initial workup, though it alone is not diagnostic given its limited sensitivity. Of note, more recently the American Cancer Society does not recommend clinical breast examination for breast cancer screening among average risk women at any age, given more advanced imaging technologies available. However, when a patient presents with a breast lump, it is important to perform a clinical breast exam. Recommendations for best practices with clinical breast examination vary, but generally follow the following guidelines: correct position, inspection, palpation of breast tissue, and lymph node exam.

For a proper breast exam, positioning that is both comfortable and appropriate for inspection will allow for a higher yield exam. Given the potential sensitivity of the breast exam, and the need to inspect both breasts at the same time, we recom-mend offering the patient a chaperone.

During the inspection portion, it is important to have the patient sit upright, and to inspect both breasts simultaneously to denote any asymmetric findings broadly. Look for any changes in the skin color, skin texture, skin dimpling/retractions, and nipple discharge of any consistency. Discharge that is outside the postpartum period is typically abnormal and should be investigated further. The patient should also be instructed to lift her arms above the head to inspect the lower part of the breasts. Then, the patient should be directed to put her hands on her hips to contract pectoral muscles that can lend insight to any abnormal puckering.

During the palpation portion, instruct the patient to lie down supine. It can be helpful to ask the patient to place her ipsilateral hand behind her head while lying supine to better expose the breast tissue in the axillary tail. Palpation of fine breast tissue is best elicited with the non-dominant hand stabilizing the breast tissue, while the free hand palpates. It is recommended to palpate delicate breast tissue with fin-ger pads and without gloves. There are different patterns to move across all four planes of the breast and axillary tail of Spence tissue, but the most evidence-based strategy is using a linear, up-and-down pattern across the tissue. When palpating the breasts, assess for shape, consistency, if the mass is fixed or immobile to the skin, and tenderness. Lastly, palpation of bulky lymph nodes in the cervical, supraclavicular, and axillary regions are recommended to complete the exam (Fig. 7.1, Table 7.1).

The differential for breast concerns is relatively limited compared to other chief concerns and can be categorized by benign and pre-malignant, and malignant entities. Over 90% of patients aged 20–50 years old with a palpable breast mass will have benign disease, however it is essential to rule out malignancy when there is sufficient clinical suspicion. An initial differential for a breast mass includes lactation mastitis, breast abscess, galactocele, simple cyst, fibroadenoma, dense breast tissue, granulomatous mastitis, atypical hyperplasia or lobular carcinoma in situ, primary breast cancer, and metastasis from other primary cancer sites to the breast. A benign mass can be either solid or cystic in nature, while a malignant mass is typically solid. In this patient's case, her personal risk factors and clinical history are extremely concerning and an urgent workup of the breast mass is recommended.

Additional diagnostic workup beyond the screening mammogram includes additional imaging with targeted breast ultrasound of the affected breast, and diagnostic mammography with or without tomosynthesis. Depending on what the ultrasound and mammogram show, she may be recommended to undergo potential biopsy with fine needle aspiration (FNA) or core needle biopsy. Imaging modalities include the breast ultrasound, which can help identify simple cysts and can also guide fine needle aspiration for sample material. While diagnostic breast mammograms are also recommended because of their increased sensitivity, breast MRIs are typically not. The imaging data is categorized based upon their likelihood of cancer according to the Breast Imaging-Reporting and Data System (BI-RADS), where higher scores

Fig. 7.1 The five areas of the breast involved in a thorough clinical breast examination

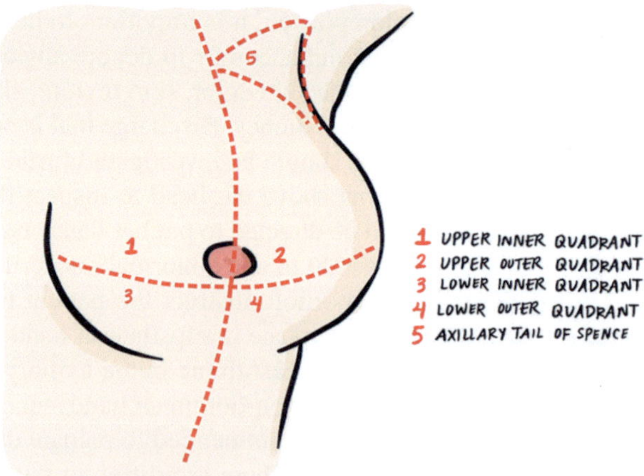

Table 7.1 Typical characteristics of a malignant and nonmalignant breast mass

	Malignant features	Nonmalignant features
Tenderness	Nontender	Tender
Shape	Irregular or spiculated (seen on imaging)	Regular borders (seen on imaging)
Consistency	Firm, rock hard	Rubbery or elastic consistency
Fixed to skin, vs. mobile	Fixed to skin	Mobile
Growth or change rate	*Rapid changes* of a lesion over weeks to months	Fluctuates in size with menstrual cycle Fixed, not growing

reflect higher suspicion for malignancy. For example, a BI-RADS score of 4 or 5 usually means that additional biopsy is indicated.

After listening to Mrs. Houston's concern and discussing our findings, we shared our assessment and concerns that her breast lump may harbor malignant features. Because of her strong family history of breast cancer, her age, and the malignant features noted on exam, we recommended she undergo urgent diagnostic mammography with L breast lump ultrasound with potential for fine needle aspiration biopsy within the next week. In our patient's case, she was diagnosed with estrogen receptor-positive breast cancer and was urgently referred to Breast Oncology to complete staging and treatment and initiation of endocrine therapy. Discussion of sentinel lymph node biopsy, staging of her cancer, and appropriate medical versus surgical treatment should be offered and managed primarily by the Breast Oncology team. Shared decision-making is critical in understanding the patient's goals and concerns about treatment.

Given the strong family history on her mother's side, we also strongly encouraged Mrs. Houston to ask her immediate family members on her mother's side, both men and women, to undergo a gene test for the *BRCA* mutation. As that point, they can be appropriate counseled about risk mitigation and appropriate screening intervals. If a family member is found to have a mutation, we would recommend early mammogram and breast MRI imaging starting at age 25.

7.4 Case 2: Appropriate Screening Intervals, Risk Assessment, Managing Modifiable Risk Factors)

While the previous case is our major concern regarding breast lumps for patients and physicians alike, the majority of breast lumps will be benign. Therefore, it is important to develop a risk stratification, management, and counseling strategy for patients with any and all breast lump concerns. Here we present a case with a more ambiguous features to practice utilization of common risk stratification tools available to the primary care physician.

7.5   Patient Case

Mrs. Huang is a 42-year-old woman with a history of hyperlipidemia and hypertension. Given that her paternal great-grandmother was diagnosed with breast cancer at age 78, Mrs. Huang wishes to discuss when to start mammogram screening given her family history. She has been told previously to get mammograms yearly, as recommended by the radiologists on her mammogram report. She prefers yearly screenings so she can feel secure that she is not missing a breast cancer diagnosis, which is one of her worst fears.

On exam, her vital signs are notable for a blood pressure of 120/67, heart rate of 81, and body mass index of 33.0 kg/m^2. She is well appearing, well nourished, with no cardiopulmonary abnormalities or neurological findings. Her breast exam is notable for scattered, firm-appearing densities across both breasts, without any fixed, large, immobile masses appreciated. There is no breast asymmetry, skin puckering, skin abnormalities on the breast, erythema, or nipple discharge.

Question: Given her history, exam findings, and personal risk, how would you counsel this patient in terms of the appropriate intervals for breast cancer screening?

7.6   Introduction of Breast Cancer Risk Assessment Models and Assessment Tools

To calculate an individual patient's risk of developing breast cancer, primary care physicians should be well versed in utilizing breast cancer risk assessment tools, which consider known and well-established breast cancer risk factors that would change an individual's risk compared to the larger population.

Risk-enhancing factors for breast cancer may be divided into non-modifiable, modifiable, and estrogen-specific categories. Unfortunately, there are no actions that patients can take to change or reverse these non-modifiable risk factors. Examples of non-modifiable risk factors include being born female, age at onset of menses, premature family history of ASCVD, family history of breast cancer, and history of cancer (e.g., Hodgkin's lymphoma) requiring chest radiation therapy. Patients should also be counseled that the number one risk factor for breast cancer is age, as lifetime accumulation of free radicals can lead to the development of aberrant cellular activity.

One popular and well validated risk stratification tool is called the GAIL Model, which was developed by scientists at the National Cancer Institute and one of its clinical trials cooperatives, the National Surgical Adjuvant Breast and Bowel Project (NSABP). With the GAIL model, an assessment for personal and family history of risk factors for breast cancer should be explored, including:

- Personal history of breast cancer
- Prior concern for breast lump indicating breast biopsy, history of in situ

- Previous radiation to chest, e.g., for prior Hodgkin lymphoma
- Known *BRCA1/BRCA2* mutation status in patient
- Any first-degree relative with breast cancer, including age at time of diagnosis, and if relative was known to have died from progression of disease
- Any environmental factors (exposure to chemicals, oil, manufacturing plants)

A clear obstetric history should be obtained, including:

- history of any pregnancies
- age at which patient had her first pregnancy
- number of previous pregnancies

Lastly, a menstrual history should also be obtained, including

- age of menarche
- age of menopause, either surgical, natural, or premature ovarian insufficiency

These questions around obstetric history and menstrual history can help estimate a patient's **lifetime estrogen exposure**, which can be a primary driver in some subtypes of breast cancer. Of note, premature ovarian insufficiency is defined as age < 40 years associated with irregular menses, negative serum human chorionic gonadotropin (hCG), and does not necessarily require presence of vasomotor symptoms or genitourinary symptoms (Fig. 7.2).

There are special considerations for risk factor assessment in patients with a history of breast cancer, given risk of recurrence, women who received radiation for the treatment of Hodgkin lymphoma, or women with known mutation in either the *BRCA1* or *BRCA2* gene. The GAIL model should not be used to assess patients in these higher risk situations (Table 7.2).

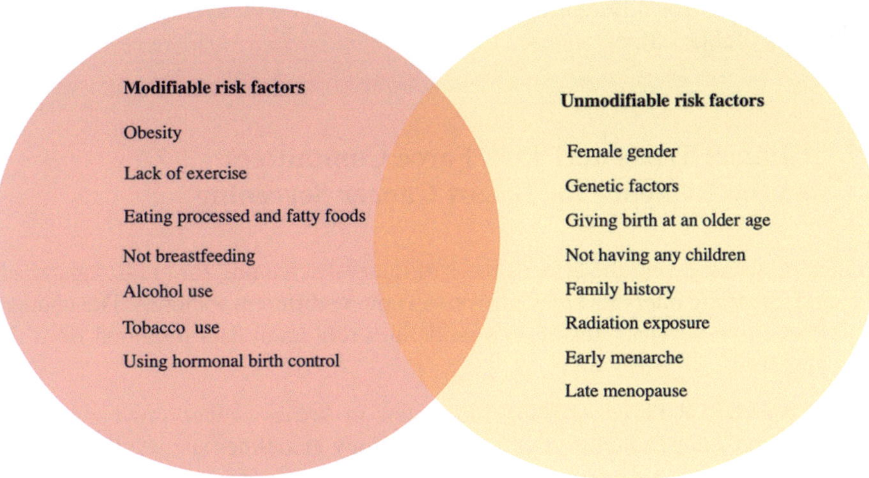

Fig. 7.2 Various modifiable and non-modifiable risk factors associated with breast cancer

Table 7.2 List of high risk features and various assessment tools for development or recurrence of breast cancer

High risk feature	Appropriate risk stratification tool/consult
History of breast cancer, ductal carcinoma in situ, lobular carcinoma in situ	IBIS breast cancer risk evaluation tool
History of prior chest radiation	Tyler Cruzick model
BRCA1 or *BRCA2* mutation	BOADICEA model
Li-Fraumeni syndrome	Medical Genetics referral

Based on her GAIL model score, our patient does not appear to have any major risk factors that would put her in a higher risk category, though her exam does have dense breast tissue. The one potential risk factor of concern is the history of breast cancer in the paternal great grandmother. Of note, family history is only positive when first-degree relatives (mother, sisters, or daughters) have been diagnosed with breast cancer. There is also increased risk in having a first-degree male relative diagnosed with breast cancer.

Screening mammograms have been the mainstay of screening interventions and are routinely offered and covered by most insurance companies. Self-breast exams were initially encouraged as part of preventative health care, but some societies such as the American Cancer Society (ACS) have discouraged this practice, as it can lead to false positive diagnoses and increased health anxiety. In 2009, the U.S. Preventive Services Task Force (USPSTF) recommended biennial screening mammography for women age 50–74 years. The decision whether to screen women age 40–49 years, or women >80 years old has been more controversial. The Task Force then based decisions for earlier screening for women 49 years and younger on *individual* patient context and values. Evidence was insufficient to recommend screening beyond age 75. The following are a summary of recommendations from the ACS, and the USPSTF for different age ranges and patients with average versus higher risk factors (Table 7.3).

7.7 Clinical Trials and Task Force Committees on the Evidence for Breast Cancer Screening

Clinical trials assessing the effectiveness of interval screening for breast cancer are few, and screening intervals are controversial among different societies. The updated U.S. Preventive Services Task Force guidelines rely upon data provided from the following trials:

- The **NSABP P-1**Trial (1998): Tamoxifen in breast cancer prevention. The American College of Obstetrics and Gynecology guidelines suggest that tamoxifen should be discussed as an option to reduce the risk of invasive breast cancer, specifically ER-positive breast cancer, in pre- and postmenopausal women who

Table 7.3 Various breast cancer screening cancer guidelines among U.S. cancer society and wellness task forces for average and high risk populations

Professional society and risk group	Criteria	Screening recommendations (Full)
United States Preventative Service Task Force for patients at **average** risk	• Patients without any risk factors per the GAIL model • No family history (first-degree relative) or personal history of breast cancer	• Age 40–49 years: Shared decision-making to start screening every 2 years • Age 50–74 years: Screening mammogram every 2 years. • Age 75 years or older: Screening not recommended
American Cancer Society recommendations for patients at **average** risk	• Patients without any risk factors per the GAIL model • No family history (first-degree relative) or personal history of breast cancer	• Age 40–44 years: shared decision-making to start screening annually • Age 45–54 years: Screening mammogram annually annually • Age 55 years and older should transition to biennial screening or have the opportunity to continue screening annually (qualified recommendation) as long as they have a life expectancy of 10 years or longer
American Cancer Society recommendations for patients at **high** risk	• Have a lifetime risk of breast cancer of about 20% to 25% or greater, according to risk assessment tools that are based mainly on family history (see risk assessment tools section) • Have a known *BRCA1* or *BRCA2* gene mutation (based on having had genetic testing) • Have a first-degree relative (parent, brother, sister, or child) with a *BRCA1* or *BRCA2* gene mutation, and have not had genetic testing themselves • Had radiation therapy to the chest when they were between the ages of 10 and 30 years • Have Li-Fraumeni syndrome, Cowden syndrome, or Bannayan-Riley-Ruvalcaba syndrome, or have first-degree relatives with one of these syndromes	• Yearly breast MRI starting at age 30 • Yearly mammogram starting at age 30

are age 35 years with a 5-year projected absolute breast cancer risk of 1.66% or with LCIS. Risk reduction benefit continues for at least 10 years.

- The **IBIS-I** trial (2001): Among women with an increased risk for breast cancer, tamoxifen reduces the risk of ER-positive breast cancer, but it provides no mortality benefit. Tamoxifen increases the risk of endometrial cancer and pulmonary embolism.

- The **Age Trial** (2006): Mammograms for 40–49 year old women. Among eligible women, initiation of mammographic screening at age 40 years, compared to initiation at age 50 years, did not reduce breast cancer mortality. Advanced breast cancer is reduced with screening for women aged 50 years or older.

7.8 Management of Breast Cancer for Primary Care: What Risk Factors Can We Mitigate?

After identifying relevant risk factors for the development of breast cancer in our patient, relevant risk factors should be appropriately managed in the primary care setting to minimize risk of breast cancer. The most important factors to address would include weight loss, abstinence from alcohol intake, smoking cessation, and management of cardiovascular risk factors such as diabetes, hypertension, cardiovascular disease.

In patients who require nuanced management of primary prevention risk factors, referral to a nutritionist, weight management expert, endocrinologist for lipid management, or substance support group for alcohol and nicotine dependence, may be appropriate (Table 7.4).

As mentioned previously, lifestyle counseling can lack the specificity to be actionable, and patients and providers alike can benefit from principles derived from motivational interviewing. It is important to provide specific, actionable steps to promote change, employing a technique called SMART goals. SMART goals are

Table 7.4 Examples of primary, secondary, and tertiary prevention of breast cancer

Primary prevention	Secondary prevention	Tertiary prevention
Identify individuals at risk for the development of breast cancer	Identify early or asymptomatic breast cancer	Prevent the recurrence or progression of existing breast cancer
Examples: • Smoking cessation • Weight management, especially following menopause • Physical activity • Taking hormones • Reproductive history • Alcohol use • Treat hypertension • Treat dyslipidemia • Treat diabetes mellitus • Treat underlying alcohol use disorder	Examples: • Mammogram screening. • Yearly breast MRI and mammogram screening in high risk patients	Examples: • Urgent referral to breast oncology for staging workup, counseling about treatment options, including surgery, chemoradiation, chemotherapy, and surveillance

defined that are **specific**, **measurable**, **actionable**, **realistic**, and **timely**. For patient encounters that are annual exams, there may not be enough time devoted to effective motivational interviewing. Therefore, it may be helpful to recommend a separate clinic encounter to focus solely on weight management, smoking and alcohol cessation, or exercise goals. For exercise, we recommend counseling patients that even a 5–10 pound weight loss can be beneficial for overall health. Nutrition recommendations may prioritize encouraging patients to eat whole foods, such as fruits, vegetables, legumes, and proteins, and avoiding boxed or processed foods. No matter which aspect of health the primary care physician chooses to address, it is imperative to maintain a welcoming, nonjudgmental perspective to promote the therapeutic, longitudinal relationship. In this way, employing motivational interviewing strategies to focus on adjusting patient's attitudes, habits, and behaviors, are all strategies to reduce these risk factors for breast cancer (Table 7.5).

After listening to Mrs. Huang's concerns and evaluating her on exam, she was informed that she has no concerning risk factors that would put her in a higher risk category. She was offered the recommendation to undergo screening mammography every two years starting at age 50, however her fears and concerns were explored, and through shared decision-making and discussion of the harms and benefits of yearly mammography compared to biennial mammography, was agreeable to undergo a mammogram every two years starting at age 47. Her mammogram resulted in a benign BIRADs-2 reading, with noted dense breast tissue obscuring

Table 7.5 Examples of concrete counseling phrases for modifying risk factors for breast cancer

Concrete examples and statements for lifestyle counseling to reduce breast cancer risk
• "Unfortunately, like most cancers, we cannot do anything differently if you or your family has higher gene risk, but we can monitor more frequently with yearly mammograms and breast MRIs."
• "Let's identify cases of breast cancer in the family that could add to your personal risk. Are there any male family members in the family with breast cancer? Of women family members, what age were they diagnosed? Did anyone have the BRCA mutation identified?"
• "We recommend 30 minutes of exercise most days of the week. To motivate yourself, try exercise with friends or family members, or use fitness tracking apps to see your progress. Habits take time, so even ten minutes consistently in the first week is better than no exercise."
• "While we cannot adjust our genes, there are some steps within our control to reduce our breast cancer risk. Avoid and cut down on alcohol, smoking. If it feels empowering, we encourage joining sobriety or support groups."
• "Eat everything, including dessert, in moderation to cultivate a positive relationship with food. When you shop for food, shop around the perimeter of the grocery store which has more whole foods, including fruits, vegetables, legumes, and proteins. This will help you avoid processed food in boxes and cans."

some of the view. She continues to seek annual mammograms with continued discussion about plans to space to every two years if yearly scans remain negative.

7.9 Conclusion

Despite advances in preventative care, increased access to screening, and advanced imaging mammogram, breast cancer remains highly prevalent among women, with significant morbidity and mortality. At the same time, many patients may have growing concerns about developing breast cancer and may feel it is therapeutic to have more frequent screening intervals for reassurance. Therefore, shared decision-making is essential to create a screening plan that is safe, rapport-building, and judicious of finite clinical resources. Primary care providers must be adept in calculating risk, interpreting up-to-date guidelines, and communicating compassionately during shared decision-making in order to be stewards of high-value care and appropriate breast cancer screening.

Although society recommendations may differ slightly, broad themes emerge with regard to general recommendations for breast cancer screening in an average risk patient. In the primary care setting, women over the age of 50 year old with average risk factors should be screened every 1–2 years, and assessed yearly for modifiable risk factors, including hypertension, dyslipidemia, tobacco use, diet, and exercise. Personal and lifestyle risk factors are largely encapsulated with a variety of risk prediction models, including the GAIL model for patients of average risk. Comprehensive obstetric, menstrual, and family histories may reveal additional risk-enhancing factors that modify the traditional GAIL risk score due to additional estrogen exposure. Investment in clinical trials around the effectiveness of low-cost/ more widely accessible screening modalities and attention to equitable enrollment in clinical trials may help develop more effective and equitable screening strategies for women moving forward in breast health.

Suggested Reading

1. Siegel RL, Miller KD, Fuchs HE, Jemal A. Cancer statistics, 2022. CA A Cancer J Clinicians. 2022;72(1):7–33.
2. Siegel RL, Miller KD, Wagle NS, Jemal A. Cancer statistics, 2023. CA A Cancer J Clinicians. 2023;73(1):17–48.
3. American Cancer Society. Cancer facts & figures 2023. Atlanta: American Cancer Society, Inc.; 2022.
4. Oeffinger KC, Fontham ET, Etzioni R, et al. Breast cancer screening for women at average risk: 2015 guidelines update from the American Cancer Society. JAMA. 2015;314(15):1599–614.
5. Malherbe F, Nel D, Molabe H, Cairncross L, Roodt L. Palpable breast lumps: an age-based approach to evaluation and diagnosis. S Afr Fam Pract. 2022;64(1):a5571. https://doi.org/10.4102/safp.v64i1.5571.

6. Rungruang B, Kelley JL. Benign breast diseases: epidemiology, evaluation, and management. Clin Obstet Gynecol. 2011;54:110–24.
7. Sickles EA, D'Orsi CJ. ACR BI-RADS®. ACR BI-RADS®-Atlas der Mammadiagnostik: Richtlinien zu Befundung, Handlungsempfehlungen und Monitoring. 2016;2:474.
8. Warner E. Screening BRCA1 and BRCA2 mutation carriers for breast cancer. Cancers. 2018;10(12):477.
9. Anderson KN, Schwab RB, Martinez ME. Reproductive risk factors and breast cancer subtypes: a review of the literature. Breast Cancer Res Treat. 2014;144:1–10.
10. Rockhill B, Spiegelman D, Byrne C, Hunter DJ, Colditz GA, Validation of the Gail, et al. Model of breast cancer risk prediction and implications for chemoprevention. https://doi.org/10.1093/jnci/93.5.358. PMID: 11238697
11. Dyrstad SW, Yan Y, Fowler AM, Colditz GA. Breast cancer risk associated with benign breast disease: systematic review and meta-analysis. Breast Cancer Res Treat. 2015;149:569–75.
12. Nelson HD, Cantor A, Humphrey L, Fu R, Pappas M, Daeges M, et al. Screening for breast cancer: a systematic review to update the 2009 U.S. preventive services task force recommendation. Rockville: Agency for Healthcare Research and Quality (US); 2016. Internet Accessed 2023 April 1.
13. Siu AL, U.S. Preventive Services Task Force. Screening for breast cancer: U.S. preventive services task force recommendation statement. Ann Intern Med. 2016;164(4):279–96.
14. Fisher B, Constantino JP, Wickerham DL, Redmond CK, Kavanah M, Cronin WM, et al. Tamoxifen for prevention of breast cancer: report of the national surgical adjuvant breast and bowel project p-1 study. J Natl Cancer Inst. 1998;90(18):1371–88.
15. Cuzick J, Sestak I, Forbes JF, Dowsett M, Cawthorn S, Mansel RE, et al. Use of anastrozole for breast cancer prevention (IBIS-II): long-term results of a randomised controlled trial. Lancet. 2020;395(10218):117–22.
16. Moss SM, Cuckle H, Evans A, Johns L, Waller M, Bobrow L, et al. Effect of mammographic screening from age 40 years on breast cancer mortality at 10 years' follow up: a randomized controlled trial. Lancet. 2006;368(9552):2053–60.
17. Tabár L, Fagerberg CJ, Gad A, Baldetorp L, Holmberg LH, Gröntoft O, et al. Reduction in mortality from breast cancer after mass screening with mammography. Randomised trial from the breast cancer screening working Group of the Swedish National Board of health and welfare. Lancet. 1985;1(8433):829–32.

Chapter 8
Diagnosis and Management of Urinary Incontinence

Amanda Artsen and Ashley Murillo

8.1 Introduction

The bladder has two primary functions: to store urine and to eliminate it by voiding. Urinary incontinence (UI) is the involuntary loss of urine due to a failure of the bladder to appropriately store urine. Although many patients consider this a normal consequence of aging, urinary incontinence is a prevalent issue that strongly impacts a woman's physical and mental health, quality of life, sexual function, and morbidity. Despite the wide range of the prevalence of urinary incontinence reported by numerous studies, often between 25% and 45%, it is important to note that the prevalence increases with increasing age. Urinary incontinence is divided into three categories: stress urinary incontinence (SUI), urgency urinary incontinence (UUI), and mixed urinary incontinence (MUI). In this chapter we will discuss all three of these diagnoses, important considerations in the differential diagnosis, and treatments with the help of case-based discussions.

8.2 Case 1

Mrs. JG is a G2P2 42-year-old female who presents with urinary incontinence. She reports she has had occasional urinary leakage that has become worse throughout the years. She states she leaks throughout the day on her way to the restroom. She reports that she has gained about 15 lbs over the last 3 years despite to changes to her diet, although she does notice she doesn't exercise or go out as much because

A. Artsen (✉) · A. Murillo
Department of Obstetrics, Gynecology & Reproductive Services, Division of Urogynecology, University of Pittsburgh Medical Center, Pittsburgh, PA, USA
e-mail: artsenam@upmc.edu; murilloa2@upmc.edu

M. Mahmoudi (ed.), *Common Cases in Women's Primary Care Clinics*,
https://doi.org/10.1007/978-3-031-48569-5_8

she is worried her peers will think she smells of urine. She drinks about 2 cups of coffee a day, a couple cans of soda and about 30 oz of water.

UUI is defined as the complaint of involuntary loss of urine associated with a sudden, compelling desire to pass urine which is difficult to defer. UUI is often seen as the sequala of overactive bladder (OAB). OAB is defined as urinary urgency, usually accompanied with frequency and nocturia, with or without urgency incontinence, in the absence of urinary tract infection or other obvious pathology. OAB is a bladder storage problem where the detrusor muscle involuntary contracts during bladder filling. The primary function of the detrusor muscle is to contract during urination and relax during bladder filling. In OAB, the detrusor muscle contracts when the bladder is not full, often randomly or in response to known triggers, such as when a patient puts their key in the front door or sees their toilet, which provoke the sudden urge that precedes incontinence.

OAB is classified into two categories, neurogenic OAB (in which any neurological process interrupts the normal function of the pontine micturition center) and non-neurogenic OAB. Non-neurogenic OAB, which occurs in the absence of a known neurologic process, remains poorly understood and poorly phenotyped. Although often thought of as myogenic, in which the increased sensitivity of the detrusor muscle to cholinergic stimulation leads to increased spontaneous activity or in which the intrinsic phasic activity of the detrusor muscle is altered (the "autonomous bladder theory"), other theories such as the afferent signaling theory or neurogenic theory suggest that increased afferent output or a reduction in inhibitory neural impulses lead to activation of the micturition reflex. These theories emphasize the complex interactions between the detrusor muscle and the central and peripheral nervous systems even in the absence of known neurologic disorder. It is also important to note that "detrusor overactivity" is the visualization of uninhibited bladder contractions seen on urodynamic testing and is not synonymous with OAB. For our discussion, we will focus on non-neurogenic OAB. If there is suspicion for neurogenic OAB as indicated by abnormal neurologic exam (signs of any upper or lower motor neuron lesions) or known neurologic diagnosis, the patient should be referred to a specialist.

Up to 33 million people are estimated to be affected by OAB, but only 15% of patients with symptoms seek medical help. Despite the impact of incontinence on a woman's quality of life, the reluctance to seek care arises from a variety of reasons which can include shame or embarrassment, and the beliefs that incontinence is natural and part of aging, incontinence is incurable, and the only treatment is surgery. Screening with validated questionnaires, the most simplest of which is 3 Incontinence Questions (3IQ), can improve the detection rates of incontinence. The American College of Obstetrics and Gynecology recommends routine screening in women for urinary incontinence. However, it should be noted that there is no evidence that demonstrates that routine screening improves women's quality of life or outweighs potential harms. Therefore, an assessment of distress or bother should always be included, and evaluation and treatment should focus on patient goals.

When addressing urinary incontinence, the first step is to obtain a through history and physical. The history should focus on when the leaking occurs, how often, what occurs before the patient leaks, and daily fluid intake as well as bowel function. A careful history is the most reliable way to determine the type of urinary incontinence experienced. A focused review of systems, review of past medical and surgical history, and review of medications (including previously tried OAB medications) are vital to the assessment of incontinence. When reviewing the patient's past medical history, questions about any neurologic conditions (such as dementia, Parkinson disease, multiple sclerosis, neoplasia, spinal cord injury, cerebrovascular disease), gynecologic and obstetric history, history of radiation or pelvic trauma should be included. DIAPPERS (delirium, infections, atrophic vaginitis, psychological causes, pharmacologic, endocrine, restricted mobility, and stool impaction) is a common mnemonic used to recall common causes of incontinence. Common medications that can cause incontinence include diuretics, alpha-1 blockers, and benzodiazepines. Surgical history should also include any pelvic surgeries, or previous treatments for incontinence. Many patients also complain of nighttime voiding, and it is important to distinguish the difference between nocturia and voiding at night when sleep is disturbed for other reasons. Nocturia specifically is defined as the complaint of interruption of sleep one or more times because of the need to micturate . A crucial detail that differentiates nocturia is that each void is preceded and followed by sleep; patients with insomnia, for example, who void because they are already awake need treatment of their underlying sleep disorder. Another type of nighttime voiding that should not be confused with nocturia is nocturnal enuresis. Nocturnal enuresis is when voiding occurs during sleep without awakening. In adults, this is often caused by sleep apnea.

The physical exam should start with a good general examination including age, stature, weight, and fragility; it should also include a neurologic examination including examination of gait, neurologic status, motor reflexes, and muscle strength. A pelvic exam is critical to rule out the following listed diagnoses, which would change treatment. The pelvic exam should include an evaluation of the vulvar skin (signs of vaginal atrophy), vagina (abnormal discharge, evidence of vesicovaginal fistula or prolapse), uterus and adnexa (space occupying lesions such as fibroids or adnexal masses), urethra (lesions, masses, or tenderness which may indicate a diverticulum), and pelvic floor muscle resting tone and strength. High pelvic muscle tone is also associated with urinary urgency and should be sought out in a patient who experiences pelvic pain or dyspareunia. Resting pelvic floor muscle tone should be assessed before insertion of a speculum to avoid reactional spasm due to the exam. Patients with high levator muscle tone who are told to perform Kegel exercises can experience worsening of symptoms. If the primary symptom is leaking urine with coughing, laughing, sneezing or activity without an urge, a cough stress test can be performed (see Sec. 4. Case 2).

During the evaluation, a urinary tract infection should also be ruled out with a urinalysis (or urine culture if inconclusive). Society guidelines and experts recommend urinalysis in the initial work up of urinary incontinence with a two-fold goal: to rule out infection and to evaluate for hematuria. A negative urinalysis has a high negative predictive value (92–100%) in those with a low-pretest probability but poor specificity and therefore when positive must be confirmed by microscopy and urine culture. Criteria for diagnosing UTI vary but must include both UTI symptoms and laboratory criteria (see chapter on UTIs for more information). Microscopic hematuria can be due to infection; foreign bodies such as kidney or bladder stones, sutures or mesh; urethral diverticulum; bladder cancer; or, most commonly, idiopathic. Referral to a urologist or urogynecologist is indicated for microscopic hematuria in the absence of a known benign cause. When available, a post-void residual (by ultrasound or straight catheterization) rules out occult voiding dysfunction, although this is not necessary for uncomplicated patients or those who will receive first-line treatment. Indications for post-void residual measurement or referral to a specialist include sensation of incomplete bladder emptying, prolapse or prior UI treatment such as midurethral sling or botox injection. If after history and physical evaluation, the diagnosis is still unclear, then a voiding diary (24–72-h documentation of fluid intake and voids) is recommended. If further advanced evaluation with cystometrics, urodynamics, cystoscopy or targeted imaging is necessary, then referral to a specialist is indicated. Other reasons to refer to a specialist includes if the patient has a lifelong history of incontinence (since childhood), recurrent urinary tract infections, pelvic organ prolapse, hematuria in the absence of infection, difficulty passing a urethral catheter or long-term history of catheterization, primary symptom of pain or if there is any uncertainty in the diagnosis or lack of improvement despite treatment (Fig. 8.1).

In this case, after a review of Mrs. JG's past medical history, surgical history and medication list, there were no medical conditions, medications or past surgeries that appeared to be contributing to her history. Her physical exam demonstrated normal external and internal genitalia, no urethral mobility and high pelvic floor muscle tone. Urinalysis did not have evidence of urinary tract infection and PVR of 40 cc. She was diagnosed with urgency urinary incontinence.

Fig. 8.1 Indications for further evaluation or referral to a specialist

- Neurologic signs or symptoms
- Incontinence since childhood
- Hematuria in the absence of a UTI
- Abnormal exam findings such as pelvic organ prolapse or inability to pass a catheter
- Recurrent UTIs
- Elevated postvoid residual
- Lack of response to treatment
- Dominant symptom of
    - Pain
      Nocturia in the absence of daytime symptoms
    - Nocturnal enuresis

8.3 Treatments

Treatments are outlined by the American Urologic Association and first-line treatments for OAB are behavioral therapies such as fluid management, bladder training, bladder control strategies, and pelvic floor muscle training (PFMT). Cure is hard to achieve, but symptom improvement is common. Setting expectations based on planned treatment regimen and reevaluation for response are important. An important initial recommendation for patients involves fluid management including avoiding excessive fluid intake, particularly in the few hours before going to bed, and avoiding bladder irritants (such as caffeine, artificial sweeteners, and citruses).

In the absence of medical contraindications, limiting total fluid intake to 40–50 oz. is also recommended. Other recommendations including voiding prior to going to bed, stopping smoking, and reducing weight. Obesity is a strong risk factor for urinary incontinence and symptoms can significantly improve with as little as a 5% weight reduction from baseline weight. Although weight can be a difficult topic to address, asking permission to discuss weight or starting with "how are you feeling about your weight?" can be a gentle way to open the discussion. Many patients who are overweight are actively managing this and congratulating successes as a first step can strengthen the therapeutic relationship.

If nocturia is the primary complaint, these lifestyle modifications including limiting excessive fluid/food intake prior to bedtime and decreasing caffeine and alcohol intake may be adequate to produce a satisfactory response. Moving diuretic timing to the early afternoon, compression stockings, and leg elevation 3 hours before bedtime can be useful if leg edema is present. If behavioral treatments are not sufficient further evaluation should be made with a bladder diary, which should also include volume and type of fluid ingested, volume and time of each voided urine, the time of retiring to bed, time of waking up and subjective evaluation of whether their sleeping pattern was good, bad, or normal. This information can lead help elicit a diagnosis of a sleep disorder (such as insomnia, obstructive sleep apnea, or sleep disorders related to medical disease like chronic obstructive lung disease or cardiac disease, etc.) or polyuria (which can be caused by diabetes mellitus or diabetes insipidus). Melatonin has been shown to reduce the number of nighttime voids. Patients with both daytime and nighttime symptoms often respond to treatments for urgency incontinence.

Bladder training has been found to decrease incontinence episodes from 60–80%. Treatment programs range from 6 to 12 weeks and focus on scheduling voids every 15–60 min (depending on the patient's baseline frequency or incontinence episodes) and increasing the voiding intervals by 15–60 min. During these programs, patients are taught how to voluntarily contract their pelvic floor when they feel urgency to inhibit a detrusor contraction. Bladder training also focuses on how patients respond to urgency; commonly, patients feel an urge and rush to the restroom therefore increasing intraabdominal pressure and setting up an environment to void. Bladder training empowers the patient to pause or sit when urgency happens, allowing greater control on when voiding will proceed.

Functional incontinence refers to incontinence secondary to the inability (or unwillingness) to get to a toilet. The most common causes are conditions that lead to immobility or mental function, such as stroke, dementia, or depression (specifically leading to psychogenic incontinence). Treatment revolves around environmental modifications (such as bedside commodes), timed voids where a patient voids at a fixed interval regardless of urge, occupational therapy to improve mobility, antidepressants, or cognitive behavioral therapy.

If the patient has poor pelvic floor muscle strength, poor coordination, high muscle tone, or inability to isolate their pelvic floor muscles, referral to a trained pelvic floor physical therapist for PFMT is recommended. During physical therapy, the patient will participate in 6–12 sessions to improve strength, range of motion and coordination of the pelvic floor muscles. There is insufficient evidence to recommend a specific program. There are also numerous online resources for pelvic muscle training which can improve patient access, however provider contact appears to be only factor in increased success so guidance in PFMT by a trained physical therapist should be encouraged if home exercises are ineffective, or if a patient has high pelvic muscle resting tone or is unable to identify the correct muscles. It should be noted that women are often instructed to stop their urine stream to identify the correct muscles but once identified, this should not be done routinely as this pelvic floor contraction can send mixed signals to the bladder as to whether it should void or store urine.

Ongoing research is investigating situational triggers for urinary urgency and incontinence. Specifically, a common phenomenon of "key in the door" incontinence and urgency upon hearing running water among patients with OAB and UUI was observed as a common trigger. This emerging research suggests a role for cognitive behavioral therapy in the treatment of incontinence.

These behavioral therapies can be combined with pharmacologic treatments. Pharmacologic management is second-line treatment for OAB. These medications fall into two categories: oral anti-muscarinic or oral β-3 adrenoceptor agonists, both of which increase storage capacity and allow for bladder relaxation during filling. Anti-muscarinic agents are darifenacin, fesoterodine, oxybutynin, solifenacin, tolterodine or trospium (listed in alphabetical order; no hierarchy is implied). These medications block muscarinic receptor stimulation by acetylcholine and reduce smooth muscle contraction of the bladder. This blockade during bladder filling results in increasing bladder capacity and decreasing urgency. Unfortunately, anti-muscarinic medications are not selective to the receptors in the bladder and common adverse effects include dry mouth, constipation, dry eye, somnolence, blurred vision, and risk for urinary retention. When prescribing these agents, often the extended release or transdermal routes are preferable to immediate release because of decreased incidence of side effects. Notably, increasing literature describes the association with anticholinergic medication and the increased risk of new onset dementia, therefore caution is recommended when prescribing these medications to middle aged and older patients who may be on other common medications with anticholinergic properties due to the cumulative total anticholinergic exposure risk. A 2020 systematic review and meta-analysis by Dmochowski et al. reported an overall rate ratio for incident dementia with anticholinergic use of 1.46 (95% CI: 1.17–1.81; number of studies = 6). The risk of incident dementia increased with increasing anticholinergic exposure (number of studies =3). Two studies from this meta-analysis reported an increased risk of dementia with ≥3 months of use of bladder antimuscarinics (adjusted odds ratios ranged from 1.21 to 1.65, depending on exposure category). Of the anticholinergics, oxybutynin has the clearest cognitive risk. Trospium does not cross the blood brain barrier and data from a multicenter, randomized, and placebo-controlled trial of trospium in elderly patients demonstrated no reports of CNS effects. Darifenacin has also been shown to not have any negative changes on cognitive and memory function in the elderly. Fesoterodine also has decreased central nervous system penetration but less robust clinical data. Therefore, if anticholinergic use is necessary in the elderly, darifenacin and trospium are recommended. In addition, these risks must be weighed against the impact of urinary incontinence on a patient's general health including risk of falls when rushing to the toilet and decreased physical and social activity.

The second class of medications are beta-3 agonists, namely mirabegron and vibegron. These medications do not carry a risk of dementia and are better tolerated due to lower rates of dry mouth and constipation. Due to reported small increases in blood pressure (1–4 mmHg) compared with placebo, mirabegron is not recommended for patients with severe or uncontrolled hypertension. The most common side effects are headache and nasopharyngitis, although both are infrequent. In addition, vaginal estrogen can improve both incontinence and irritative voiding in women with genitourinary syndrome of menopause/vaginal atrophy and is safe even for many with contraindications to oral estrogen. Prescription should be in collaboration with a patient's oncologist in the setting of a personal history of breast cancer.

Third line treatments include intravesicular onabotuliniumtoxin A (BTX-A or BOTOX®) injections, posterior tibial nerve stimulation (PTNS) and Sacral Neuromodulation (SNM). Intravesicular BOTOX® injections are most often done in the office (although can be performed in the operating room if patient prefers) and involves the use of a cystoscope to inject the bladder walls with 100–200 units of BTX-A. Adverse events include urinary retention requiring clean intermittent catheterization and increased risk of UTI. SNM is a two-stage procedure: Stage 1 (or the initial trial phase) can be performed in the operating room or in the office and involves placement of a wire lead into the S3 foramen, which connects to a stimulation device. The patient then monitors their symptoms over 1–2 weeks and if symptoms improve by >50% then implantation of the internal battery (stage 2) is performed. Adverse events include infection, migration of the lead, or lack of efficacy. PTNS is non-surgical nerve modulator treatment that is performed by percutaneous electrical stimulation of the posterior tibial nerve (a branch of the sciatic nerve) which is involved in the voiding reflex. This treatment involves 12 weekly 30-minute sessions where a small needle (34-guage) electrode is placed into the lower leg and an electrical current travels to the sacral nerve plexus via the tibial nerve. The main side effect is pain at the needle site. Therefore, if the time commitment is feasible, this is a good alternative to surgery.

8.3.1 Case 1 Conclusion

Mrs. JG was diagnosed with urgency urinary incontinence with high pelvic floor tone. She was counseled on behavioral modifications, physical therapy and if she is interested, she can start a beta-3 agonist such as mirabegron. If after 6 weeks, symptoms continue, patient should be referred to a specialist (urogynecologist or urologist).

8.4 Case 2

Ms. R is a 55-year -old-female with a history of two vaginal deliveries who presents with urinary incontinence for the last 10 years. She reports that she leaks every day with coughing, sneezing, or lifting heavy objects. She used to exercise more but is now limiting this because she leaks with moderate levels of activity. She also leaks on the way to the bathroom with a strong urge once per week. She denies acutely worsening symptoms, dysuria, and gross hematuria. She drinks 1 cup of coffee and 60 oz of water during the day. She has normal bowel movements.

8.5 Discussion

Stress urinary incontinence (SUI) is defined by the International Continence Society as the "complaint of involuntary loss of urine on effort or physical exertion (e.g., sporting activities), or on sneezing or coughing." This can be due to either lack of support of the urethra or intrinsic urethral sphincter deficiency. This usually occurs without an urge, although urgency can be generated when urine enters the urethra. Frequency in the setting of stress incontinence may also occur to a protective desire to void rather than with an associated urge to void. SUI effects 30–49% of women. The evaluation for stress incontinence is the same as discussed above for urgency incontinence and the addition of a cough stress test, in which the urethral meatus is observed for hypermobility and leakage while asking the patient to cough with a comfortably full bladder. Although urethral hypermobility is classically defined using the Q-tip test where a lubricated Q-tip is inserted into the urethra and the displacement angle at maximum strain is measured to be at least 30 degrees, this can be uncomfortable and unnecessary; visual inspection is generally sufficient.

In this case, Ms. R demonstrates mild vaginal atrophy; no urethral, vaginal, or pelvic masses; a normal appearing cervix and a uterus with normal size and contour without vaginal or uterine prolapse; poor pelvic floor muscle tone and squeeze, no urine present in the vagina. Urine can be seen coming from the urethra when asked to cough with a comfortably full bladder. Urinalysis is clear and a PVR is performed by ultrasound showing 20 mL 10 minutes after voiding. She is diagnosed with mixed urinary incontinence, stress predominant.

The treatments for stress urinary incontinence include behavioral therapies, which are similar to those employed for urgency incontinence. Specifically, avoiding bladder irritants and excessive fluid intake as discussed above can decrease SUI. Pelvic floor muscle training can be particularly effective for stress urinary incontinence as it strengthens the pelvic floor muscles that support the urethra. Similarly, with a combination of behavioral therapy and PMFT, up to 75% of women reported treatment satisfaction at 3 months and 50% at 1 year.

An incontinence pessary, a silicone ring that goes in the vagina and serves to support the urethra is a second treatment option. This is particularly useful for women with predictable leakage, such as leakage with exercise, who learn to insert and remove it themselves; however, it can also be worn continuously with regular office exams. A large, randomized control trial has shown better treatment satisfaction and fewer bothersome incontinence symptoms with behavioral therapy with PFMT compared to a pessary, however, a pessary is a good option for women who do not have the time or financial means to attend regular PFMT sessions. Although there was no benefit of adding a pessary to behavioral therapy with PFMT, a pessary can also provide immediate relief for some patients and therefore both modalities may still prove beneficial for some. Alternatives to traditional pessaries that do not require fitting by a physician include Impressa®, an over-the-counter nonabsorbable tampon-like vaginal insert, Revive®, an over-the-counter silicone one-size-fits-most vaginal insert, and Uresta®, a resuable prescription device made of a medical grade resin. Both Impressa® and Uresta® start with a fitting kit that is used at home and all of these are managed by the patient.

Surgical treatments include autologous fascial sling procedures, colposuspension procedures, a synthetic midurethral sling, which can be placed through a retropubic (Fig. 8.2) or transobturator approach, single incision midurethral slings, or periurethral bulking. An autologous sling uses fascia lata or abdominal fascia to support the vagina and is placed through vaginal and suprapubic incisions after fascial harvest. The Burch colposuspension procedure can be performed laparoscopically or robotically and uses a suture bridge from the vagina on either side of the urethra to Cooper's ligament on the pubic bone to support the urethra. Since the advent of polypropylene midurethral slings, autologous fascial slings and Burch colposuspension procedures have been performed less frequently due to their increased invasiveness with over 80% of procedures for SUI being a midurethral sling.

Polypropylene midurethral slings have been found to be safe and effective, with cure rates of approximately 85%. FDA warnings regarding mesh implantation pertain only to vaginally placed mesh used to repair prolapse and not to midurethral slings. Nonetheless there is a 3–5% risk of mesh complications with these procedures, leading some patients to seek non-mesh alternatives. The least invasive of these is periurethral bulking, which can be done in the office and provides about a 60–90% improvement rate at 12 month follow-up with up to 7 years of durability.

In women with MUI, it is useful to explain the symptoms of stress versus urgency incontinence and to determine the frequency and severity of each. This can help set expectations for which treatments will improve which symptoms. Patient with MUI

Fig. 8.2 The approximate position of a midurethral sling in relation to the bony pelvis, bladder, and urethra. 3D printed model of the bony pelvis and bladder and urethra which are shown in blue. Used with permission from the Translational Research Laboratories in Urogynecology and Pamela Moalli MD, PhD

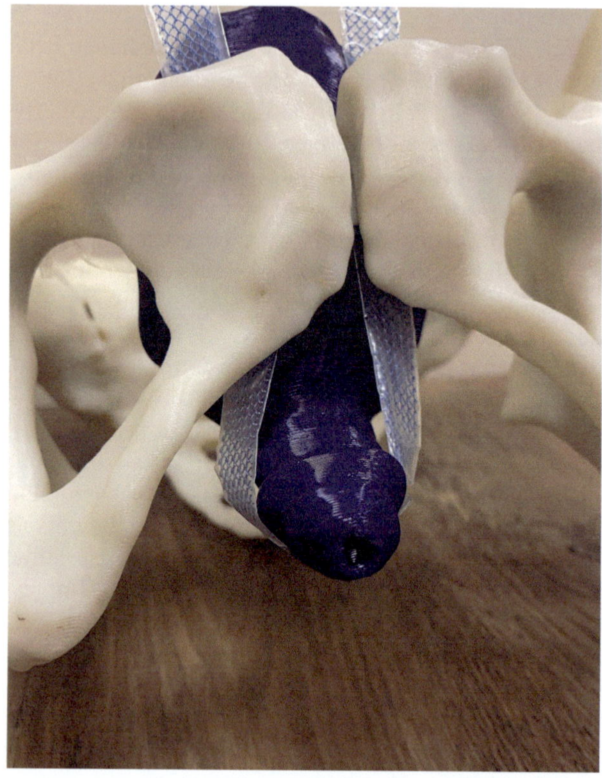

Fig. 8.3 Take-home points and clinical pearls

- Urinary incontinence affects up to 30% of women and can be extremely bothersome
- Careful history and physical exam including pelvic exam can reveal treatment-changing conditions
- Distinguishing between UUI, SUI and MUI guides initial treatment
- Most women with urinary incontinence benefit from lifestyle modifications and pelvic muscle training
- Referral is necessary for atypical features or lack of response

are considered candidates for both stress and urgency incontinence therapies and initial treatment is often focused on the most bothersome component (Fig. 8.3).

Ms. R is counseled on her treatment options and experiences significant relief with behavioral interventions and pelvic floor muscle training. She may benefit from a midurethral sling if her symptoms worsen with age and are no longer controlled with conservative therapy.

Suggested Reading

1. Huang P, et al. Urinary incontinence is associated with increased all-cause mortality in older nursing home residents: a meta-analysis. J NursScholarsh. 2021;53(5):561–7. https://doi.org/10.1111/jnu.12671.
2. Haylen BT, et al. An International Urogynecological Association (IUGA)/International Continence Society (ICS) joint report on the terminology for female pelvic floor dysfunction. Int Urogynecol J. 2010;21(1):5–26. https://doi.org/10.1007/s00192-009-0976-9.
3. Leron E, Weintraub AY, Mastrolia SA, Schwarzman P. Overactive bladder syndrome: evaluation and management. Current Urol. 2018;11(3):117–25. https://doi.org/10.1159/000447205. S. Karger AG
4. Brown JS, Bradley CS, Subak LL, Richter HE, Kraus SR, Brubaker L, Lin F, Vittinghoff E, Grady D. Diagnostic Aspects of Incontinence Study (DAISy) Research Group. The sensitivity and specificity of a simple test to distinguish between urge and stress urinary incontinence. Ann Intern Med. 2006;144(10):715–23. https://doi.org/10.7326/0003-4819-144-10-200605160-00005. PMID: 16702587; PMCID: PMC1557357.
5. Lukacz ES, Santiago-Lastra Y, Albo ME, Brubaker L. Urinary incontinence in women: a review. JAMA. 2017;318(16):1592–604. https://doi.org/10.1001/jama.2017.12137.
6. Burgio KL, et al. Behavioral vs drug treatment for urge urinary incontinence in older women: a randomized controlled trial. JAMA. 1998;280(23):1995–2000. https://doi.org/10.1001/jama.280.23.1995.
7. Dmochowski RR, et al. Increased risk of incident dementia following use of anticholinergic agents: a systematic literature review and meta-analysis. Neurourol Urodyn. 2021;40(1):28–37. https://doi.org/10.1002/nau.24536.
8. Sand PK, Johnson Ii TM, Rovner ES, Ellsworth PI, Oefelein MG, Staskin DR. Trospium chloride once-daily extended release is efficacious and tolerated in elderly subjects (aged ≥ 75 years) with overactive bladder syndrome. BJU Int. 2011;107(4):612–20. https://doi.org/10.1111/j.1464-410X.2010.09519.x.
9. Richter HE, et al. Continence pessary compared with behavioral therapy or combined therapy for stress incontinence: a randomized controlled trial. Obstet Gynecol. 2010;115(3):609–17. https://doi.org/10.1097/AOG.0b013e3181d055d4.
10. Nager C, Tulikangas P, Miller D, Rovner E, Goldman H. Position statement on mesh midurethral slings for stress urinary incontinence. Female Pelvic Med Reconstr Surg. 2014;20(3):123–5. https://doi.org/10.1097/SPV.0000000000000097. Erratum in: Female Pelvic Med Reconstr Surg. 2014 May-Jun;20(3):125. PMID: 24763151

Chapter 9
Intimate Partner Violence in Primary Care: Screening, Recognition, and Contingency Planning

Emily Harris and Molly Heublein

9.1   Introduction

Intimate partner violence (IPV) is a term used to describe a range of behaviors that lead to aggression, fear, or abuse within a romantic relationship. IPV includes four main categories of behavior: physical violence, sexual violence, stalking, and psychological aggression (Table 9.1). While many physically violent behaviors are well-recognized forms of IPV, other behaviors such as reproductive coercion (preventing access or controlling access to contraception) or exerting financial control over a partner are less commonly thought of as forms of IPV.

9.2   Epidemiology

IPV is common, and while typically thought of within the paradigm of heterosexual relationships with male perpetrators and female victims, it can take many forms. It is estimated that 33% of women and 28% of men have experienced physical violence, sexual violence, or stalking by an intimate partner. An even higher number—approximately 50%—experience other forms of psychological aggression within romantic relationships. It is difficult to fully characterize the epidemiology and

E. Harris (✉)
Department of Pulmonary and Critical Care, University of Washington, Seattle, WA, USA
e-mail: Emily.Harris@ucsf.edu

M. Heublein
Department of General Internal Medicine, UCSF Women's Health Primary Care,
San Francisco, CA, USA
e-mail: Molly.Heublein@ucsf.edu

M. Mahmoudi (ed.), *Common Cases in Women's Primary Care Clinics*,
https://doi.org/10.1007/978-3-031-48569-5_9

Table 9.1 Types of IPV

Physical violence	– Hitting/slapping – Kicking – Pushing – Strangulation
Sexual violence	– Rape – Other unwanted sexual contact – Unwanted sexual communication (e.g., texting) – Reproductive coercion
Stalking	– Physical stalking – Electronic monitoring or tracking
Psychological abuse	– Insulting – Manipulating – Financial control

patterns of IPV due to underreporting, but the survey data suggests that most people first experience IPV in adolescence and that behavior usually begins as psychological aggression such as insults and manipulation, with escalation to physical or sexual violence occurring later. Research suggests that IPV often begins or escalates during pregnancy or the postpartum period.

Given the prevalence of IPV, it is experienced by people in all segments of the population. Historically the paradigm of IPV has been thought of as something that is perpetrated by heterosexual men and experienced by their heterosexual female partners. Data shows that IPV is experienced by heterosexual men and queer people as well. However, some are more at risk than others, and the factors that increase risk of experiencing IPV track closely with social determinants of health for many other diseases. Minority patients are generally at higher risk for IPV than white patients, with Native American women being at particularly high risk. Patients who identify as lesbian, gay, bisexual, queer, transgender, or intersex (LGBTQI) are also at elevated risk.

9.3 Case 1

Bethany is a 23-year-old woman with no significant past medical history who is seen in clinic for new headaches which occur daily. She has not had headaches in the past. She tells her physician that she has also been experiencing new abdominal pain and anxiety related to her new symptoms. Despite a high symptom burden, she tells her physician that she is still doing chores around the house in addition to working two part-time jobs because her male partner becomes angry if she doesn't "keep up with housework."

9.4 Morbidity and Mortality

IPV carries risk of significant injury and death for victims. Physical and sexual violence can lead to significant injury that interferes with work or daily activities. Furthermore, an estimated 13.5% of homicides worldwide are attributed to IPV. This number increases to 38.6% in homicides of females. In addition to direct health consequences of IPV behaviors such as traumatic injury and sexual transmitted infections, IPV carries high morbidity and has been associated with a wide range of sequelae (Table 9.2). In the primary care setting, patients may present with symptoms related to one of these comorbid conditions, such as abdominal pain, pelvic pain, or substance use disorder. Recognizing constellations of such comorbidities may allow primary care providers to increase suspicion for IPV in some patients. In Bethany's case, her headaches, abdominal pain, and anxiety may be comorbidities of her experience with IPV.

Table 9.2 Sequelae of IPV

Neurologic	– Headaches – Stroke – Insomnia
Cardiac	– Chest pain – Myocardial infarction – Hypertension/gestational hypertension
Pulmonary	– Respiratory infections – Asthma – Emphysema
Gastrointestinal	– GERD – Irritable bowel syndrome
Genitourinary	– Pelvic pain/dyspareunia – Sexually transmitted infections – Urinary tract infections – Preterm delivery – Unplanned pregnancy – Menstrual disorders – Incontinence
Musculoskeletal	– Back pain – Arthritis
Endocrine	– Diabetes
Psychiatric	– Depression – Anxiety – Schizophrenia – Substance use disorder – Eating disorders – PTSD – Suicide

9.5   Case 1B

Bethany's physician becomes concerned for IPV and asks a few more open-ended questions. Bethany does not feel ready to discuss in detail at this time. Her physician responds with "thank you for sharing with me. I know it isn't easy to talk about these things. This is a safe space to discuss more if you ever need to talk in the future." Bethany agrees to return to clinic in one month to follow-up on her symptoms.

9.5.1   Screening for IPV

The high prevalence and significant morbidity of IPV necessitates screening in order to detect cases early and allow providers to intervene in a meaningful way. Despite the importance of screening for IPV, data suggests that screening rates are low relative to the prevalence of IPV in the population. Screening for IPV should be conducted frequently, and ideally take place at every annual exam, prenatal visit, and obstetrics visit. Screening should not be limited to ambulatory visits and should be considered in the inpatient and emergency department setting as well. Optimizing the screening environment and using appropriate screening questions increase patient comfort with the process and may lead to more effective screening.

Providers and clinic staff should work to create a clinical environment aimed at patient comfort during screening. Asking patients' preferred name and pronouns early in the patient-provider relationship is an important step in establishing rapport with patients, particularly prior to screening for sensitive topics like IPV. Because patients experiencing IPV may feel stigma, framing screening is also important. Providers may begin with phrasing such as "I ask all patients about other factors that affect health and safety." Patients should be made physical comfortable during screening, including being fully clothed and sitting in a chair rather than on an exam table. Patients may also prefer that screening occur without direct involvement of a healthcare professional, for example, by answering written survey questions.

There is no one rule for formulating screening questions for IPV. In general, open-ended questions without stigmatizing language are most effective (e.g., Do you feel safe at home?). Several screening tools have been created and validated, though the USPSTF does not strongly recommend any specific tool and no one tool has been shown to be more effective in meta-analyses. In the absence of a clearly superior screening tool, it is most important that providers choose questions or a tool that they are comfortable with using and can remember easily. A single question asked routinely to all patients can increase the detection of IPV in primary care.

9.5.2 Screening Tools

General open-ended screening questions

- How are things at home?
- Do you feel safe at home?
- How does your partner treat you?
- What happens when you and your partner have disagreements?

  Abuse Assessment Screen (AAS)
  Developed to screen pregnant women
  Positive response to any question is positive screening
  Sensitivity: 93–94% Specificity: 55–99%

1. Have you ever been emotionally or physically abused by your partner or someone important to you?
2. Within the last year, have you been hit, slapped, kicked, or otherwise physically hurt by someone? If yes, by whom? How many times?
3. Since you have been pregnant, have you been hit, slapped, kicked, or otherwise physically hurt by someone? If yes, by whom? How many times and where?
4. In the last year, has anyone forced you to have sexual activities? If so, whom? How many times?
5. Are you afraid of your partner or anyone you listed above?

  Partner Violence Screen (PVS)
  Positive response to any question is a positive screen
  Sensitivity 35–71% Specificity 80–94%

1. Have you been hit, kicked, punched, or otherwise hurt by someone in the past year? If so, by whom?
2. Do you feel safe in your current relationship?
3. Is there a partner from a previous relationship who is making you feel unsafe now?

9.6 Case 2

Casey is a 20-year-old male patient who is seen in clinic for an annual exam. As part of his annual exam, his primary care physician performs IPV screening by asking a single standardized question ("What happens when you and your partner have disagreements?"). Casey responds that his partner often becomes very angry and yells and has even broken dishes and damaged the walls of their shared apartment during arguments. During one incident, Casey's partner pushed him, and he bruised his forehead on the corner of a wall.

A disclosure of IPV from a patient either during screening or during other parts of a clinical encounter can feel overwhelming. While many providers wish to act in order to protect patients, validation of a patient's experience and listening to understand more can lead to more effective and patient-centered care.

9.6.1 Validation and Listening

In many cases, patients may not have discussed their experience with IPV with anyone. Thanking the patient for sharing the information and asking if it is okay to discuss further during the visit can help to reassure the patient that their partner will not be told about the disclosure by creating an environment of confidentiality. Examples of phrasing are listed in Table 9.3.

Validating a patient's experience and the injustice of their situation is also vital to maintaining a strong patient-provider relationship when discussing sensitive topics. Reassuring a patient that they are not at fault for the IPV that they are experiencing and that no one should be treated that way can help maintain this relationship (Table 9.3).

Lastly, respecting patient autonomy is crucial. In addition to asking patients if they are open to discussing IPV, reassuring them that they do not need to share all details right away helps maintain autonomy.

9.7 Evaluating for Risk of Immediate Harm

While IPV leads to significant morbidity and mortality, the pattern of violence typically escalates over time and not every patient is necessarily at risk of immediate harm. Most patients do not consider leaving their relationship despite what many may consider to be a dangerous level of frightening experiences. However, detecting cases in which a patient is currently unsafe can help prevent significant injury or death. Several tools have been developed and validated for the purposes of detecting risk of serious harm, including the Danger Assessment Tool (a 20-item questionnaire) and the brief Danger Assessment Tool (DA-5). Both tools are predicated on the association of certain behaviors with increased risk of future harm. While the

Table 9.3 Responses to patient disclosure of IPV

Express thanks	"Thank you for sharing what has been happening."
Validate	"You have been through a lot and I am sorry this has been happening to you."
Acknowledge the injustice	"No one deserves to be treated this way." "This is not your fault."
Respect patient autonomy	"Thank you for sharing with me. I know it isn't easy to talk about these things. This is a safe space to discuss more if you ever need to talk in the future."

formal danger assessment tool is more comprehensive, the 5-question version may be easier to remember in busy clinic settings.

Danger assessment tool 5
Has violence increased over the past 6 months? Has your partner used a weapon or threatened you with a weapon? Do you believe your partner is capable of killing you? Have you been hit while pregnant? OR has your partner ever tried to strangle you? Is your partner violently and constantly jealous of you?
A "yes" response to three or more questions on the questionnaire indicates a high risk of harm, with a sensitivity of 83%. Outside of the above questionnaire, data shows that prior strangulation by a partner is associated with a ten-fold increased risk of death. Presence of a gun in the home is associated with a five-fold increased risk of death.

9.8 Case 2B

After Casey's disclosure of his partner's behavior at home, he tells his physician that he is willing to further discuss IPV. His physician uses the DA-5 to evaluate for risk of serious harm. Casey says that his partner owns a gun and with which he has threatened Casey, has tried to strangle him in the past, and that these episodes seem to be occurring more frequently in the past several months.

9.8.1 High Risk Planning

If a patient screens positively for high risk of harm, providers should engage the patient in immediate safety planning. Informing patients that they are at high risk of harm is a component of safety planning, as it allows providers to contextualize the discussion with their patient. Immediate safety planning should consist of asking whether the patient feels safe to return home that day, and whether they would like to speak with someone about resources during the clinic visit.

If patients state that they do not feel safe returning home that day, they may be able to identify another safe location (e.g., the home of a friend or family member). Ensuring that patients have access to important documents, items such as cell phones, and keys should also be considered. Engaging other clinical staff such as

Table 9.4 Safety planning resources for IPV

National Domestic Violence Hotline	Web: www.thehotline.org Phone: 1–800-799-SAFE
National Coalition against Domestic Violence	Web: www.ncadv.org
United stated Department of Health & human services Office of Women's Health	Web: https://www.womenshealth.gov/relationships-and-safety/relationships-and-safety-resources

social workers and case managers, if present in clinic, can assist in this process. Furthermore, clinical social workers can provide additional information regarding shelter resources and support for patients. Some clinics may not have ancillary support on site, in which case providing information about nationwide hotlines and websites can be helpful (Table 9.4). It is important to avoid judging or pressuring patients experiencing IPV who are not yet ready to leave the abusive partner. Reasons patients continue to stay in abusive relationships are complex, and can include a valid fear that leaving will trigger further harm to the patient or family. Continuing to offer support and resources can allow the patient to feel comfortable reaching out to the provider when they are ready.

9.8.2 Mandatory Reporting

Physicians and other healthcare providers are mandated reporters of IPV. Laws regulating mandatory reporting vary by state. In most states, providers are mandated to report any injury resulting from IPV. Further, in most of those states victims are not able to decline reporting. Remaining open and honest with patients regarding mandatory reporting responsibilities is best practice when caring for those experiencing IPV. In the case that reporting is required, discussing the situation with patients and finding out how they would like their provider to advocate for them can facilitate more patient-centered care.

Documentation in the electronic medical record does not constitute formal documentation of IPV where mandatory reporting is concerned. Formal documentation should be filed with the appropriate government agency. While documentation of IPV is a necessary part of medical care for patients, providers should be mindful of documenting only necessary information. Furthermore, in an age when most parts of the medical record are accessible by patients via web portal, providers should use whatever option exists in the EMR to avoid sharing notes with patients, as perpetrators of IPV may have access to these web portals.

9.8.3 Safety Planning

Even in cases in which patients are not at high risk of harm or death, safety and contingency planning is a first line intervention for IPV. In fact, safety planning and contingency planning during these times can help patients prepare for potential future escalations of IPV.

Many resources exist to assist patients and providers in safety planning (Table 9.4), but all safety plans should involve contingencies to prepare a patient to leave a situation if IPV escalates or worsens. Other components of safety plans include:

- Copies of important documents and keys
- Securing cash
- Creating a bag with personal necessities
- Identifying a safe place to go
- Plan for notifying family/friends of immediate danger (e.g., code words)
- Providing resources such as domestic violence shelters and hotlines

Providers should inquire about whether patients would like to talk about safety planning prior to asking about details and providing resources in order to avoid overwhelming patients. Generally, establishing a plan regarding where a patient might go, how they would get there, and who would come with them (e.g., children and pets) are the basic components of a safety plan. Locating and storing important documents should also be discussed, and many patients benefit from obtaining cash and storing it in a secure place with other important items.

Efforts should be made to avoid giving patients written materials that may be discovered by a perpetrator. Saving important phone numbers and hotlines under alternate names in a cell phone is a way to discretely provide information to patients. Some patients may prefer to memorize phone numbers. When information is accessed via the internet, patients should be reminded that they may want to erase their browser history so that it cannot be discovered by their perpetrator. Many websites with resources for those experiencing IPV, such as the National Domestic Violence Hotline website, allow visitors to erase the website from their browsing history prior to closing a browser window.

9.9 Case 2c

Casey and his physician discuss safety further, and Casey feels safe returning to his partner today, and can identify a friend he could stay with if he felt unsafe at home. He plans to obtain copies of important documents and keep them in a safe place. Casey declines to talk with the social worker today, but accepts a hotline number for further support.

9.10 Conclusion

IPV is prevalent in primary care patients and leads to significant morbidity. Detection in the primary care setting can help identify cases early in an effort to reduce harm. Screening for IPV in a patient-centered way should be a routine part of all wellness exams and annual visits. When patients screen positive or disclose IPV to providers, evaluating for high risk of harm or death is an important next step. Discussing both immediate and future safety planning allows providers and patients to collaboratively develop plans to leave situations that become dangerous. With incorporation into routine screening and discussion, providers can incorporate these patient-centered strategies for care into their general practice.

Suggested Reading

1. Fast facts: preventing intimate partner violence |violence prevention|injury center|CDC. Published March 24, 2022. Accessed April 29, 2022. https://www.cdc.gov/violenceprevention/intimatepartnerviolence/fastfact.html
2. Breiding MJ, Smith SG, Basile KC, Walters ML, Chen J, Merrick MT. Prevalence and characteristics of sexual violence, stalking, and intimate partner violence victimization – national intimate partner and sexual violence survey, United States, 2011. Morb Mortal Wkly Rep Surveill Summ Wash DC 2002. 2014;63(8):1–18.
3. Gazmararian JA, Lazorick S, Spitz AM, Ballard TJ, Saltzman LE, Marks JS. Prevalence of violence against pregnant women. JAMA. 1996;275(24):1915–20.
4. Risk and Protective Factors|Intimate Partner Violence|Violence Prevention|Injury Center|CDC. Published November 5, 2021. Accessed April 29, 2022. https://www.cdc.gov/violenceprevention/intimatepartnerviolence/riskprotectivefactors.html
5. Stöckl H, Devries K, Rotstein A, et al. The global prevalence of intimate partner homicide: a systematic review. Lancet Lond Engl. 2013;382(9895):859–65. https://doi.org/10.1016/S0140-6736(13)61030-2.
6. Miller E, McCaw B. Intimate partner violence. N Engl J Med. 2019;380(9):850–7. https://doi.org/10.1056/NEJMra1807166.
7. O'Doherty L, Hegarty K, Ramsay J, Davidson LL, Feder G, Taft A. Screening women for intimate partner violence in healthcare settings. Cochrane Database Syst Rev. 2015;(7):CD007007. https://doi.org/10.1002/14651858.CD007007.pub3.
8. Rabin RF, Jennings JM, Campbell JC, Bair-Merritt MH. Intimate partner violence screening tools. Am J Prev Med. 2009;36(5):439–445.e4. https://doi.org/10.1016/j.amepre.2009.01.024.
9. Paterno MT, Draughon JE. Screening for intimate partner violence. J Midwifery Womens Health. 2016;61(3):370–5. https://doi.org/10.1111/jmwh.12443.
10. Snider C, Webster D, O'Sullivan CS, Campbell J. Intimate partner violence: development of a brief risk assessment for the emergency department. Acad Emerg Med. 2009;16(11):1208–16. https://doi.org/10.1111/j.1553-2712.2009.00457.x.
11. Messing JT, Campbell JC, Snider C. Validation and adaptation of the danger assessment-5: a brief intimate partner violence risk assessment. J Adv Nurs. 2017;73(12):3220–30. https://doi.org/10.1111/jan.13459.

Chapter 10
Women and the Immune System

Jacquelyn Nestor and Marcy B. Bolster

10.1　Introduction

The human immune system is designed to protect the body from outside intruders, such as bacteria, viruses and foreign bodies, but in some cases the immune system is misdirected and "attacks" its own body (or "self"), resulting in the development of autoimmune disease. Most autoimmune diseases occur more commonly in women, such as systemic lupus erythematosus, systemic sclerosis (scleroderma), and rheumatoid arthritis (RA). Rheumatoid arthritis is the most common autoimmune disease, characterized by inflammation in the joints, which can lead to substantial joint stiffness and functional limitations; it can be debilitating, severely affecting quality of life. Continued poorly-controlled joint inflammation can, over time, lead to permanent joint destruction that not only causes pain and deformity, but leads to significant functional loss as well. Here we use RA to illustrate the predisposition in women for autoimmune diseases and how their management requires consideration of several conditions and comorbidities, specific to women.

J. Nestor (✉)
Division of Rheumatology, Allergy and Immunology, Department of Medicine, Massachusetts General Hospital, Boston, MA, USA

Harvard Medical School, Boston, MA, USA

Broad Institute, Cambridge, MA, USA
e-mail: JNESTOR@mgh.harvard.edu

M. B. Bolster
Division of Rheumatology, Allergy and Immunology, Department of Medicine, Massachusetts General Hospital, Boston, MA, USA

Harvard Medical School, Boston, MA, USA
e-mail: mbolster@mgh.harvard.edu

M. Mahmoudi (ed.), *Common Cases in Women's Primary Care Clinics*, https://doi.org/10.1007/978-3-031-48569-5_10

The reasons for a female predilection of autoimmune diseases, and more specifically RA, remain uncertain. Most agree that the pathogenesis of RA is likely multifactorial involving a combination of both genetic predisposition and environmental exposures. The mechanisms behind these influences have not yet been fully elucidated. Given the differences in incidence between sexes, it has been proposed that estrogen may be an important contributor to disease development. Interestingly, it has been suggested that it is not just the elevated levels of estrogen, but it is also the fluctuations in estrogen levels throughout a woman's lifetime that contribute to the increased incidence of RA in women. The role of estrogen as a risk factor can seem contradictory. The time during which a woman is pregnant may be protective against RA for some, but increased parity has also been associated with augmented RA incidence. The initial period after beginning lactation has been shown to be a high-risk time for RA development, but increased duration of breastfeeding has been demonstrated to be protective against RA. The impact of hormone replacement therapy and oral contraceptives on disease incidence and activity remains controversial. Further elucidation of the mechanism behind the development of RA and its increased incidence in women will be helpful in the development of new treatment strategies to better manage the disease in both sexes.

Because autoimmune disease, and more specifically RA, affects women more than men, there are additional factors including those associated with contraception, pregnancy, and lactation in women of child-bearing age, which must be taken into consideration for disease management. Beyond the joints, patients with RA are also at high risk for developing atherosclerotic cardiovascular disease (ASCVD) and osteoporosis, requiring a comprehensive approach to patient care that acknowledges the interplay between multiple comorbidities in women. These considerations add to the complexity of managing this autoimmune disease. Because RA is the most common autoimmune disease, we present the cases of RA in two women at different stages of life, and we discuss how the presentation and management interplays with each woman's overall health.

10.2 Case 1

AB is a 27-year-old woman with no significant medical history who is seen for an urgent appointment after experiencing several weeks of pain and swelling of her hands and feet. She first noticed her symptoms a few weeks prior when she was getting dressed in the morning and was having difficulty applying her makeup because she was unable to grip items with her fingers. When asked which part of her hands hurt her the most, she describes the pain as being worst over her knuckles on the back of both hands, and she has noticed that when the swelling is worst, she cannot distinguish her knuckles at all. At first, she managed her pain by running warm water over her hands until they "loosened up," but this is no longer helpful. The pain has continued to worsen, now lasting several hours in the mornings, such that she is experiencing difficulties at work. Over the last few weeks, she has also noticed wrist pain when brushing her hair or picking up dishes. She is recently married and has been having difficulty putting her rings on and off due to finger swelling, so she has stopped wearing them. Over the last few weeks, she has taken acetaminophen and ibuprofen for her pain, but she reports that these medications have provided minimal relief, prompting her to schedule her urgent appointment today.

On interview she denies skin rash, oral ulcers, alopecia, fever, recent infections, or new medications. She has not traveled and denies known tick exposures. The review of systems is otherwise unremarkable. She has no allergies and takes no medications. She remembers her grandmother had "arthritis," but is unsure of the type. She is a never smoker, drinks alcohol socially, and is sexually active in a mutually monogamous relationship with her husband. She denies history of sexually transmitted infections.

Her physical exam is notable for swelling, tenderness, erythema, and warmth of bilateral metacarpophalangeal (MCP) and proximal interphalangeal (PIP) joints, with limited ability to fully make a fist with each hand. Her wrists are also swollen, and there is tenderness over the ulnar styloid bilaterally; limited wrist flexion and extension is noted due to pain. Her elbows, shoulders, knees, and ankles are without joint swelling and are nontender. Metatarsophalangeal (MTP) squeeze elicits tenderness. There are no skin rashes.

Given the presence of symmetric synovitis on exam, with small joint involvement, you are concerned she has developed RA, and you recognize the importance of prompt diagnosis and initiation of treatment. You request same-day lab testing. Her labs are notable for elevated inflammatory markers, including the erythrocyte sedimentation rate (ESR) at 48 mm/h, c-reactive protein (CRP) at 75 mg/L. Other labs include an elevated rheumatoid factor (RF) at 100 IU/mL and an elevated anti-cyclic citrullinated peptide (CCP) at 200 U/mL. X-rays obtained of her hands and feet do not show erosions or joint space narrowing, but comment is made of periarticular osteopenia at the MCP joints. You discuss the role of prednisone with her, including its risks and benefits. As this is the medication that is most likely to help her quickly, you initiate prednisone 15 mg daily. She returns to the office for follow-up 1 week later, and reports significant improvement in her symptoms, though she has not experienced complete resolution. Morning stiffness persists, but it now lasts less than an hour; she is also able to wear her rings again. You discuss that although prednisone acts quickly, it has many significant potential risks, thus she would benefit from another medication that will be "steroid sparing" and, importantly, treat her underlying inflammatory arthritis.

10.3 Case 1 Discussion

The first step in RA management requires quick recognition of the disease in order to limit inflammation and potential joint damage. This starts with differentiating inflammatory and non-inflammatory arthritis (Table 10.1). On history, patients with inflammatory arthritis typically endorse significant morning stiffness, lasting more

Table 10.1 Factors differentiating inflammatory and non-inflammatory arthritis

		Inflammatory	Non-inflammatory
AM stiffness		>1 h	<1 h
Joint exam			
	Temperature	Warm	Cool
	Color	Erythematous	Non-erythematous
	Enlargement	Soft tissue swelling	Bony prominence
	Effusions	Present	Present or absent

than 1 h after awakening; at times the stiffness can persist all day. On examination, involved joints will exhibit synovitis, characterized by joint swelling, tenderness, erythema, and warmth. In those with joint inflammation, it is not requisite to detect each of these features; swelling and tenderness are most characteristic. Inflammation can also severely limit joint range of motion both in the short term due to the degree of swelling and pain, and in the long term, due to chronic inflammatory destructive changes to the joints. Several types of inflammatory arthritis exist, including RA, spondyloarthropathies, reactive arthritis, and systemic lupus erythematosus among others, and often, features elucidated on history or physical examination can lead the clinician to the correct diagnosis. Rheumatoid arthritis is further differentiated from other types of inflammatory arthritis by its predilection for symmetric involvement of the small joints of the hands and feet, particularly the MCP, PIP, and MTP joints. AB's presentation represents a convincing case of a patient with an inflammatory arthritis. The swelling, tenderness, warmth, and erythema overlying her MCP joints are characteristic of synovitis and in association with several hours of morning stiffness, her presentation is consistent with a symmetric polyarticular inflammatory arthritis, more specifically, RA.

Her laboratory evaluation lends further support for a diagnosis of RA, with elevated RF, anti-CCP antibody, and inflammatory markers. Patients can be characterized as seropositive or seronegative based on laboratory testing being positive for RF and/or anti-CCP antibody. Anti-CCP antibodies are highly specific for the diagnosis of RA. Higher titers of these antibodies are associated with more difficult to control disease and can signal a provider to be more aggressive in their initial management as shown in the 2004 TIRA study. The inflammatory findings in the joints may be reflected in laboratory results including elevated inflammatory markers, such as ESR and CRP.

The effects of this disease can be further characterized by erosions on plain film imaging, which in RA occur predominantly in the MTPs, MCPs, and PIPs. It can be helpful to obtain baseline hand and foot X-rays in patients with newly-diagnosed RA to use for future comparison, but erosions can be seen in early disease as well. Fortunately, AB's imaging does not show erosions, but there is radiographic evidence of periarticular osteopenia. This is a characteristic early change that can often be seen in patients with RA.

Rheumatoid arthritis often requires a combined approach when selecting therapeutics. Acutely, symptoms can be managed with corticosteroids, such as prednisone or methylprednisolone, in order to reduce joint inflammation. Corticosteroids should not be used indefinitely given their array of potential adverse effects, including but not limited to, increased risk of infection, cataracts, skin thinning, osteonecrosis, and bone loss. AB will benefit from the addition of a steroid-sparing agent, specifically a disease-modifying antirheumatic drug (DMARD). DMARDs can be separated into synthetic and biologic (bDMARD) agents, with synthetics further delineated as conventional synthetic (csDMARD) or targeted synthetic (tsDMARD) (Table 10.2). It is crucial to be aggressive in the initial treatment of RA, as early intervention in patients with RA is associated with limited progression of radiographic findings, superior disease outcomes and most importantly, improved quality of life. Patients are typically first started on the csDMARD, methotrexate, which is considered the backbone of RA treatment regimens. If patients have an inadequate response to monotherapy with methotrexate, one could consider switching to an alternative csDMARD, such as sulfasalazine or leflunomide in specific cases, or combining methotrexate, sulfasalazine and leflunomide for "triple therapy." Commonly, providers will add a biologic agent to the regimen, such as a tumor necrosis factor (TNF) inhibitor, interleukin-6 (IL-6) inhibitor, or a tsDMARD such as a janus kinase (JAK) inhibitor. Most clinical trials for evaluating new RA medications are completed in patients who are concomitantly on methotrexate.

Given a female predominance of RA, it is important for providers to consider the implications of DMARDs on reproductive health in women of child-bearing age. Unfortunately, methotrexate, the medication most commonly used as first-line

Table 10.2 DMARDs commonly used in the management of rheumatoid arthritis

Conventional synthetic (csDMARD)	
	Hydroxychloroquine[a]
	Leflunomide
	Methotrexate[a]
	Sulfasalazine[a]
Biologic (bDMARD)	
TNF inhibitor	Adalimumab
	Certolizumab
	Etanercept
	Golimumab
	Infliximab
IL-6R inhibitor	Sarilumab
	Tocilizumab
T-cell costimulation inhibitor	Abatacept
B-cell inhibitor	Rituximab
Targeted synthetic (tsDMARD)	
JAK inhibitor	Baricitinib
	Tofacitinib
	Upadacitinib

[a]Medications that are utilized together as triple therapy

treatment of RA, is a teratogen and therefore should not be used in patients desiring pregnancies in the near future. Family planning, thus, must be thoroughly discussed prior to methotrexate initiation. Given the teratogenic nature of methotrexate, one must ensure the use of an effective form of contraception in all premenopausal patients on methotrexate, preferably with an intrauterine device or oral contraceptive pills. Although discussion of pregnancy planning and contraception are important, the diagnosis of RA and its medications do not preclude safe and healthy pregnancies. It is critical for there to be an honest relationship between patient and provider regarding pregnancy wishes and planning. It should also be emphasized that well-controlled disease has a positive impact both on conception and on the ability to carry out a healthy pregnancy. Treatment of RA is not fixed and can vary over time, with changes not only in arthritis disease activity, but also in the context of life milestones. In order to overcome these challenges, patients may need to change their treatment during pregnancy and lactation.

Once the arthritis is well-controlled and the patient desires a pregnancy, medications can be adjusted to those better suited for pregnancy. In 2020 the American College of Rheumatology (ACR) released Reproductive Health Guidelines, which assist in finding appropriate medications for female patients with rheumatic disease during pregnancy and lactation. For patients taking methotrexate, the first step includes tapering off methotrexate, which is considered unsafe in pregnancy, with plans for conception to be delayed for 1–3 months after methotrexate cessation. Other medications such as TNF inhibitors are commonly utilized for disease management through the first two trimesters of pregnancy and during lactation. Many providers will choose to transition their patients specifically to certolizumab, a TNF inhibitor that can be utilized throughout all three trimesters. Certolizumab is often preferred as it is the only pegylated TNF inhibitor and with its large size and lack of an Fc receptor, it is unable to transition through the placenta to the fetus. Therefore, this structural design minimizes potential exposure to the fetus.

Although there are many implications of rheumatic disease medications on conception and pregnancy, it is also important to consider the effect of pregnancy on RA disease activity. The Pregnancy-induced Amelioration of Rheumatoid Arthritis (PARA) study in 2008, showed that many patients with RA will have remission of their disease during pregnancy, and even require less use of medications for their rheumatic disease. Unfortunately, this study also showed that many of these same patients experienced increased RA disease activity postpartum. This increase in disease activity can have implications on the newborn, particularly if the patient intends to breastfeed their baby for the first year of life. Many of the medications used for RA management are shown to not only accumulate in breast milk, but subsequently in the newborn as well. As such, TNF inhibitors, not just certolizumab, are the treatment of choice during lactation. The data regarding the use of methotrexate is limited and therefore this medication is not recommended for treatment while a patient is breastfeeding.

Unfortunately, the switching and titration of alternate medications, especially in the postpartum period, can lead to flares that may be difficult to control, typically requiring corticosteroids to control symptoms. While not contraindicated, corticosteroid dosing should be limited during both pregnancy and lactation to ideally less than 20 mg daily. It is also recommended that corticosteroid dosing be temporally separated from breastfeeding by at least 4 h in an effort to limit infant exposure. Once the patient has completed breastfeeding, they can be maintained on their current regimen if it is adequately controlling their symptoms, or they can be transitioned back to their pre-pregnancy regimen with appropriate contraception.

10.4   Case 2

MN is a 72-year-old woman with obesity, hypertension, hyperlipidemia, atrial fibrillation, gastroesophageal reflux disease (GERD), and type 2 diabetes, and presents for her annual follow-up. Throughout the last year it has been difficult for her to manage her multiple medical conditions, and the last 6 months have been complicated by the development of significant pain and swelling of her wrists and hands that has made it difficult for her to open pill bottles at times, leading to her missing several doses of her medications. She feels extremely stiff in the mornings and depends on her husband to make her coffee, but even then, she still finds it challenging to pick up her coffee cup. Sometimes she feels like her morning stiffness "lasts all day." She has also struggled with sleeping due to numbness and aches in her hands that wake her up throughout the night. She felt that this was all just part of "getting old," so she did not seek help sooner. Acetaminophen has not significantly helped her joint pains, and she has been told to avoid NSAIDs given her atrial fibrillation medications and symptoms of acid reflux. She borrowed cannabidiol (CBD) salve from her granddaughter, and she found this to be helpful though costly.

On review of symptoms, she denies any other symptoms including rash. For medications she is currently taking atorvastatin, lisinopril, apixaban, omeprazole, and metformin. She denies a family history of arthritis, but she notes that her mother recently broke her hip after a fall at home. She currently uses tobacco and has a 50-pack-year history. She has intermittently tried nicotine patches, but has struggled with smoking cessation. She reports social alcohol use. She is married and has three children and one grandchild.

When reviewing her vital signs, she is surprised by her height, noting that she has lost one inch in height. Her physical examination is notable for a normal pulmonary and cardiovascular exam. She does not have any spinous process or paraspinal muscle tenderness, but there is slight accentuation of the thoracic kyphosis. Her musculoskeletal examination is notable for swelling and tenderness of the MCP joints and wrists, with the wrist swelling causing limited range of motion. She has bony enlargement of several DIP joints, and there is squaring of the first carpometacarpal (CMC) joints. Tinel's sign is positive bilaterally, replicating the numbness sensation she experiences at night when trying to sleep.

You discuss that while some of her symptoms represent osteoarthritis (OA), you are also concerned about a concomitant inflammatory arthritis. Moreover, you are concerned that her symptoms represent RA given the symmetric synovitis of the wrists and MCP joints. Her new bilateral carpal tunnel symptoms with positive Tinel's sign are further consistent with synovitis of each wrist causing compression of the median nerves. Laboratory testing and radiographic findings support your suspicions with a high positive RF and anti-CCP antibody; inflammatory markers, ESR and CRP, are also elevated. You start her on prednisone 15 mg daily and refer her to a rheumatology provider to help guide DMARD selection, recognizing the complexity of her care in light of her multiple comorbidities. When you place the referral, you make sure to share her cardiac and diabetes history. You predict that she will likely need several months of corticosteroids, thus addressing her bone health is a high priority. A dual X-ray absorptiometry (DXA) scan reveals osteopenia with elevated FRAX scores based on prednisone use, tobacco use, RA, and her mother's recent hip fragility fracture. Using shared-decision making, you initiate treatment with annual zoledronic acid infusions, start calcium and vitamin D supplementation, and recommend varenicline for smoking cessation.

10.5 Case 2 Discussion

MN's diagnosis of RA is less straightforward than the previous case, as the new joint symptoms are superimposed on OA. Early intervention is an important aspect in the management or RA, so it is crucial to make a timely differentiation between OA and RA (Table 10.3). The simplest way to differentiate the two is by presence or absence of inflammation, as RA is an inflammatory arthritis, and OA is predominantly a non-inflammatory arthritis (Table 10.1). One difficulty in differentiating RA from OA arises in the cases of inflammatory OA. On history, timing of symptoms throughout the day can help with differentiation, as the morning stiffness in

Table 10.3 Factors differentiating rheumatoid arthritis and osteoarthritis

	Rheumatoid arthritis	Osteoarthritis
History		
AM stiffness >30 min	Yes	No
Time of day most symptomatic	Morning	Evening
Association with activity	Worst after rest	Worst after activity
Joint exam		
Distribution	MCPs, PIPs, MTPs	PIPs, DIPs
Deformities	Swan neck	Heberden nodes
	Boutonniere's	Bouchard nodes
	Ulnar deviation	First CMC squaring
Labs		
Inflammatory markers	Elevated	Normal
Radiographic findings		
Joint space narrowing	Yes	Yes
Erosion location	At the joint margin	Central

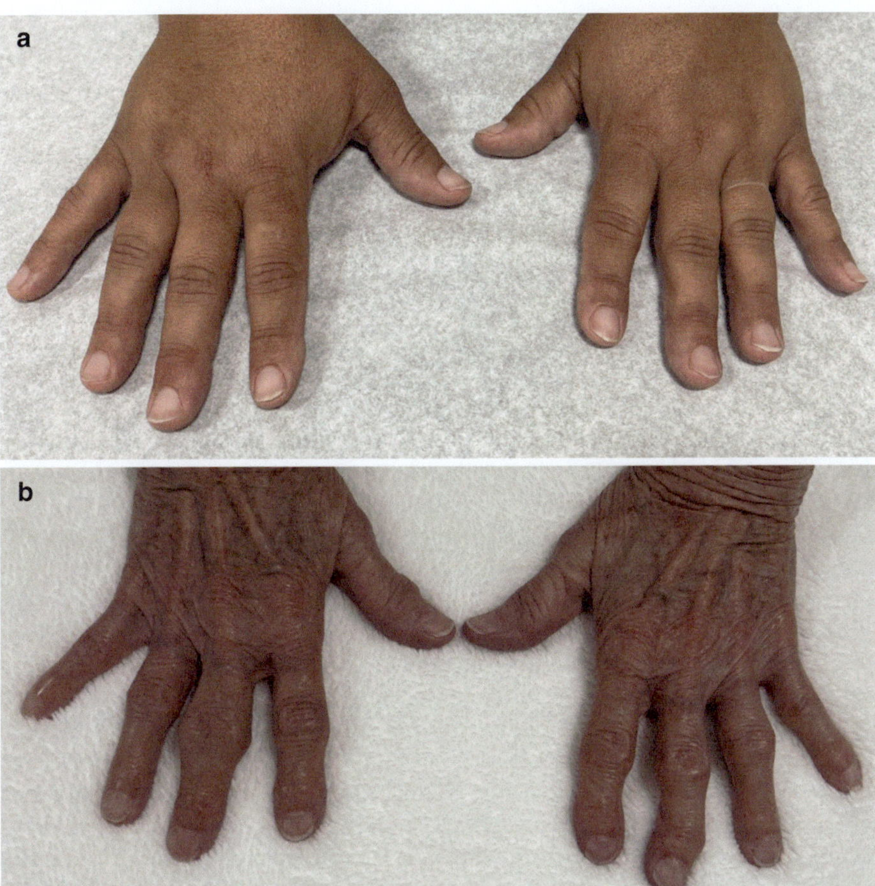

Fig. 10.1 Representative images of the hands of patients with rheumatoid arthritis (**a**) and osteo-arthritis (**b**)

patients with RA is worst and prolonged in the morning, while morning stiffness tends to be brief in those with OA. In contrast to RA, OA-related pain is most symptomatic in the evening and is augmented by an increased activity level involving the affected joint(s). This differentiator blurs somewhat in severe cases of RA, such as in the case of MN, where the "morning stiffness" never resolves and unfortunately progresses to become "all day stiffness." Another crucial differentiator is the distribution of joints involved, with RA involving the MCP and PIP joints (Fig. 10.1a), whereas OA involves the PIP and DIP joints (Fig. 10.1b). It is also important to consider involvement of joints in the feet when differentiating OA and RA. MTP involvement in patients with OA typically affects the great toe rather than all the toes as is more typically seen in RA. Great toe involvement in OA is characterized by bony enlargement and a hallux valgus deformity. While both forms of arthritis can cause joint enlargement, in OA this is typically characterized by hard, bony enlargement characteristically seen in Bouchard and Heberden nodes (Fig. 10.1b). Alternatively, RA causes joint effusions and synovitis, causing the joints to appear larger (Fig. 10.1a), but the involved joints are softer to touch on joint examination reflecting the synovial swelling. MN's exam is a combination of the two types of arthritis with the presence of Heberden nodes related to OA; however, it is the additional finding of MCP and wrist synovitis that suggests RA as the primary diagnosis driving her symptoms.

Once a diagnosis of RA is made there are many comorbidities to be considered in a patient in their 70s when compared to one in their 20s, with cardiovascular health being prime among them. RA is associated with an increased risk of cardiovascular disease, which has been highlighted in women in particular in the analysis of the Nurses' Health Study data. This study showed that women with RA had twice the risk of myocardial infarction compared to women without RA, even when adjusted for other risk factors associated with cardiovascular disease. Although these results have yet to change guidelines in cardiovascular screening for patients with RA, it is a point that should be kept in mind when the primary care provider is managing other cardiovascular risk factors such as hypertension and hyperlipidemia. For the rheumatologist, the increased risk of cardiovascular disease becomes a particular issue in patients who have high disease activity and may require trials of multiple DMARDs beyond methotrexate to control their disease. This becomes problematic, specifically when considering JAK inhibitors, which were recently shown to have an additional increased risk of cardiovascular events when compared to patients on TNF inhibitors, leading to a Black Box warning from the U.S. Food and Drug Administration. These results make it unappealing to start JAK inhibitors in patients with RA and known cardiovascular disease. In patients already on JAK inhibitors, it is crucial to aggressively treat cardiovascular-associated comorbidities and to even consider switching to a different DMARD class in patients with prior cardiovascular events. MN has multiple comorbidities to consider when determining management. In her case, a JAK inhibitor would be a less appealing option given her comorbidities of hypertension, hyperlipidemia, diabetes, and tobacco use.

Osteoporosis is another comorbidity that must be highly considered in patients with RA, especially given the increased total exposure to corticosteroids during their lifetimes. This can be particularly impactful in both male and female patients who are on corticosteroids for long periods of time because of difficult to control disease and can lead to glucocorticoid-induced osteoporosis (GIOP). Based on this increased risk, the ACR recommends bone density screening on all adult patients on 2.5 mg or more of prednisone daily for greater than 3 months, regardless of age or sex. Beyond increased corticosteroid exposure, RA itself places patients at higher risk for developing osteoporosis. Other factors intrinsic to RA must be considered including CCP antibody positivity, increased inflammation, and decreased functional status, which can all increase bone loss risk. Furthermore, chronic inflammatory changes can lead to decreased mobility complicated by increased falls, putting patients with RA at significantly higher risk for osteoporotic fractures. All patients with RA, and in general, any patient taking long-term corticosteroids, need adequate calcium and vitamin D intake for bone health management. When osteoporosis treatment is indicated, bisphosphonates remain the first-line treatment in patients with normal kidney function. Bone health is an often overlooked, but crucial aspect of the comprehensive care of patients with RA.

10.6 Conclusion

Rheumatoid arthritis is an important example of an inflammatory autoimmune disease to which women are predisposed to develop. The management of RA requires a multifaceted approach, starting with the primary care provider who strives for the early identification of patients with RA, by differentiating between inflammatory and non-inflammatory arthritis presentations. Once diagnosed, medical management must be balanced with the patient's stage of life, with consideration given to reproductive health and comorbidities. In younger women, the DMARDs used for disease management have many implications for reproductive health, from contraception to pregnancy to lactation. Across the spectrum of ages, there is an increased risk of cardiovascular disease in patients with RA. Additionally, patients with RA have an increased risk of osteoporosis, which must be balanced with the use corticosteroids that can also negatively impact bone health. Corticosteroids and immunosuppressive medications are critical aspects of the management of all autoimmune diseases, not just RA, making the recognized effects of these drug classes on women's health applicable across the spectrum of autoimmune diseases. This complexity requires integrated co-management and collaboration between primary care and rheumatology providers to optimize successful management of women with RA as well as other autoimmune diseases.

Suggested Reading

1. Alpízar-Rodríguez D, Pluchino N, Canny G, et al. The role of female hormonal factors in the development of rheumatoid arthritis. Rheumatology. 2017;56(8):1254–63. https://doi.org/10.1093/rheumatology/kew318.
2. Humphrey MB, Russell L, Danila MI, et al. 2023 American College of Rheumatology guideline for the prevention and treatment of glucocorticoid-induced osteoporosis. Arthritis Rheum. 2023;1–15.
3. de Man Y, Dolhain J, van de Geijn SP, et al. Disease activity of rheumatoid arthritis during pregnancy: results from a nationwide prospective study. Arthritis Rheum. 2008;59(9):1241–8. https://doi.org/10.1002/art.24003.
4. Grigor C, Capell H, Stirling A, et al. Effect of a treatment strategy of tight control for rheumatoid arthritis (the TICORA study): a single-blind randomised controlled trial. Lancet. 2004;364(9430):263–9. https://doi.org/10.1016/S0140-6736(04)16676-2.
5. Kastbom A, Strandberg G, Lindroos A, et al. Anti-CCP antibody test predicts the disease course during 3 years in early rheumatoid arthritis (the Swedish TIRA project). Ann Rheum Dis. 2004;63:1085–9. https://doi.org/10.1136/ard.2003.016808.

6. Sammaritano L, Bermas B, Chakravarty E, et al. 2020 American College of Rheumatology guideline for the management of reproductive health in rheumatic and musculoskeletal diseases. Arthritis Rheum. 2020;72(4):529–56. https://doi.org/10.1002/acr.24130.

7. Smolen J, Aletaha D, Barton A, et al. Rheumatoid arthritis. Nat Rev Dis Primers. 2018;4:1–23. https://doi.org/10.1038/nrdp.2018.1.

8. Solomon D, Karlson E, Rimm E, et al. Cardiovascular morbidity and mortality in women diagnosed with rheumatoid arthritis. Circulation. 2003;107:A1303–7. https://doi.org/10.1161/01.CIR.0000054612.26458.B2.

9. U.S. Food and Drug Administration. FDA requires warnings about increased risk of serious heart-related events, cancer, blood clots, and death for JAK inhibitors that treat certain chronic inflammatory conditions; 2021.

10. Wysham K, Baker J, Shoback D. Osteoporosis and fractures in rheumatoid arthritis. Curr Opin Rheumatol. 2021;33(3):270–6. https://doi.org/10.1097/BOR.0000000000000789.

11. Ytterberg S, Bhatt D, Mikuls T, et al. Cardiovascular and cancer risk with tofacitinib in rheumatoid arthritis. N Engl J Med. 2022;386:316–26. https://doi.org/10.1056/NEJMoa2109927.

Chapter 11
Cardiovascular Disease in Women

Jessica Holtzman and Rita Redberg

11.1   Introduction

Cardiovascular disease remains the primary cause of morbidity and mortality for women in the USA. Despite dramatic improvements in cardiovascular outcomes for both men and women since the 1980s, reduction in annual cardiovascular morbidity and mortality has plateaued and even slightly worsened for women over the past decade since 2010. In the USA, it is estimated that more than $350 billion is spent annually on the direct and indirect costs associated with cardiovascular disease, including medication payments, healthcare expenditures, disability, and lost productivity. Increasing attention has been paid to the delineation of sex-based differences in the presentation of cardiovascular disease. Both gender (relating to a sociocultural role and identity) and sex (relating to biologic differences arising from gene expression) have been demonstrated to impact health outcomes. However, sex-specific risk factors, disease progression, and treatment differences remain inadequately understood. Research has demonstrated that clinicians, including primary care physicians and subspecialists, and patients are yet to fully appreciate the risk factors for and burden of cardiovascular disease in women. Clinical trials assessing the effectiveness of medications and medical devices enroll and retain inadequate numbers of women relative to the prevalence of disease, leading to treatment recommendations that may not hold external validity for women as they are from predominantly male populations.

Recent (2019) guidelines by the American Heart Association and the American College of Cardiology for the primary prevention of atherosclerotic cardiovascular disease (ASCVD) include recommendations for management of hypertension,

J. Holtzman · R. Redberg (✉)
University of California, San Francisco, San Francisco, CA, USA
e-mail: Jessica.holtzman@ucsf.edu; Rita.redberg@ucsf.edu

M. Mahmoudi (ed.), *Common Cases in Women's Primary Care Clinics*,
https://doi.org/10.1007/978-3-031-48569-5_11

hyperlipidemia, and diabetes. These include optimizing lifestyle measures including tobacco cessation, exercise, nutrition, and managing psychosocial stressors to delay the development and progression of cardiovascular disease. This chapter seeks to explore cardiovascular prevention broadly, emphasizing sex-specific differences in guideline-directed management.

11.2 Case 1

Ms. Smith is a 48-year-old perimenopausal woman with a history of obesity, preeclampsia, major depressive disorder, and hypertension who presents to primary care clinic for an annual physical. She has smoked three cigarettes per day for the past 5 years and previously smoked 1 pack of cigarettes daily for 15 years. She does not drink alcohol or use any other recreational substances. She can ascend five flights of stairs without experiencing chest pain, shortness of breath, or light headedness. She lives with her partner and two healthy children, with who she feels safe and supported. She takes no medications and uses a levonorgestrel-containing intra-uterine device for contraception. Her vital signs are notable for a blood pressure of 148/92, heart rate of 76, and body mass index of 33.0 kg/m^2. Her exam is otherwise unremarkable. Lab testing reveals a total cholesterol of 256 mg/dL, HDL 52 mg/dL, triglycerides 265 mg/dL, with a calculated LDL 151 mg/dL. Her hemoglobin A1c is 6.4%. Given that her father experienced a myocardial infarction at age 48, Ms. Smith wishes to discuss how to optimize her risk factors to prevent the development of cardiovascular disease.

11.3 Discussion

11.3.1 Risk Factors for Atherosclerotic Cardiovascular Disease

The burden of cardiovascular disease among men and women in the USA is striking. According to the National Health and Nutrition Examination Survey from 2015 to 2018, 44.4% of women and men in the USA aged 20 years or older reported a diagnosis of cardiovascular disease, including hypertension, coronary artery disease, heart failure, and stroke. Extrapolated to the US population, cardiovascular disease would, therefore, be estimated to impact more than 60 million women—12.4 million women if hypertension is excluded—and account for more than 420,000 deaths in women annually. According to data presented in the 2021 Heart Disease and Stroke Statistics update from the American Heart Association, coronary artery disease, affects an estimated 18 million individuals in the United States or about 6.7% of adults over the age of 20. There is a corresponding age-adjusted prevalence of coronary artery disease of 7.4% in men and 4.1% in women. Despite these staggering statistics, reassuringly, the annual death rate attributable to coronary artery disease has declined 31.8% from 2006 to 2016.

Atherosclerotic cardiovascular disease (ASCVD) may be used to describe a wide variety of clinical syndromes including coronary artery disease, aortic atherosclerosis, peripheral artery disease, as well as cerebrovascular disease. The burden of ASCVD may be reduced through a preventative health strategy, seeking to identify and mitigate modifiable risk factors for atherosclerosis. The early identification and modification of risk factors not only serves to prevent the development and progression of coronary artery disease, but also is a cost-effective strategy to prevent the downstream expenses associated with long-term complications of ischemia. This section will explore both traditional risk factors, as well as risk-enhancing factors in order to best identify individuals at highest risk for the development of cardiovascular disease (Fig. 11.1).

- **Identification of Traditional Risk Factors**

Traditional, modifiable risk factors for atherosclerotic cardiovascular disease apply to both men and women. However, sex-specific differential effects have been demonstrated due to underlying biologic differences, as well as sociocultural differences. The traditional risk factors for ASCVD include hypertension, diabetes mellitus, hyperlipidemia, tobacco use, obesity, and physical inactivity. In our clinical case, there is no indication of pre-existing cardiovascular disease, given that she can climb five flights of stairs without angina or exertional limitation. It is important to

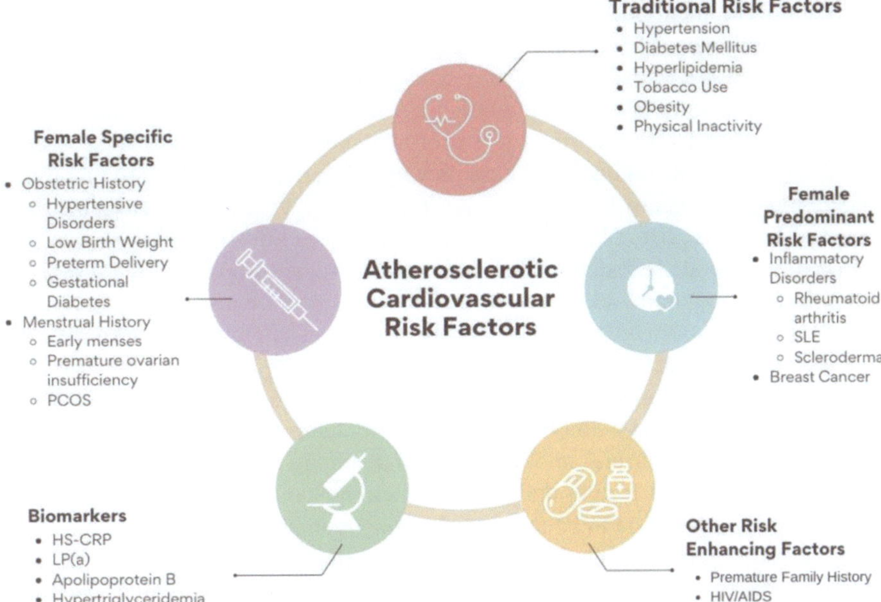

Fig. 11.1 Risk factors for atherosclerotic disease in women

screen for and identify modifiable risk factors in the primary care setting for the primary prevention of cardiovascular disease in order to counsel her on lifestyle interventions, including dietary changes, exercise recommendations, smoking cessation, and the benefit of weight loss.

Hypertension is defined by the 2017 American College of Cardiology (ACC)/American Heart Association (AHA) hypertension guidelines as systolic blood pressure ≥130 mmHg or diastolic blood pressure ≥80 mmHg. Previously, the Eighth Joint National Committee (JNC8) Guidelines defined hypertension at a higher level of >140/90 mmHg and recommended treatment initiation over a target of 150/90 mmHg. Likewise, the International Society of Hypertension (ISH) guidelines, adopted by the American Academy of Family Physicians, uses a diagnostic threshold of >140/90 mmHg in the office, with the ISH categorizing grade 1 hypertension as <160/100 mmHg and grade 2 hypertension as >160/100 mmHg. Studies have demonstrated a slightly lower prevalence of diagnosed hypertension in women (42%) versus men (49%) aged <65 years and have estimated comparable risk of adverse cardiovascular event associated with hypertension in both sexes. Notably, the prevalence of hypertension worldwide and associated projected healthcare costs have markedly increased with more stringent definitions of hypertension.

Diabetes mellitus, diagnosed as a hemoglobin A1c measurement of ≥6.5%, has been shown to have a differential effect on risk of coronary artery disease, tripling the risk for incident coronary artery disease in women and only doubling the risk in men. Adequate control of diabetes is also lower among women (30%) than men (20%).

Dyslipidemia, in particular LDL-C level, has been demonstrated to be associated with the development of ASCVD in both men and women. However, the evidence of any clinical benefit from LDL lowering by statins for women is not well established. Women are under-enrolled in primary prevention studies and have lower baseline CV risk until age 70, so are less likely to benefit from statins. Additionally, women are more likely than men to suffer medication-associated adverse events. This constellation of findings may explain why women are less likely to be offered guideline-directed statin therapy and are more likely to decline and discontinue therapy. There are post-menopausal changes in lipid profile, with known increases in LDL-C and total cholesterol following menopause, accompanied by fat redistribution leading to central adiposity. In the USA, women are also more likely to be diagnosed with overweight (BMI 25–29.0 kg/m^2), obesity (BMI ≥30.0 kg/m^2), and high-risk obesity (BMI ≥40.0 kg/m^2), as well as to exhibit behavioral patterns consistent with physical inactivity. In total, an age-adjusted prevalence of 41.1% of females were diagnosed with obesity in 2018. Epidemiologic studies have demonstrated that rates of current smoking are lower among women than men (13.5% versus 17.5%), though former and current smoking status as well as readiness for cessation should continue to be addressed among men and women at routine clinic visits. Nicotine replacement therapy should be offered routinely to patients with ongoing tobacco use. The absolute use of tobacco products worldwide, including e-cigarette use and smokeless tobacco, continues to climb despite a decline in incident traditional cigarette use.

The 2019 ACC/AHA Primary Prevention Guidelines recommend the use of the sex-specific Pooled Cohort Equations for the assessment of risk for development of ASCVD and to guide treatment recommendations. Possible results of this calculator are stratified as follows for 10-year risk of ASCVD: low risk (<5.0%), borderline risk (5.0–7.4%), intermediate risk (7.5% to 19.9%), and high risk (≥20%).

Based upon the results of the Pooled Cohort Equations, as per the 2019 ACC/AHA guidelines, a patient-clinician discussion should be undertaken to discuss the risks and benefits of initiating pharmacologic therapy including lipid lowering medications, antihypertensive agents, and aspirin. Traditional risk factors should be reviewed with patients to raise awareness of factors that may impact cardiovascular risk. It should be noted that use of the Pooled Cohort Equations has less data to support its accuracy in women as compared to men. In individuals at low risk of ASCVD, lifestyle interventions encouraging a healthy diet, adequate physical activity, weight loss, and smoking cessation may be adequate.

The 2019 ACC/AHA guidelines further specify that in individuals at intermediate risk, or selected individuals with borderline risk, coronary artery calcium score may be considered to help guide a discussion of the risks and benefits of initiating preventative therapy. However, it must be noted that there is no data supporting clinical outcomes improvement from the addition of the coronary artery calcium score and there are harms to the test including high rate of incidental findings requiring subsequent follow-up, radiation associated with the CT scan, cost often directly transmitted to the patient given limited insurance coverage, and increased anxiety associated with getting this test. In all individuals at high risk, lifestyle interventions can reduce risk. Risks and benefits of pharmacologic therapy should be discussed. Of note, lifestyle intervention should remain a cornerstone of cardiovascular preventative therapy, regardless of estimated risk for disease.

The social determinants of health should also be addressed when considering traditional risk factors for ASCVD. Social determinants of health are defined as environmental conditions – including place of birth, work environment, race or ethnicity, socioeconomic status, or gender – that contribute to health outcomes. A screening interview may include attention to routine screening for psychosocial stressors, identification of barriers to the consumption of a heart healthy diet including food scarcity and cost, location of safe and accessible facilities for physical activity, and assessment of work schedules that may be associated with short sleep duration or poor-quality sleep. According to the National Health Interview Survey in 2016, 53.6% of white females, 39.1% of black females, and 41.8% of Hispanic females currently meet the physical activity aerobic guidelines that recommend more than 150 min of aerobic physical activity weekly during leisure-time.

Using the Pooled Cohort Equations, our patient Ms. Smith would have a calculated 10-year ASCVD risk of 6.0%, which falls within the borderline risk category. She does also have history of premature family heart disease, major depressive disorder, and preeclampsia, all of which are considerations that will be discussed below. Lifestyle interventions should be recommended including a weight loss, diet rich in vegetables, fruits, legumes, nuts, whole grains, and fish and low in saturated fats, a minimum of 150 min per week of moderate intensity aerobic physical activity, decreasing sedentary behaviors, and smoking cessation.

- **Identification of Risk-Enhancing Factors**

Risk-enhancing factors for atherosclerotic cardiovascular disease may be divided into universal, female-specific, and female-predominant categories. Growing attention has been paid to emerging risk factors and biomarkers that extend beyond the traditional risk factors to better encapsulate an individual patient's risk of developing clinical cardiovascular disease in the future. It should be noted that there is little evidence to support that risk-enhancing factors improve risk prediction or long-term cardiovascular outcomes. Furthermore, there are no actions that patients can take to change or reverse most risk-enhancing factors, including age at onset of menses, premature family history of ASCVD, history of preeclampsia, and more. Thus, the inclusion of non-modifiable risk markers and risk enhancers may be costly to the healthcare system and detrimental to patients without leading to actionable treatment modification.

Family history of premature ASCVD, defined as a first degree relative with clinical coronary artery disease or sudden cardiac death (men <55 years of age and women <65 years of age), has long been known to modify predicted risk of developing atherosclerosis. In particular, the strength of association increases with decreasing age of parental coronary artery disease diagnosis. Laboratory biomarkers may also be measured to further risk stratify patients based upon lipid profile and inflammatory milieu. Relevant biomarkers to consider, if measured, may include elevated high sensitivity C-reactive protein ($\geq$2.0 mg/L), elevated lipoprotein (a) ($\geq$50 mg/dL), elevated apolipoprotein B ($\geq$130 mg/dL) often measured in the setting of triglycerides $\geq$200 mg/dL, or persistently elevated primary hypertriglyceridemia ($\geq$175 mg/dL).

Specific attention should be paid to the role that fluctuation in sex hormones and the resultant physiologic states play through menarche, pregnancy, and menopause to elevate a woman's risk of subsequent cardiovascular disease. A clear obstetric history should be obtained including (1) history of hypertensive disorders of pregnancy (eclampsia, preeclampsia, and gestational hypertension), (2) history of low birth weight (<2500 grams), (3) history of preterm delivery (<37 weeks gestation), (4) history of gestational diabetes, and (5) number of previous pregnancies. A menstrual history should also be obtained including (1) age of menarche, (2) the presence of premature ovarian insufficiency defined as age <40 years associated with irregular menses, negative serum hCG, with or without the presence of vasomotor symptoms or genitourinary symptoms, and (3) if applicable, surgical versus natural development of premature menopause (Fig. 11.2). A thorough menstrual and obstetric history may guide the assessment of female-specific risk-enhancing factors.

Adverse pregnancy outcomes including hypertensive disorders of pregnancy, preterm delivery, and gestational diabetes all increase the risk of developing cardiovascular disease. Hypertensive disorders of pregnancy, discussed further below, are associated with a diverse array of long-term cardiovascular conditions, including hypertension, coronary artery disease, stroke, heart failure, and ultimately mortality.

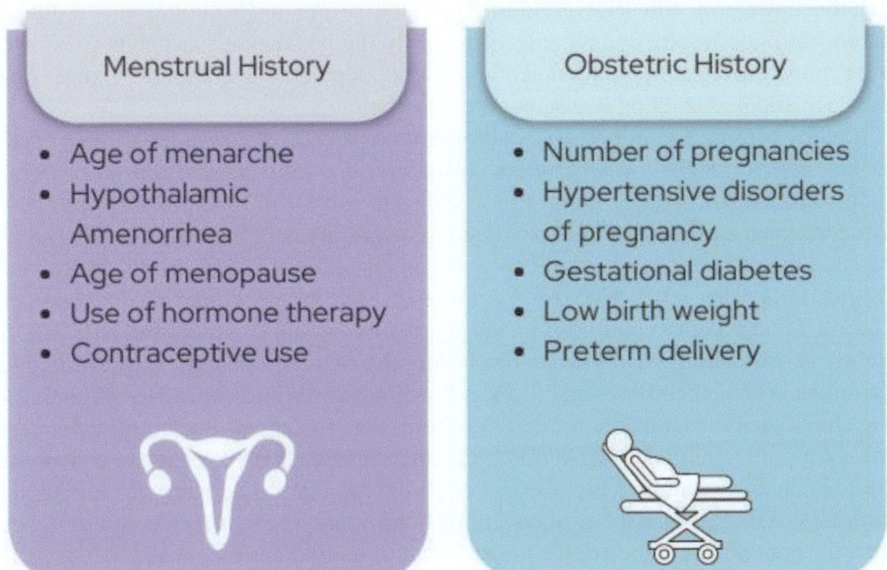

Fig. 11.2 Components of obstetric and menstrual history in cardiovascular disease

Several large studies have demonstrated that preeclampsia is associated with cardiovascular mortality (1.5-fold increase), coronary artery disease (2.2-fold increase), and subsequent chronic hypertension (3.7-fold increase). For this reason, the 2019 ACC/AHA primary prevention guidelines include preeclampsia as a risk-enhancing factor to consider when discussing the initiation of statin therapy in borderline and intermediate risk groups, though there is limited evidence to support the use of statins in primary prevention of cardiovascular disease. Preterm birth prior to 37 weeks, and to a greater extent prior to 32 weeks, has been independently associated with increased risk of cardiovascular disease. Likewise, giving birth to a small for gestational age infant and pregnancy loss have also been found to be associated with increased risk for maternal development of cardiovascular disease. Gestational diabetes has been found to be associated with a sevenfold lifetime increase in the subsequent risk of developing type II diabetes mellitus compared to women without gestational diabetes, which correlates to a nearly 50% lifetime risk for the development of diabetes, as well as a 2.8-fold increase in the risk of ischemic heart disease.

Other disease states associated with hormonal imbalance, including polycystic ovarian syndrome and functional hypothalamic amenorrhea, have been associated with increased ASCVD risk. Postulated mechanisms associated with polycystic ovarian syndrome include insulin resistance and hyperinsulinemia, as well as endothelial dysfunction. Studies have also found that early menarche, comparing age 10 versus 12, was associated with increased risk of cardiovascular disease. Both surgical and natural early menopause have also been found to be associated with cardiovascular risk, perhaps related to hormonal changes including an increase in total serum cholesterol and triglycerides, increased serum testosterone, and reduced serum estrogen levels. Endogenous estrogen in the pre-menopausal state is known to promote nitric oxide production and prevent endothelial dysfunction. Exogenous estrogen supplementation is discussed further below.

Lastly, certain diseases, such as autoimmune, such as rheumatoid arthritis, systemic lupus erythematosus, psoriatic disorders, and scleroderma are more commonly found in women and are associated with pro-inflammatory milieus. Observational studies have demonstrated associations with increased cardiovascular risk, including both epicardial coronary artery disease as well as microvascular dysfunction. The 2019 ACC/AHA guidelines encourage clinicians to consider chronic inflammatory conditions including rheumatologic disorders and HIV/AIDS to be risk-enhancing factors when discussing the risks and benefits of preventative therapies. Again, incorporation of risk-enhancing factors into clinical decision making should acknowledge the limited long-term data to support meaningful changes in risk modification and long-term cardiovascular outcomes. Studies have demonstrated that the cumulative lifetime risk of cardiovascular disease among individuals with HIV/AIDS is 44% for women and 65% for men, which is significantly higher than the general population and similar to that of individuals diagnosed with type II diabetes mellitus.

Though our patient Ms. Smith falls in the borderline risk category based upon the Pooled Cohort Equations with an ASCVD risk score of 6.0%, her history of pre-eclampsia, premature family history of cardiovascular disease, and perimenopausal state should be noted when undertaking shared decision making regarding preventative therapies and lifestyle modification.

11.3.2 Management of Cardiovascular Risk Factors

After identifying relevant risk factors for the development of cardiovascular disease in our patient, relevant risk factors may be appropriately managed in the primary care setting to minimize risk of progression to clinical cardiovascular disease. In patients who require further risk stratification or nuanced management of primary prevention, referral to a preventative cardiologist or lipid expert, either in the field of cardiology or endocrinology based upon the medical center, may be appropriate. The American Heart Association has proposed the ABCDE Guide to guide clinicians managing the primary prevention of cardiovascular disease. While all components may not apply to each individual patient, each category should be considered to optimize risk management. The components to this guide, discussed in detail below, include (1) **a**ntiplatelet therapy, (2) **b**lood pressure management, (3) **c**holesterol treatment, (4) **c**igarette or tobacco cessation, (5) **d**iet and weight management, (6) **d**iabetes prevention and treatment, and (7) **e**xercise (Fig. 11.3). **E**motion, to represent psychosocial stressors and disorders of mental health, may be added as a reminder to screen for major depression, anxiety disorders, and post-traumatic stress disorder.

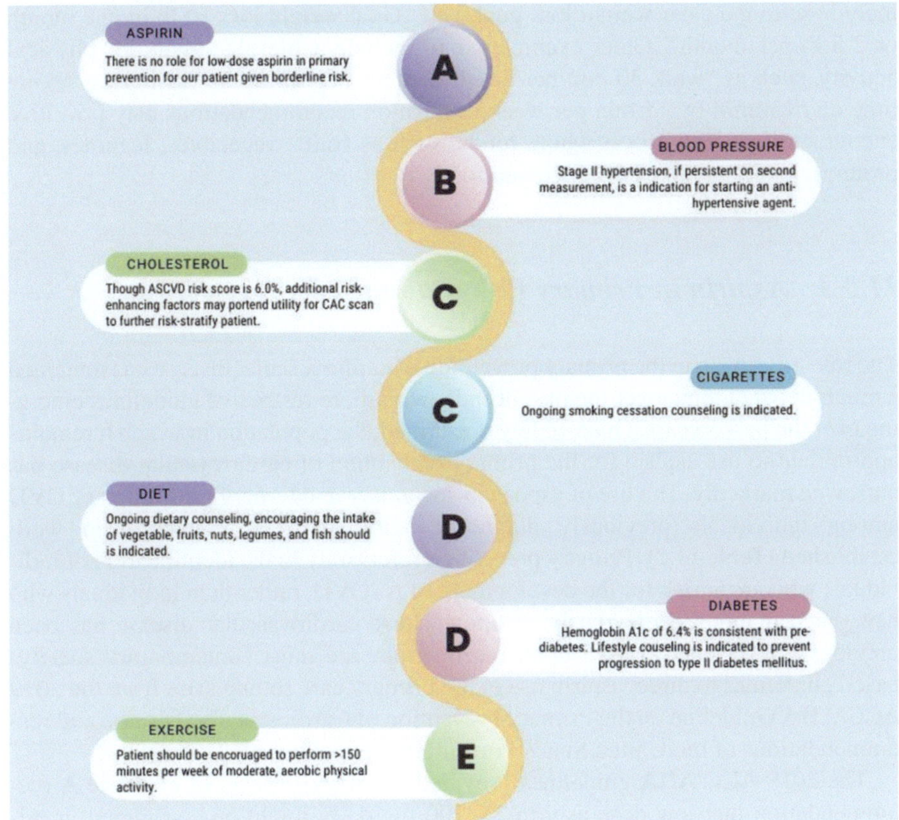

Fig. 11.3 Management of cardiovascular risk factors in a clinical case

Table 11.1 Examples of concrete lifestyle counseling

Examples of lifestyle counseling
Perform 30 min of exercise most days of the week.
It is acceptable to divide 30 min of exercise into 10 min increments spread throughout the day if more manageable
Exercise with friends and family members
Use pedometers or other activity trackers if they are motivating
Eat whole foods including fruits, vegetables, legumes, and proteins, avoiding processed food out of boxes and cans
Shop around the perimeter of the grocery store rather than the center aisles that have more processed food
Eat everything, including dessert, in moderation to cultivate a positive relationship with food

Lifestyle counseling presents a challenge as it may lack the specificity to be actionable. Vague recommendations for weight loss and exercise without tangible goals may be challenging for patients to implement. It is important to provide specific, actionable steps to promote change (Table 11.1). Examples of such steps may include setting a clear weight loss goal, i.e., "Goal weight loss 10 lb in one month or 2.5 lb per month." Other examples may include achievable goals for physical activity, such as "walk 30 min per day five times per week" or "increase walking time on treadmill by 15 min per week." Nutrition recommendations may prioritize encouraging patients to eat whole foods, such as fruits, vegetables, legumes, and proteins, avoiding boxed or processed foods.

11.3.3 Aspirin in Primary Prevention

The role for aspirin in the primary prevention of cardiovascular disease has remained a much-debated topic over the past decade, with more restrictive guidelines emerging over the past 5 years. Once widely prescribed, the population in which it remains appropriate to use aspirin for the primary prevention of cardiovascular disease has narrowed markedly. The use of aspirin in secondary and tertiary prevention of CVD among individuals previously diagnosed with ASCVD remains been well-established (Table 11.2). Primary prevention refers only to the identification of individuals who are at risk for the development of ASCVD, rather than individuals who have been diagnosed previously or upon whose cardiovascular disease has been previously intervened. Based upon recent trials, the most contemporary society-based guidelines to direct aspirin use in the primary care setting arise from the 2019 ACC/AHA Guideline on the Primary Prevention of Cardiovascular Disease and recommendations of the United States Preventative Task Force.

The 2019 ACC/AHA guidelines provided a Class IIB, level of evidence A recommendation that low-dose aspirin 75–100 mg daily might be considered in primary prevention among individuals aged 40–70 years of age who are at high ASCVD risk (>10% 10-year risk), but who are not at increased bleeding risk. The same guidelines provided a Class III, level of evidence B recommendation that daily low-dose aspirin should not be administered on a routine basis in individuals over the age of 70 or who are at increased risk of bleeding. However, in 2022, the United States Preventative Task Force (USPTF) finalized a statement that individuals aged

Table 11.2 Primary, secondary, and tertiary prevention

Primary prevention	Secondary prevention	Tertiary prevention
Identify individuals at risk for the development of CVD	Identify early or asymptomatic CVD	Prevent the recurrence or progression of existing CVD

Examples:
  Smoking cessation
  Weight management
  Physical activity
	Examples:
	  Treat hypertension
	  Treat dyslipidemia
	  Treat diabetes mellitus
	  Aspirin with known CAD
		Examples:
		  Aspirin and statin after myocardial infarction
		  ACE inhibitor, beta blocker, mineralocorticoid receptor antagonist in heart failure

60 or older should not start taking aspirin for heart disease or stroke prevention. They recommended that only individuals aged 40–59 who are at higher risk for CVD and do not have a history of bleeding complications should decide with their clinician whether to start taking aspirin.

The updated USPTF guidelines rely upon data provided from three trials published in 2018. The ARRIVE trial demonstrated that in moderate risk, non-diabetic patients without prior ASCVD events, there was no difference in ASCVD endpoint but increased risk of GI bleeding with aspirin. Next, the ASCEND trial demonstrated that in patients with diabetes who were >40 years of age without prior ASCVD events, aspirin provided a risk neutral profile, with a NNT =59 and NNH = 77. Lastly, the ASPREE trial demonstrated that in patients >70 year of age without prior ASCVD events, there was no difference in ASCVD events, though there was a significant increase in bleeding (NNH = 42) and higher all-cause mortality (due to cancer) with the use of aspirin.

Therefore, based on the sum of these three trials, current recommendations suggest that aspirin for primary prevention should be considered only among individuals at high ASCVD risk with poorly controlled risk factors who are aged 40–59. With the expanding use of advanced cardiovascular imaging, including the coronary artery calcium score, the detection of subclinical coronary artery disease has blurred the line between primary and secondary prevention. A coronary artery calcium score of >100 may provide additional evidence supportive of poorly controlled risk factors placing a patient at risk for the progression of coronary artery calcium to overt clinical coronary artery disease and therefore may warrant the use of aspirin. Outside of these criteria, clinicians should undertake risk-benefit discussions regarding the deprescribing of aspirin for primary prevention. Of note, careful attention should be pain to patients taking aspiring for secondary or tertiary prevention of ASCVD, as these patients should still be counseled to continue taking aspirin based upon a broad evidence base.

According to these guidelines, aspirin therapy for the primary prevention of cardiovascular therapy would not be indicated for this patient.

11.3.4 Management of Blood Pressure

- **Essential Hypertension**

According to the 2017 ACC/AHA hypertension guidelines, hypertension remains the leading cause of death and disability-adjusted life years worldwide, accounts for a majority of deaths from coronary artery disease and stroke, and is associated with prevalent non-cardiovascular conditions including end-stage renal disease. The ACC/AHA Primary Prevention guidelines newly modify the definition of stage I hypertension as systolic blood pressure of 130–139 mmHg or diastolic blood pressure of 80–89 mmHg. The guidelines were updated to reflect that stage II hypertension is now defined as systolic blood pressure ≥140 mmHg and diastolic blood pressure $\geq$90 mmHg. Hypertension must be documented using $\geq$2 readings obtained using proper technique on $\geq$2 occasions to formally establish a diagnosis. The 2017 ACC/AHA guidelines additionally recommend ambulatory blood pressure monitoring to establish a diagnosis of hypertension in both men and women. In contrast, the International Society of Hypertension (ISH) guidelines, adopted by the American Academy of Family Physicians, continue to use a less aggressive diagnostic threshold of >140/90 mmHg in the office, >135/85 mmHg at home, or >130/80 mmHg using a 24-hour ambulatory monitor. In contrast to the ACC/AHA guidelines, the ISH categorizes grade 1 hypertension as <160/100 mmHg and grade 2 hypertension as >160/100 mmHg. Similarly, the prior JNC8 guidelines defined hypertension over the threshold over 140/90 mmHg.

Attention should be paid to ingested substances including alcohol, caffeine, and herbal supplements as well as medications including oral estrogen-containing contraceptives, NSAIDs, systemic corticosteroids, and antidepressants that may induce hypertension, particularly when superimposed upon a diagnosis of pre-existing chronic hypertension. For previously normotensive women who develop hypertension after the initiation of oral contraceptives, alternative forms of birth control including long-acting reversible contraception (i.e., intrauterine device), barrier methods, or progestin-only contraception. In women who develop sudden onset, pharmacologically resistant, or severe hypertension, secondary causes may be considered including renovascular disease, primary aldosteronism, obstructive sleep apnea, or endocrinopathy such as hyperthyroidism or Cushing's syndrome.

In individuals with stage I hypertension in the absence of a $\geq$10% 10-year risk of ASCVD or pre-existing clinical cardiovascular disease, nonpharmacological interventions may be considered in the treatment of hypertension. All individuals with hypertension regardless of pharmacologic therapy should be encouraged to pursue nonpharmacological interventions in conjunction with other therapies. Such interventions may include weight loss, a heart healthy diet such as the DASH (Dietary Approaches to Stop Hypertension diet, sodium reduction, potassium supplementation in the absence of renal disease, increased physical activity, and reduction in alcohol consumption.

In individuals with stage II hypertension or greater, or stage I hypertension with ASCVD score of $\geq$10% or pre-existing cardiovascular disease, pharmacologic treatment is recommended by the current 2017 ACC/AHA hypertension guidelines. Though these recommendations were based upon the results of the SPRINT trial, this trial enrolled only 36% women and demonstrated lower cardiovascular event rates among women than men. As such, the SPRINT trial was underpowered to detect heterogeneity of effects between sexes and optimal blood pressure goals for women as compared to men have yet to be established.

Primary classes of antihypertensive agents that should be considered include thiazide diuretics, ACE inhibitors, angiotensin receptor blocking (ARB) agents, or calcium channel blockers. In women of reproductive age, ACE inhibitors and ARBs should be used with caution as they are rated pregnancy category D and should be promptly discontinued if pregnancy is expected or desired due to risk for fetal harm.

Clinicians should be sure to discuss safe contraception options, including long-acting reversible contraception, with women of reproductive age if considering treatment with ACE inhibitors or ARBs to avoid teratogenicity. Based upon the SPRINT trial results, no clear guidelines exist to direct differential use of antihypertensive therapeutics in men versus women. Calcium channel blockers are safe and effective in women though may be associated with increased risk of peripheral edema as compared to men.

In this patient, if she were demonstrated to have a repeat blood pressure at second time point with sustained blood pressures of systolic blood pressure ≥ 140 mmHg and diastolic blood pressure ≥ 90 mmHg, this would be consistent with a diagnosis of stage II hypertension. Lifestyle interventions such as weight loss, dietary modification, and tobacco cessation are all indicated. However, it would also be recommended to start an antihypertensive agent; a calcium channel blocker, thiazide diuretic, or ACE inhibitor or ARB would all be appropriate first-line choices. If laboratory work-up reveals any additional abnormalities including electrolyte derangement, renal dysfunction, or proteinuria, results could influence the first-line choice of antihypertensive agent accordingly.

- **Hypertensive Disorders in Pregnancy**

Women who become pregnant may develop a variety of hypertensive disorders, with an estimated prevalence of 5–10% of all pregnancies. Adverse pregnancy outcomes occur in up to 10–20% of pregnancies and are associated with a 1.8–4.0-fold increase in the risk of cardiovascular disease in the future. In normal pregnancy physiology, blood pressure is often lower in the first and second trimesters due to reduced systemic vascular resistance as a result of estrogen-mediated vasodilation. Due to the reduced systemic vascular resistance, the renal angiotensin-aldosterone system is activated to maintain blood pressure, resulting in a 50–75% increase in plasma volume by the second trimester of pregnancy to meet the increased circulatory demands of the placenta. As above, to establish a diagnosis of hypertension, blood pressure during pregnancy should be taken using appropriate technique on two separate occasions separated by a minimum of 4 h.

Chronic hypertension may be diagnosed on the basis of blood pressure measurements with systolic blood pressure ≥ 130 mmHg or diastolic blood pressure ≥ 80 mmHg taken before pregnancy, before 20 weeks of gestation, or taken during pregnancy that persists a minimum of 12-weeks beyond delivery (Table 11.3). Gestational hypertension is diagnosed as a minimum of two measurements demonstrating systolic blood pressure ≥ 140 mmHg or diastolic blood pressure ≥ 90 mmHg after 20-weeks gestation in a woman who was previously normotensive, indicating a pregnancy-induced process. Notably, patients may not demonstrate proteinuria or other features of severe pre-eclampsia including thrombocytopenia, acute kidney injury, elevated hepatic transaminases, pulmonary edema, altered mental status, or visual changes to establish this diagnosis, which would change the diagnosis to preeclampsia.

Preeclampsia is diagnosed in previously normotensive women who develop new onset hypertension ($\geq 140/90$ mmHg on two separate occasions or $\geq 160/110$ mmHg

Table 11.3 Summary of hypertensive disorders of pregnancy

Hypertensive disorder	Diagnosis
Chronic hypertension	SBP ≥130 mmHg or DBP ≥80 mmHg Requires two measurements at least 4 h apart Diagnosed <20 weeks gestation or persists 12-weeks beyond delivery
Gestational hypertension	SBP ≥140 mmHg or DBP ≥90 mmHg Requires two measurements at least 4 h apart unless severe Diagnosed >20 weeks gestation Without proteinuria or features of severe preeclampsia

Preeclampsia	SBP ≥140 mmHg or DBP ≥90 mmHg twice; or SBP ≥160 mmHg or DBP ≥110 mmHg once
	Diagnosed after 20 weeks gestation
	Presence of
	    Proteinuria
	    OR
	    End organ dysfunction including pulmonary edema, thrombocytopenia, elevated transaminases, renal insufficiency, or cerebral or visual disturbances

Preeclamptic syndromes	Preeclampsia with severe features: SBP ≥160 mmHg or DBP ≥110 mmHg on two measures 4 h apart before treatment or end organ injury HELLP: Syndrome of hemolysis, elevated liver enzymes, and low platelets associated with preeclampsia or eclampsia Eclampsia: Generalized tonic-clonic seizure with preeclampsia
Chronic hypertension with preeclampsia	If chronic hypertension, sudden increase in blood pressure that was previously well controlled If chronic hypertension, new onset of worsening proteinuria

SBP systolic blood pressure, *DBP* diastolic blood pressure

on one occasion) associated with end-organ dysfunction as evidence by proteinuria (>300 mg/24-h urine collection). Alternatively, in the absence of proteinuria, patients may experience one of the following: thrombocytopenia (platelets <100,000/microL), acute kidney injury (creatinine >1.1 mg/dL or twice the baseline measurement), elevated transaminases (more than twice the upper limit of normal), pulmonary edema, or cognitive symptoms. Preeclampsia may then progress to have severe features, as well. Established risk factors for the development of preeclampsia including personal or family history of preeclampsia, chronic hypertension, older age, multiple gestation, and obesity. Preeclampsia may also increase in severity of presentation if superimposed upon chronic hypertension.

The primary care clinician may play a role in monitoring blood pressure closely in the postpartum period, either through in-person visits or home blood pressure monitoring initiatives (Fig. 11.4). Clinicians should counsel patients following a diagnosis of a hypertensive disorder of pregnancy regarding the increased long-term risk for cardiovascular disease, as discussed above. Patients should be monitoring soon after discharge from the hospital, ideally within 1 week, for persistent or recrudescent hypertension. This may be performed through in-office visit or ambulatory blood pressure monitoring with virtual visits, which may reduce barriers to women presenting to clinic for follow-up soon after delivery. Care coordination for women

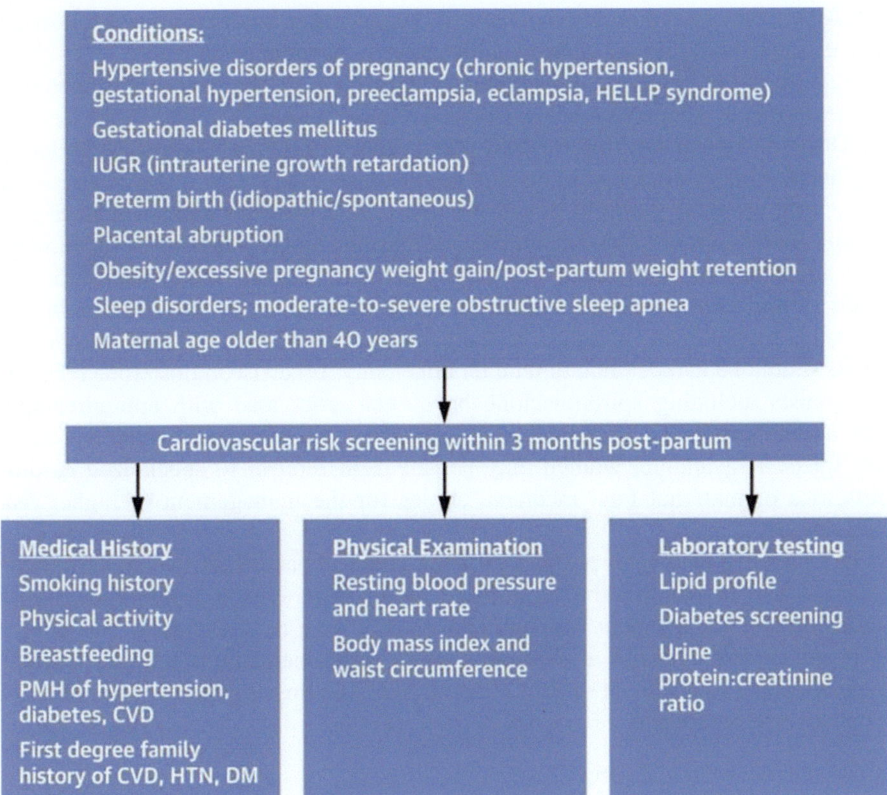

Fig. 11.4 Cardiovascular risk screening after adverse pregnancy outcomes
Reprinted from Journal of the American College of Cardiology, Cho L et al., Summary of Updated Recommendations for Primary Prevention of Cardiovascular Disease in Women: JACC State-of-the-Art Review, Pages 2602–2618, VOL 75, No. 20, Copyright 2020, with permission from Elsevier

who experienced preeclampsia during pregnancy, either with a primary care provider or cardiologist, is of utmost importance to avoid long-term complications. Within 3 months of delivery, patients should be monitored for the development of additional risk factors for cardiovascular disease including dyslipidemia and diabetes. Regular aerobic exercise and healthy weight maintenance should be encouraged. Recent reports suggest that currently ~7.2% of women smoke cigarettes during pregnancy, which may be an additional risk factor is consider in the discussion of hypertensive disorders of pregnancy.

Both the United States Preventative Task Force and the American College of Obstetricians and Gynecologists recommend the use of low-dose aspirin 81 mg daily starting at 12-weeks gestation and continuing through delivery for women at high risk for preeclampsia, including those with a personal history of preeclampsia, multiple gestation, chronic hypertension, diabetes, renal disease, or autoimmune disease for the prevention of preeclampsia. Aspirin may be discontinued following delivery and should not be continued barring any secondary indication.

Regarding the treatment of hypertensive disorders of pregnancy, both maternal and fetal risks and benefits must be weighed. Online resources including the Centers for Disease Control Treating for Two portal, Food and Drug Administration labeling, and the LactMed database may be used to assess the safety of medications for use during pregnancy and lactation. Optimal blood pressure management targets systolic blood pressure 130–150 mmHg and diastolic blood pressure 80–100 mmHg. Safe antihypertensive agents in pregnancy may include calcium channel blockers (such as amlodipine and nifedipine), thiazide diuretics, beta blockers including labetolol, methyldopa, hydralazine, and nitrates. As above, ACE inhibitors and ARBs should be avoided due to fetal teratogenicity. Likewise, aldosterone receptor antagonists including spironolactone have been associated with anti-adrenergic activity and permanent anatomical derangement of the male and female reproductive tracts. If available, women may benefit from referral to specialized cardio-obstetrics or maternal fetal medicine clinics for the management of higher risk pregnancies.

Our patient's history of preeclampsia may have impacted her overall cardiovascular risk and the risk that she developed essential hypertension. It is unknown what screening and management were undertaken following her pregnancy. The history of preeclampsia does not change our current recommendations that her stage II hypertension should be treated in order to avoid downstream cardiovascular and renal adverse outcomes.

11.3.5 Management of Disorders of Cholesterol

The ACC/AHA Guidelines for cholesterol management indicate the benefit of statin therapies in four main subgroups: (1) individuals with the known existence of clinical ASCVD; (2) individuals with LDL-C >190 mg/dL; (3) individuals with diabetes mellitus aged 40–75 years with LDL-C levels between 70 mg/dL and 189 mg/dL, and (4) individuals without ASCVD or diabetes mellitus with LDL-C between 70 mg/dL and 189 mg/dL with a 10 year risk of ASCVD >7.5%. In some cases, ezetimibe and proprotein convertase subtilisin/kexin type 9 (PCSK-9) inhibitors may be considered as adjunctive therapy to reach goal cholesterol levels, although it should be noted that clinical trials have consistently under-enrolled women based on the overall disease prevalence and that most data is extrapolated from secondary prevention trials. The high cost of PCSK-9 inhibitors limits more wide spread use outside of the secondary prevention arena.

Among individuals in the fourth category, a 10-year risk of ASCVD of >7.5% does not suggest that statin therapy should be initiated immediately. A risk-benefit discussion including a role for patient preference should be undertaken with patients, emphasizing the benefits of lifestyle modification including dietary changes, smoking cessation, and augmentation of aerobic and anaerobic exercise regimens and the risks including adverse effects and drug interactions. These risks of statin therapy must also be considered including limited evidence base in women for primary prevention, as well as increased risk of diabetes.

With a 10-year ASCVD risk score of 6.0%, our patient Ms. Smith does not currently meet the criteria for which statin therapy would be recommended. She will get the most lifetime benefit from changes in her diet to include more fruits, vegetables, and whole foods, smoking cessation, increased physical activity and weight loss. These will also reduce her chances of developing diabetes or worsening obesity, which will modify her risk of developing cardiovascular disease. If her hemoglobin A1c were to cross the threshold to $\geq$6.5%, consistent with a diagnosis of diabetes mellitus, it would be reasonable to discuss use of a moderate intensity statin regardless of her 10-year ASCVD estimated risk. A discussion of the risks and benefits of statin therapy should acknowledge potential adverse effects, drug interactions, and patient preferences when undertaking shared decision making. It should be noted that statin therapy is pregnancy category X, indicating either animal or human studies that have demonstrated fetal abnormalities associated with this therapy and are therefore contraindicated in pregnancy (Fig. 11.5). Statin therapy should be stopped a minimum of 2 months prior to pregnancy to avoid risk of teratogenicity and is rarely indicated in women of childbearing age.

In select asymptomatic, borderline risk and intermediate risk patients with risk-enhancing factors, the 2019 ACC/AHA Primary Prevention statement suggests that clinicians consider obtaining a coronary artery calcium score to assist a treatment decision. A coronary artery calcium scan is a low-radiation, non-contrast, gated CT scan that calculates the coronary artery calcium content as a function of plaque area and density. This modality allows for the measurement of subclinical disease, improving traditional risk prediction models. As compared to a CT coronary angiogram, a coronary artery calcium score should not be used independently for diagnosis or localization of clinically significant coronary artery disease among individuals experiencing angina or symptoms consistent with myocardial ischemia. It should be noted that beneficial clinical outcomes have not been demonstrated to be associated with use of coronary artery calcium scores. The extent of population level data does not yet exist so as to warrant wide implementation of this test. The potential harms of the CAC score must be considering, as well, including but not limited to anxiety associated with additional testing, financial harm to the patient due to cost that is rarely covered by insurance, radiation exposure, and risk of incidental findings. Therefore, it may be reasonable to discuss the risks and benefits of a CAC score in a select group of intermediate risk patients, though little data supports the clinical utility of this test at this time.

If a coronary artery calcium score is obtained, the results may help inform subsequent treatment decisions. Per the 2019 ACC/AHA guidelines, if a coronary artery calcium score is zero Agatston units, it is reasonable to defer initiation of statin therapy in the absence of significant risk-enhancing factors. If the coronary artery calcium score is 100 Agatston units or higher, or in the 75th percentile for a given age range and sex, the guidelines suggest that it may also be reasonable to

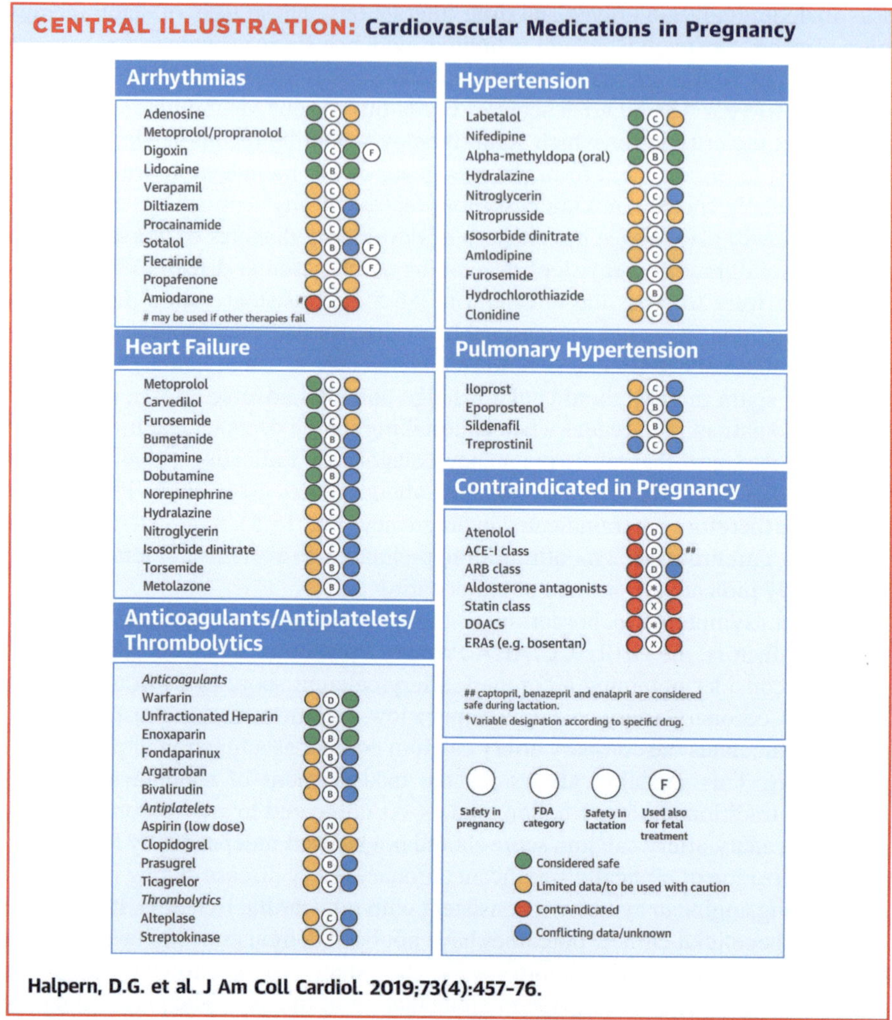

Fig. 11.5 Overview of cardiovascular medications in pregnancy
Reprinted from Journal of the American College of Cardiology, Halpern DG et al., Use of Medication for Cardiovascular Disease During Pregnancy JACC State-of-the-Art Review, Pages 457–476, VOL 73, No. 4, Copyright 2019, with permission from Elsevier

initiate statin therapy. If a score is greater than 400 Agatston units, this result would be consistent with severe atherosclerotic disease.

For our patient with borderline risk of developing atherosclerotic cardiovascular disease with ongoing tobacco use, obesity, and a history of preeclampsia, it would be reasonable to consider obtaining a coronary artery calcium score if the patient were interested in further risk stratification, though the risks and benefits of this test should be addressed with the patient. An elevated coronary artery calcium score may both guide recommendations regarding lipid lowering therapy and may provide tangible evidence to demonstrate the importance of lifestyle modification, including weight loss and smoking cessation, for Ms. Smith.

11.3.6 Management of Diabetes Mellitus in Cardiovascular Disease

Diabetes mellitus is well documented as one of the greatest risk factors for the development of cardiovascular disease in both men and women. Per the 2019 ACC/AHA primary prevention guidelines, all individuals with a hemoglobin A1c $\geq 6.5\%$ consistent with a diagnosis of diabetes mellitus should undergo dietary counseling and should be encouraged to engage in a minimum of 150 min per week of aerobic physical activity, along with the aggressive treatment of other cardiovascular risk factors. The guidelines suggest that metformin should remain the first-line pharmacologic agent for glycemic control and to reduce risk of cardiovascular disease. However, should a patient's hemoglobin A1c remain $\geq 7.0\%$ despite first-line therapy and lifestyle modification, in the presence of other cardiovascular risk factors, an sodium-glucose cotransporter 2 (SGLT-2) inhibitor or a glucagon like peptide-1 (GLP-1) receptor agonist should be considered both to further improve glycemic control and independently reduce cardiovascular risk.

Of note, recent studies of SGLT-2 inhibitors have demonstrated a reduction in heart failure adverse events and progression of chronic kidney disease independent of glycemic control. Therefore, SGLT-2 inhibitors and GLP-1 agonists may both be considered as cardiovascular prevention agents for second-line therapy after metformin and lifestyle interventions in individuals at elevated risk for cardiovascular disease in both men and women. No sex-specific disparity in benefit has been noted between men and women with regard to SGLT-2 inhibitor in the primary prevention of cardiovascular disease. Some reports have demonstrated improved glycemic control among men using GLP-1 agonists as compared to increased weight loss among women using GLP-1 agonists.

11.3.7 Psychosocial Stressors and Mental Health

The interplay between cardiovascular disease and psychosocial stressors reflects a complex dynamic among biologic, social, behavioral, and psychological factors. Disparities in health are underscored through the association of socioeconomic status, race, gender, stress, and social isolation with cardiovascular disease. Further, a robust literature links the Diagnostic and Statistical Manual of Mental Disorders (DSM-5) diagnoses of major depressive disorder and generalized anxiety disorder to increased development and progression of cardiovascular disease. Of note, it is estimated that up to 45% of patients with cardiovascular disease demonstrate symptoms of depression and that 15–20% of patients with cardiovascular disease meet the full DSM-5 diagnostic criteria for major depressive disorder. Depression is an independent risk factor for the development of cardiovascular disease and is associated with increased major cardiac events, hospitalizations, and all-cause mortality. Post-traumatic stress disorder has also been shown to be associated with an increased risk of developing cardiovascular disease likely through changes in the neurobiological stress response. In women, hormonal fluctuations associated with oral contraceptive use, pregnancy, and a menopausal state may further exacerbate both changes in mood and risk of depression, as well as a pro-inflammatory state that increases risk of cardiovascular disease. Associations between mental health and cardiovascular disease have been proposed both through associated maladaptive behavioral and lifestyle changes, as well as hormonal changes in stress response.

Therefore, women should be routinely screened using the Patient Health Questionaire-2 or -9 (PHQ-2, PHQ-9) for major depression and the Generalized Anxiety Disorder-2 or -7 (GAD-2, GAD-7) to identify early signs of depression and anxiety. Patients should be adequately treated with selective serotonin reuptake inhibitors and referred for cognitive behavioral therapy, as appropriate. It would be appropriate to incorporate brief screening tools into the workflow of this primary care visit in order to ensure that psychiatric risk factors are adequately addressed.

11.3.8   Hormone Therapy and ASCVD

The discussion of hormone replacement therapy commonly arises in the primary care setting among perimenopausal women like the clinical case presented. Cardiovascular and metabolic changes perimenopause should be acknowledged, including increased rates of dyslipidemia and body fat redistribution associated with estrogen withdrawal, impaired glucose tolerance, and hypertension associated with changes endothelial function and vascular tone. Though a higher percentage of men are diagnosed with hypertension before the age of 65, conversely a higher percentage of females over the age of 65 are diagnosed with hypertension as compared to men. However, based upon available evidence, there is no recommendation for the use of menopausal hormone therapy in the primary prevention of cardiovascular disease.

Menopause is a retrospective diagnosis made after 12 months of amenorrhea without other pathologic or physiologic causes. Per the National Institutes of Health Consensus Statement on menopause, in the USA, the average age range for onset occurs between 40 and 58 years of age, with a median age of 51.4 years. Women are diagnosed with primary ovarian insufficiency if the onset of menopause occurs before the age of 40. Secondary causes of amenorrhea including pregnancy, hypo- or hyperthyroidism, and hyperprolactinemia should be considered among women aged 40–45 years. Over the age of 45, menopause is a clinical diagnosis that does not require the measurement of follicular stimulating hormone (FSH) for formal

Table 11.4 Common Clinical Symptoms of Menopause

Vasomotor symptoms	Genitourinary symptoms	Cognitive symptoms
Hot flashes (80%)	Dyspareunia	Mood changes and depression
Night sweats	Urinary frequency	Decreased libido
	Vaginal dryness	Sleep disturbance
	Vaginal pruritis	Irritability

diagnosis. In the late reproductive years, hormonal levels may fluctuate based upon first shortening then lengthening of the follicular stage of menses, and therefore hormone levels may be challenging to interpret throughout the reproductive cycle.

As our patient Ms. Smith ages, she may soon expect the onset of menopausal symptoms, with irregular menses often beginning 4 years prior to the final menstrual period. Classic symptoms of menopause may include vasomotor symptoms (hot flashes, night sweats), genitourinary symptoms (dyspareunia, urinary frequency, vaginal dryness, and vaginal pruritis), and cognitive changes (mood changes and depression, decreased libido, sleep disturbance, irritability) (Table 11.4). Menopause may be more challenging to diagnosis in patients using oral or long-acting reversible contraception and in individuals with underlying menstrual cycle disorders, including polycystic ovarian syndrome. Our patient currently uses a levonorgestrel-containing intrauterine device for contraception and therefore likely experiences oligomenorrhea or amenorrhea. Clinicians may consider removing the contraceptive device by age 51 years. An FSH level may be measured 2–4 weeks after removal of the device with a level of >25 IU/L typically indicating a menopausal state, though no biomarker provides absolute reassurance that a patient has achieved a clinical diagnosis of menopause.

If our patient develops bothersome vasomotor symptoms associated with menopause, non-hormonal treatment may be considered including selective serotonin reuptake inhibitors (such as paroxetine, escitalopram, citalopram, or fluoxetine), serotonin and norepinephrine reuptake inhibitors (such as venlafaxine or desvenlafaxine), gabapentinoids (pregabalin, gabapentin), or clonidine. Patients starting serotonin and norepinephrine reuptake inhibitors should be monitoring closely for the development of hypertension that may exacerbate underlying cardiovascular risk. Similarly, patients using clonidine may experience severe rebound hypertension if this therapy is abruptly stopped. Non-hormonal therapies are discussed in greater detail elsewhere in this text.

If our patient develops bothersome genitourinary symptoms of menopause, including dyspareunia or vaginal dryness, both non-hormonal and hormonal therapies may be appropriate. The North American Menopause Society recommends a trial of non-hormonal therapies as the first-line treatment for genitourinary symptoms of menopause before considering hormone-based therapies. Non-hormonal therapies may include topical vaginal moisturizers and lubricants. Vaginal estrogen preparations are available in several different preparations in the United States, including vaginal rings, vaginal inserts, and vaginal creams based upon patient preference, therapy availability, and insurance coverage. Topical vaginal estrogen has been demonstrated to result in minimal changes in serum estrogen concentration, with circulating estrogen levels most often remaining in the post-menopausal range of 3–10 pg/mL, without evidence of endometrial proliferation or hyperplasia.

If patients continue to demonstrate bothersome vasomotor, genitourinary, or cognitive symptoms, it may be appropriate to consider hormone therapy. In the absence of surgical hysterectomy, our patient would require hormone therapy with the use of both progesterone as well as estrogen in order to protect against the risk of endometrial hyperplasia that accompanies unopposed estrogen therapy. Systemic estrogen preparations include oral pills, estrogen or estrogen/progestin combine patches, topical gels, and intrauterine gels. Prior to initiation of hormone therapy, the cardiovascular and non-cardiovascular risks of therapy must be discussed with patients. Such risks include invasive breast cancer, venous thromboembolism, and ongoing controversy regarding risk of cardiovascular disease and stroke. Guidelines suggest that hormone therapy may be appropriate for consideration among women less than 60 years of age who are within 10 years of onset of menopause for the shortest tolerated duration, in the absence of strict contraindications.

The evidence regarding hormone therapy and cardiovascular disease has vacillated widely since the early 1990s and remains controversial. The Nurse Health Study published in 1991 first demonstrated in an observational, retrospective study of more than 48,000 women a statistically significant decrease in the relative risk of major coronary artery disease among current and former uses of post-menopausal estrogen therapy. The Heart and Estrogen/Progestin Replacement Study published in 1998 failed to demonstrate a statistical difference in cardiovascular death or myocardial infarction among women randomized to either combine estrogen/progestin therapy or placebo. To the opposite extreme, the Women's Health Initiative published in 2002 and enrolling more than 16,000 women was stopped early due to signal for harm among women randomized to combined estrogen/progestin therapy due to excess cardiovascular death, myocardial infarction, and invasive breast cancer. More recently, the Early versus Late Intervention Trial with Estradiol study published in 2016 demonstrated slowing of the progression of carotid intimal-medial thickness among women received combined estrogen/progestin therapy early after the onset of menopause. This representative sample of studies demonstrates ongoing clinical uncertainty regarding the safety and effectiveness of combined hormone therapy with regard to cardiovascular disease. However, evidence currently suggests no role for menopausal hormone therapy in the primary prevention of cardiovascular disease.

Prior to initiating hormone therapy, a risk assessment for cardiovascular disease and breast cancer must be undertaken. In individuals with known atherosclerotic cardiovascular disease, peripheral arterial disease, prior thromboembolic event, prior stroke, genetic or acquired hypercoagulable state, liver disease, or breast and/or endometrial cancer, hormone therapy is contraindicated. A Pooled Cohort Eqs. 10-year ASCVD risk of $\geq 7.5\%$ in the absence of clinical atherosclerotic disease may also be considered a contraindication. Caution and rigorous risk counseling should be undertaken in women desiring to start hormone therapy with borderline

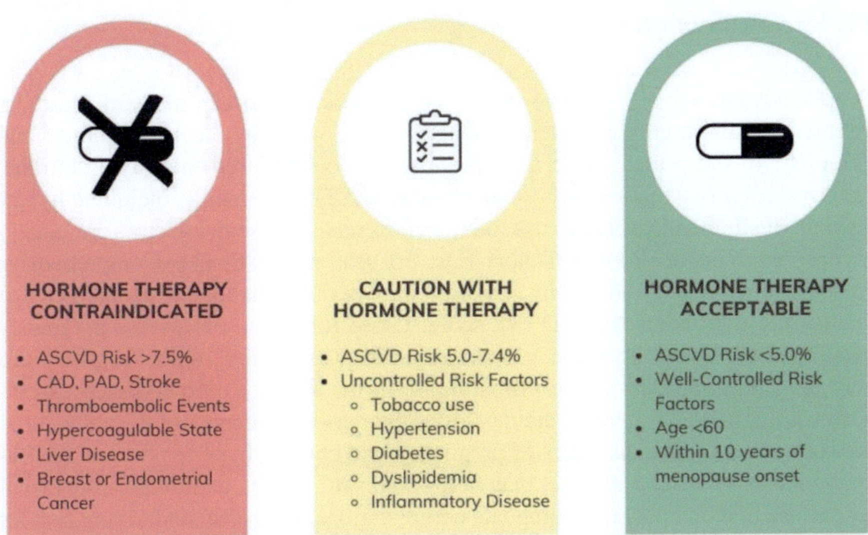

Fig. 11.6 Cardiovascular risk assessment for hormone therapy initiation. *ASCVD* atherosclerotic cardiovascular disease

ASCVD risk of 5.0–7.4% or uncontrolled risk factors for ASCVD including ongoing smoking, obesity, sedentary lifestyle, uncontrolled hypertension, poorly controlled diabetes, poorly controlled dyslipidemia, and inflammatory disorders (such as systemic lupus erythematosus, rheumatoid arthritis, psoriatic disorder, or scleroderma) that serve as risk-enhancing factors for cardiovascular disease, discussed above. A 10-year ASCVD risk score of <5% may be consistent with an appropriate cardiovascular risk profile in the absence of other contraindications (Fig. 11.6). Though no professional organizations recommend hormone therapy for the primary or secondary prevention of coronary artery disease, there is some evidence to suggest reduced risk of cardiovascular disease in women if hormone therapy is started soon after the onset of menopause.

Though there are no clear guidelines for when to stop hormone therapy, the American Association of Clinical Endocrinology recommends using hormone therapy for the shortest duration possible. Hormone dosage may be tapered after 5–7 years and if risks exceed the benefits of ongoing therapy. In the event that our patient Ms. Smith wishes to start hormone therapy following the development of vasomotor or genitourinary symptoms, a frank discussion must be undertaken regarding her cardiovascular risk factors. With a Pooled Cohort Eqs. 10-year ASCVD risk of 6.0% and ongoing smoking, non-hormonal and local estrogen therapy may be preferable over systemic hormone therapy. If she expresses a strong preference to proceed with hormone therapy despite the known cardiovascular risks, she should be counseled regarding lifestyle interventions to minimize risk including weight loss, physical activity, nutrition, and smoking cessation.

11.4 Conclusion

Despite advances in preventative cardiovascular care, atherosclerotic cardiovascular disease remains highly prevalent among women, with significant morbidity and mortality. In the primary care setting, women should be screened for traditional cardiovascular risk factors, represented by the ABCDE mnemonic, including hypertension, dyslipidemia, tobacco use, diet, and exercise. These risk factors are largely encapsulated in the Pooled Cohort Eqs. 10-year risk estimate. Comprehensive obstetric, menstrual, and family histories may reveal risk-enhancing factors that modify the traditional ASCVD risk score. Close follow-up of adverse pregnancy outcomes to prevent immediate readmission as well as long-term complications may fall under the purview of primary care in the absence of specialized cardio-obstetrics or maternal fetal medicine clinics. Increased awareness of the association between hypertensive disorders of pregnancy and chronic hypertension, as well as incident cardiovascular disease, may help to prevent, detect, and treat cardiovascular disease in women who develop late complications. Likewise, underlying risk for cardiovascular disease should be considered when counseling women regarding the risks and benefits of menopausal hormone therapy. Growing awareness of sex-specific risk factors and attention to equitable enrollment in clinical trials may help tailor precise, preventative therapies for women moving forward.

Suggested Reading

1. Virani SS, Alonso A, Aparicio HJ, Benjamin EJ, Bittencourt MS, Callaway CW, et al. Heart disease and stroke Statistics-2021 update: a report from the American Heart Association. Circulation. 2021;143(8):e254–743. https://doi.org/10.1161/CIR.0000000000000950.
2. Arnett DK, Blumenthal RS, Albert MA, Buroker AB, Goldberger ZD, Hahn EJ, et al. 2019 ACC/AHA guideline on the primary prevention of cardiovascular disease: a report of the American College of Cardiology/American Heart Association task force on clinical practice guidelines. Circulation. 2019;140(11):e596–646. https://doi.org/10.1161/CIR.0000000000000678.
3. Grundy SM, Stone NJ, Bailey AL, Beam C, Birtcher KK, Blumenthal RS, et al. 2018 AHA/ACC/AACVPR/AAPA/ABC/ACPM/ADA/AGS/APhA/ASPC/NLA/PCNA guideline on the management of blood cholesterol: a report of the American College of Cardiology/American Heart Association task force on clinical practice guidelines. Circulation. 2019;139(25):e1082–e143. https://doi.org/10.1161/CIR.0000000000000625.
4. Okunrintemi V, Valero-Elizondo J, Patrick B, Salami J, Tibuakuu M, Ahmad S, et al. Gender differences in patient-reported outcomes among adults with atherosclerotic cardiovascular disease. J Am Heart Assoc. 2018;7(24):e010498. https://doi.org/10.1161/JAHA.118.010498.
5. Force USPST, Krist AH, Davidson KW, Mangione CM, Barry MJ, Cabana M, et al. Behavioral counseling interventions to promote a healthy diet and physical activity for cardiovascular disease prevention in adults with cardiovascular risk factors: US preventive services task force recommendation statement. JAMA. 2020;324(20):2069–75. https://doi.org/10.1001/jama.2020.21749.
6. Cho L, Davis M, Elgendy I, Epps K, Lindley KJ, Mehta PK, et al. Summary of updated recommendations for primary prevention of cardiovascular disease in women: JACC state-of-the-art review. J Am Coll Cardiol. 2020;75(20):2602–18. https://doi.org/10.1016/j.jacc.2020.03.060.

7. Redberg RF, Katz MH. Statins for primary prevention: the debate is intense, but the data are weak. JAMA. 2016;316(19):1979–81. https://doi.org/10.1001/jama.2016.15085.
8. Daly B, Toulis KA, Thomas N, Gokhale K, Martin J, Webber J, et al. Increased risk of ischemic heart disease, hypertension, and type 2 diabetes in women with previous gestational diabetes mellitus, a target group in general practice for preventive interventions: a population-based cohort study. PLoS Med. 2018;15(1):e1002488. https://doi.org/10.1371/journal.pmed.1002488.
9. Teede HJ, Misso ML, Costello MF, Dokras A, Laven J, Moran L, et al. Recommendations from the international evidence-based guideline for the assessment and management of polycystic ovary syndrome. Clin Endocrinol. 2018;89(3):251–68. https://doi.org/10.1111/cen.13795.
10. Honigberg MC, Zekavat SM, Aragam K, Finneran P, Klarin D, Bhatt DL, et al. Association of premature natural and surgical menopause with incident cardiovascular disease. JAMA. 2019;322(24):2411–21. https://doi.org/10.1001/jama.2019.19191.
11. Mosca L, Benjamin EJ, Berra K, Bezanson JL, Dolor RJ, Lloyd-Jones DM, et al. Effectiveness-based guidelines for the prevention of cardiovascular disease in women – 2011 update: a guideline from the American Heart Association. J Am Coll Cardiol. 2011;57(12):1404–23. https://doi.org/10.1016/j.jacc.2011.02.005.
12. Guirguis-Blake JM, Evans CV, Perdue LA, Bean SI, Senger CA. Aspirin use to prevent cardiovascular disease and colorectal cancer: an evidence update for the U.S. preventive services task Force, Evidence synthesis no. 211. Rockville: Agency for Healthcare Research and Quality; 2021. AHRQ publication no. 21-05283-EF-1
13. Aggarwal NR, Wood MJ. Sex differences in the pathophysiology, presentation, diagnosis and management of cardiac disease. 1st ed. Waltham: Elsevier; 2021.
14. Whelton PK, Carey RM, Aronow WS, Casey DE Jr, Collins KJ, Dennison Himmelfarb C, et al. 2017 ACC/AHA/AAPA/ABC/ACPM/AGS/APhA/ASH/ASPC/NMA/PCNA guideline for the prevention, detection, evaluation, and management of high blood pressure in adults: executive summary: a report of the American College of Cardiology/American Heart Association task force on clinical practice guidelines. Circulation. 2018;138(17):e426–e83. https://doi.org/10.1161/CIR.0000000000000597.
15. Wenger NK, Ferdinand KC, Bairey Merz CN, Walsh MN, Gulati M, Pepine CJ, et al. Women, hypertension, and the systolic blood pressure intervention trial. Am J Med. 2016;129(10):1030–6. https://doi.org/10.1016/j.amjmed.2016.06.022.
16. Culver AL, Ockene IS, Balasubramanian R, Olendzki BC, Sepavich DM, Wactawski-Wende J, et al. Statin use and risk of diabetes mellitus in postmenopausal women in the Women's Health Initiative. Arch Intern Med. 2012;172(2):144–52. https://doi.org/10.1001/archinternmed.2011.625.
17. Khera A. Texas atherosclerosis imaging bill: quiet origins, broad implications. Arch Intern Med. 2011;171(4):281–3. https://doi.org/10.1001/archinternmed.2011.25.
18. Zelniker TA, Wiviott SD, Raz I, Im K, Goodrich EL, Furtado RHM, et al. Comparison of the effects of glucagon-like peptide receptor agonists and sodium-glucose cotransporter 2 inhibitors for prevention of major adverse cardiovascular and renal outcomes in type 2 diabetes mellitus. Circulation. 2019;139(17):2022–31. https://doi.org/10.1161/CIRCULATIONAHA.118.038868.
19. Marjoribanks J, Farquhar C, Roberts H, Lethaby A, Lee J. Long-term hormone therapy for perimenopausal and postmenopausal women. Cochrane Database Syst Rev. 2017;1:CD004143. https://doi.org/10.1002/14651858.CD004143.pub5.
20. Pinkerton JV. Hormone therapy for postmenopausal women. N Engl J Med. 2020;382(24):e91. https://doi.org/10.1056/NEJMc2005199.

Chapter 12
Birth Control

Charlotte Chaiklin

12.1 Introduction

Contraception is the deliberate use of a medication, device, or behavior that allows people with child bearing potential to play an active role in family planning by preventing pregnancy. Given the wide variety of contraceptive methods, clinicians must consider benefits, risks, patient preferences, and efficacy of each contraceptive method when providing contraceptive counseling. The following chapter will discuss the various types of contraceptive methods. This chapter will not include information about postpartum care, abortion care, or emergency contraception.

12.2 Clinical Case

A 24-year-old woman presents to your primary care clinic to establish care. At the start of the visit, she states she wants to discuss contraception options as she has become sexually active with a new male partner. She was recently screened for sexually transmitted infections, is up to date with her cervical cancer screening, and has no genitourinary complaints. She reports having regular periods with 5 days of menstruation every 30 days. She has no children but would like to preserve her fertility for the future. Her past medical history includes migraine headaches with aura for which she takes topiramate for prophylaxis and sumatriptan as needed and

C. Chaiklin (✉)
Division of General Internal Medicine, Department of Medicine, University of Florida, Gainesville, FL, USA
e-mail: cchaiklin@ufl.edu

M. Mahmoudi (ed.), *Common Cases in Women's Primary Care Clinics*, https://doi.org/10.1007/978-3-031-48569-5_12

obesity class II with a body mass index of 37 kg/m². She smokes a quarter pack of cigarettes daily. She has never had any surgeries and denies a personal or family history of breast cancer. How would you counsel this patient about her contraceptive options?

12.3 Discussion

This clinical case emphasizes the importance of first obtaining a thorough patient history. Past medical history, surgical history, family history, social history, and current medications should all be reviewed prior to initiating a conversation about contraception as certain methods may be contraindicated. When discussing contraceptive methods, it is important that the clinician takes into consideration not only the patient's history but also patient preference in order to determine the optimal contraceptive method.

The efficacy of the various contraceptive methods in preventing pregnancy ranges from 76% to greater than 99%. Additionally, user dependent contraceptive methods such as pills, patches, vaginal rings, condoms, and fertility awareness require correct use to achieve maximal efficacy. The reported efficacy of user dependent contraceptive methods varies significantly when evaluating typical versus perfect use. For example, patients who receive progestin intramuscular injections will experience unintended pregnancy within the first year of use at a rate of 6% with typical use versus 0.2% with perfect use. Patients who utilize combined oral contraceptives will experience unintended pregnancy within the first year of use at a rate of 9% with typical use versus 0.3% with perfect use. When discussing various contraceptive methods, the clinician should emphasize the differences in efficacy with typical versus perfect use amongst the user dependent contraceptive methods and encourage patients to practice perfect use. When initiating a conversation about contraceptive options, clinicians should consider starting with the most effective user independent contraceptive options and then proceeding sequentially to the least effective user dependent methods. The following discussion will similarly review contraceptive methods from most to least effective starting with user independent options (Fig. 12.1).

12.3.1 Tubal Occlusion

Tubal occlusion often referred to as female sterilization is a highly effective permanent user independent method of contraceptive that is best suited for patients who have completed childbearing, understand the permanence of the procedure, and/or have medical contraindications to reversible contraceptive methods. Tubal occlusion can be performed as a laparoscopic outpatient procedure or via a minilaparotomy. In randomized controlled trials, there was no difference in major morbidity

Efficacy of Contraceptive Methods

<u>User Independent Methods</u>

Tubal Occlusion	>99%
Copper Intrauterine Device	>99%
Levonorgestrel Intrauterine Device	>99%
Progestin Implant	>99%

<u>User Dependent Methods</u>

Progestin Injectables	Typical Use: 94%	Perfect Use: >99%
Progestin-Only Pills	Typical Use: 91%	Perfect Use: >99%
Combined Hormonal Contraception	Typical Use: 91%	Perfect Use*: >99%
External Condom Barrier Contraception	Typical Use: 82%	Perfect Use: 98%
Internal Condom Barrier Contraception	Typical Use: 79%	Perfect Use: 95%
Fertility Awareness	Typical Use: 76%	Perfect Use: Unknown

*Efficacy rate for combined hormonal contraception pills only

**Efficacy rates are based on number of pregnancies within the first year of use of the contraceptive method

Fig. 12.1 Efficacy of contraceptive methods

noted between the two tubal occlusion methods. That being said, minilaparotomy is generally utilized in the postpartum setting or in patients at high risk of laparoscopy associated complications.

Tubal occlusion is highly effective as demonstrated by the United States Collaborative Review of Sterilization (CREST) study which was a large, prospective, multicenter observational study of more than 10,500 patients with childbearing potential. Per the CREST study, the 5-year cumulative pregnancy rate or failure rate of tubal occlusion is 13 per 1000 for all sterilization methods. It is important to note that vasectomy procedures and intrauterine devices (IUDs) have similar efficacy in preventing pregnancy. Per the CREST study, the 5-year cumulative failure rate of the copper IUD is 14 per 1000 procedures, the 5-year cumulative failure rate of the levonorgestrel-releasing IUD is 5–11 per 1000 procedures, and the 5-year cumulative failure rate of partner vasectomy is 11 per 1000 procedures.

In addition to high efficacy, tubal occlusion offers non-contraceptive benefits. Multiple observational trials have demonstrated a reduced incidence of ovarian cancer in patients who undergo tubal occlusion. This protective effect is noted even after adjusting for age, history of oral contraceptive use, and parity. Even in patients at high risk of developing ovarian cancer due to breast cancer susceptibility gene 1 (BRCA1) and breast cancer susceptibility gene 2 (BRCA2) mutations, the protective effect is maintained. The proposed mechanism of this protective effect is derived from research that suggests ovarian cancer arises from the fimbriae of the fallopian tube and therefore complete salpingectomy, an increasingly common tubal occlusion technique, prevents its development. While tubal occlusion does not protect against sexually transmitted infections (STIs), it has been shown to decrease the rates of pelvic inflammatory disease (PID) by preventing the spread of organisms from the lower genital tract to the peritoneal cavity.

Even though morbidity and mortality of tubal occlusion procedures are quite low, the healthcare provider should counsel patients about possible risks. There are an estimated 1–2 deaths per 100,000 laparoscopic sterilization procedures performed in the United States. Death rates are largely driven by complications associated with general anesthesia including hypoventilation and cardiopulmonary arrest. The overall complication rate of tubal occlusion procedures of all types is estimated at 0.9–1.6 per 100 procedures. Complications include conversion to laparotomy, unplanned major surgery as a result of the tubal occlusion procedure, blood transfusion, a life-threatening event, febrile morbidity, and rehospitalization. Independent predictors of tubal occlusion surgery complications include a history of diabetes mellitus, previous abdominal or pelvic surgery, and the use of general anesthesia. Healthcare providers should consider a patient's surgical risk when discussing tubal occlusion as a possible contraceptive method.

Beyond morbidity and mortality, sterilization is often associated with regret and therefore, comprehensive counseling should take place prior to the procedure. Risk factors for post tubal occlusion regret include young age (less than 30 years old) at time of sterilization, having received little information about the procedure, having less access to alternative forms of contraception, pressure from a spouse, being in an unstable relationship, low parity, and undergoing the procedure because of a medical indication. Per the results of the CREST study, the 14-year cumulative probability of requesting reversal information was as high as 40.4% in patients who were between the ages of 18–24 years old at time of tubal occlusion. The request for tubal occlusion reversal information from patients 18–24 years old at the time of the procedure was almost four times higher than for patients older than 30 years at the time of tubal occlusion. Interestingly, the number of living children has not been shown to be associated with requests for tubal occlusion reversal information (Fig. 12.2).

Healthcare providers should include tubal occlusion as an option when discussing contraceptive methods with their patients especially if the patient has completed childbearing and is greater than 30 years old. It is important that the healthcare provider stresses the permanence of this contraceptive method and highlights the fact that long-acting reversible contraceptive methods (intrauterine devices and implants) provide similar efficacy.

Tubal Occlusion Quick Facts

Advantages	**Disadvantages**
Efficacy: >99%	Requires a surgical procedure
Non-hormonal	Permanent contraceptive method
User independent	Risk of regret
Decreases ovarian cancer risk	Does not protect against STIs
Decreases the risk of PID	

Fig. 12.2 Tubal occlusion quick facts

For our patient in the clinical case, tubal occlusion is not an appropriate contraceptive method given her young age and desire for future fertility. Once our patient no longer desires fertility and is older than 30 years old, tubal occlusion may become an appropriate contraceptive option. Instead, the healthcare provider should focus on reversible contraceptive methods starting with the most efficacious options such as the long-acting reversible contraception methods.

12.3.2 Long-Acting Reversible Contraception

Long-acting reversible contraception methods (LARC) are long term, dependable, and highly effective user independent options for preventing pregnancy after a one-time placement procedure. LARCs have been shown to be approximately 20 times as effective as user dependent contraceptive methods. In the United States, the types of LARCs include the non-hormonal copper IUD, the levonorgestrel-releasing IUD (LNG-IUD) which comes in multiple forms, and the subdermal etonogestrel implant.

12.4 Copper IUD

The copper IUD prevents fertilization by means of copper toxicity to sperm, is >99% effective, and provides effective contraception for 10 years following placement. The copper IUD is an appropriate contraceptive option for patients who take medications that affect the function of liver enzymes such as antiepileptics and rifampin and can interfere with the metabolism of hormonal contraception. For patients who have a history of breast cancer, the copper IUD is recommended given its non-hormonal mechanism of action. The copper IUD is the only LARC that is recommended in patients with severe decompensated cirrhosis, hepatocellular adenoma, or hepatic malignancy. In patients with systemic lupus erythematosus (SLE), the copper IUD can be used regardless of antiphospholipid antibody status. However, in patients with SLE with severe thrombocytopenia (<50,000 platelets/microliter) the copper IUD should generally not be used due to an increased risk of heavy bleeding during menses as the copper IUD is known to cause menorrhagia. This method of contraception is contraindicated in patients with a hypersensitivity to copper, a known current pelvic infection or STI, unexplained vaginal bleeding, distorted uterine cavity incompatible with IUD placement, patients with gestational trophoblastic disease with persistently elevated human chorionic gonadotropin (hCG) levels or malignant disease, known or suspected pregnancy, and cervical or endometrial cancer (however, if the copper IUD has been previously placed, the patient may continue to use the IUD while awaiting cancer treatment). The copper IUD may change menstrual bleeding patterns and has specifically been shown to increase menstrual bleeding. Therefore, this option may not be suitable for patients

Copper IUD Quick Facts	
Advantages	**Contraindications**
Efficacy: >99%	SLE with severe thrombocytopenia
Non-hormonal	Hypersensitivity to copper
User independent	Current pelvic infection or STI
Provides 10 years of contraception	Unexplained vaginal bleeding
after placement	Distorted uterine cavity incompatible with IUD placement
	Gestational trophoblastic disease with persistently
Disadvantages	elevated hCG levels or malignant disease
Does not protect against STIs	Known or suspected pregnancy
Menorrhagia and/or hypermenorrhea	Cervical or endometrial cancer[*]

*If copper IUD previously placed, the patient may continue to use the IUD while awaiting cancer treatment

Fig. 12.3 Copper IUD quick facts

with known menorrhagia or hypermenorrhea. Prior to copper IUD placement, the healthcare provider should make the patient aware of this possible change in menstruation (Fig. 12.3).

12.5 LNG-IUD

The LNG-IUD prevents fertilization by inhibiting ovulation and thickening cervical mucus to obstruct the penetration of sperm, is >99% effective, and provides contraception for 3–8 years depending on the type used. Similar to the copper IUD, the LNG-IUD is an appropriate contraceptive option for patients who take medications that affect liver enzyme function such as antiepileptics and rifampin as IUD efficacy is not decreased with such medications. The LNG-IUD is an acceptable contraceptive option for patients with a history of or at risk for venous thromboembolism (VTE), myocardial infarction (MI), or stroke. In patients with known thrombogenic mutations such as prothrombin G20210A mutation, factor V Leiden, protein C, protein S, or antithrombin deficiency, the LNG-IUD can be used. When discussing the use of the LNG-IUD with patients with SLE, the healthcare provider should first clarify whether the patient has positive antiphospholipid antibodies (lupus anticoagulant, anticardiolipin antibody, and anti-beta2-glycoprotein antibody). If this information is unavailable, the healthcare provider should either obtain antiphospholipid antibody testing or treat as if the patient has positive antiphospholipid antibodies. In patients with SLE and positive antiphospholipid antibodies, the LNG-IUD should not generally be used due to concerns for increased risk of both arterial and venous thrombosis. In patients with SLE with negative antiphospholipid antibodies and severe thrombocytopenia (<50,000 platelets/microliter), the LNG-IUD can generally be used with careful follow-up. The LNG-IUD has been shown to be safe and effective without increased risk of contraceptive failure, infection, or other adverse events in patients with SLE on immunosuppressants with negative antiphospholipid antibodies. For patients with cardiovascular risk factors (smoking, obesity, diabetes, hypertension, or migraine with aura), the LNG-IUD is an appropriate contraceptive option. In patients with gynecologic malignancy, the use of a previously placed LNG-IUD for contraception is appropriate as the patient awaits treatment or if sterility does not result from treatment. In patients with treated gestational trophoblastic disease with falling or undetectable hCG levels or elevated hCG levels with no evident or suspected intrauterine disease, the LNG-IUD is considered an appropriate form of contraception. The LNG-IUD can be used in patients with long standing diabetes mellitus (more than 20 years) or evidence of diabetes related microvascular disease (nephropathy, retinopathy, or neuropathy). All LNG-IUDs work locally on the uterus. Therefore, efficacy is not affected by body mass index and can be utilized in patients with obesity. Obese patients are at increased risk of abnormal uterine bleeding (AUB) and endometrial hyperplasia. The use of the LNG-IUD in obese patients may provide the added benefit of stabilizing the endometrium and protect against AUB and endometrial hyperplasia. Because the LNG-IUD decreases menstrual blood loss by endometrial stabilization, it is also a good contraceptive option for patients taking anticoagulant medications.

There are multiple contraindications to LNG-IUD use. Similar to the copper IUD, the LNG-IUD is contraindicated in patients with hypersensitivity to any components of the LNG-IUD, a known current pelvic infection or STI, unexplained vaginal bleeding, distorted uterine cavity incompatible with IUD placement, gestational trophoblastic disease with persistently elevated hCG levels or malignant disease, known or suspected pregnancy, and cervical or endometrial cancer (however, if the LNG-IUD has been previously placed, the patient may continue to use the IUD while awaiting cancer treatment). Unlike the copper IUD, the LNG-IUD should not be used in patients with active or treated breast cancer given concerns for worse prognosis with progestin exposure (Fig. 12.4).

Before the insertion of either the copper IUD or the LNG-IUD, patients generally do not need to undergo STI screening as long as they have had appropriate STI screening per the Centers for Disease Control and Prevention (CDC) guidelines. The CDC recommends annual chlamydia trachomatis screening for women less than 25 years old and for older women with increased risk for STIs. No blood pressure monitoring is required for patients using the LNG-IUD for contraception. Patients that have no signs or symptoms suggestive of cervical malignancy and are up to date with routine cervical cancer screening do not require additional screening prior to IUD insertion.

Levonorgestrel-releasing (LNG) IUD Quick Facts

Advantages	**Appropriate for the following Medical Conditions**
Efficacy: >99%	History of VTE, MI, or stroke
User independent	Thrombogenic mutations
Provides 3-8 years of contraception after placement	SLE with negative antiphospholipid antibodies and severe thrombocytopenia[*]
	Smoking
	Obesity
Can be used with medications that affect liver enzyme function	Diabetes mellitus for any duration with or without microvascular disease
	Hypertension
	Migraine with aura
Protection against AUB and endometrial hyperplasia due to stabilization of the endometrium	History of gynecologic malignancy if sterility does not result from treatment
	Gestational trophoblastic disease with falling or undetectable hCG levels or elevated hCG levels with no evident or suspected intrauterine disease

Contraindications

SLE with positive or unknown antiphospholipid antibodies

Disadvantages

Hypersensitivity to any components of the LNG-IUD

Does not protect against STIs

Current pelvic infection or STI

Unexplained vaginal bleeding

Distorted uterine cavity incompatible with IUD placement

Gestational trophoblastic disease with persistently elevated hCG levels or malignant disease

Known or suspected pregnancy

Cervical or endometrial cancer[**]

Current or history of breast cancer

*Clinicians should consider careful follow up when using in such patients
**If the LNG-IUD previously placed, the patient may continue to use the IUD while awaiting cancer treatment

Fig. 12.4 Levonorgestrel-releasing (LNG) IUD quick facts

12.6 Subdermal Etonogestrel Implant

In the United States, only one type of subdermal implant is offered for contraception purposes. This progestin-only implant continually releases low amounts of progestin to thicken cervical mucus and inhibit ovulation and provides up to 3 years of contraception with a failure rate of 0.05% within the first year of use. The subdermal implant can be placed any time during the menstrual cycle as long as pregnancy has been ruled out and works within 24 hours of insertion. This form of contraception is suitable for patients who cannot take estrogen, have long standing diabetes (more than 20 years duration) or evidence of diabetes related microvascular disease, have a history of or are at risk of VTE, MI, or stroke, and have cardiovascular risk factors including migraine with aura, hypertension, diabetes, and/or obesity. In patients taking medications that affect liver enzyme function (such as antiepileptics, rifampin, etc.), the subdermal implant can be utilized. Prior to implant placement, patients should be counseled that there are case reports of pregnancy in patients using the implant and taking enzyme inducing medications but given the high contraceptive efficacy the implant is deemed to have a low failure rate even with enzyme inducing medications. The subdermal implant is an ideal contraceptive option for patients who wish to immediately return to fertility upon implant removal. After implant discontinuation, patients have been shown to have similar rates of pregnancy as patients who do not use contraception with a reported pregnancy rate of 60% within 6 months, 80% at 1 year, and 90% at 2 years. Given the quick return to fertility, patients should be counseled about the importance of keeping track of the removal date and possibility of contraception failure at the end of 3 years of use. The subdermal implant should not be used in patients with the presence or history of breast cancer, unexplained vaginal bleeding, known or suspected pregnancy, and the presence or history of severe liver disease.

Prior to subdermal implant placement, there is no indication for pelvic examination, laboratory testing, breast examination, or cervical cancer screening outside of recommended routine care. Additionally, blood pressure monitoring is not required prior to or during implant use. Patients should be counseled that there is limited evidence to support weight gain amongst implant users. In one study looking at weight gain in patients using implants versus non-hormonal IUDs, the average weight gain noted in the implant group was 1–2.4 pounds. Patients should also be informed that all types of hormonal contraception, including the subdermal implant, can be utilized in patients with depressive disorders as depressive symptoms have not been shown to worsen with the use of hormonal contraception. Finally, it is important the healthcare provider provide anticipatory guidance in regards to changes in menstrual bleeding patterns (i.e., lighter or heavier bleeding, prolonged or irregular bleeding, or amenorrhea) with the use of the subdermal implant. Patients should be advised that menstrual irregularities while common with the subdermal implant usually improve with time (Fig. 12.5).

For our patient in the clinical case, any LARC option is medically appropriate and can be used to provide her with highly effective user independent contraception for 3–10 years duration depending on the type of LARC selected. In helping our patient make an informed decision, the healthcare provider should discuss the advantages and potential disadvantages of each type of LARC. For the copper IUD,

Etonogestrel Implant Quick Facts

Advantages
Efficacy: >99%
User independent
Provides 3 years of contraception after placement
Can be used with medications that affect liver enzyme function
Quick return to fertility after removal
Progestin only contraception

Disadvantages
Does not protect against STIs
Menstrual irregularities

Appropriate for the following Medical Conditions
History or at risk of VTE, MI, or stroke
Obesity
Diabetes mellitus for any duration with or without microvascular disease
Hypertension
Migraine with aura

Contraindications
Presence or history of severe liver disease
Unexplained vaginal bleeding
Known or suspected pregnancy
Current or history of breast cancer

Fig. 12.5 Etonogestrel implant quick facts

the healthcare provider should emphasize that this method is hormone free, provides contraception for up to 10 years, and is associated with menorrhagia and/or hypermenorrhea. When discussing the LNG-IUD, the healthcare provider should highlight that the LNG-IUD provides protection against AUB and endometrial hyperplasia due to stabilization of the endometrium and contraception for 3–8 years after placement depending on the type of LNG-IUD selected. Finally, the healthcare provider should counsel our patient about the etonogestrel implant as a 3-year contraceptive option with quick return to fertility after removal and possible menstrual irregularities with use. Once all LARC options have been discussed, the healthcare provider should assess our patient's preferences with respect to changes in menstruation and IUD versus subdermal implant in order to identify the best possible LARC method for our patient.

12.6.1 Progestin-Only Injections

The two forms of progestin-only injectables offered in the United States include the depot medroxyprogesterone acetate intramuscular (DMPA-IM) injection and the depot medroxyprogesterone acetate subcutaneous (DMPA-SC) injection. Both prevent pregnancy by suppressing ovulation, thickening cervical mucus, and thinning the endometrial lining and can be started any time during the menstrual cycle provided pregnancy has been ruled out. DMPA-IM and DMPA-SC are administered every 3 months (or every 13 weeks) and are user dependent forms of contraception. In the United States, 6% of patients with typical use and 0.2% of patients with perfect use experience pregnancy within 1 year of progestin-only injection use. It is important that healthcare providers emphasize the difference in efficacy of progestin-only injections with typical versus perfect use when counseling patients about this contraceptive method.

The benefits of progestin-only injections include a discrete form of contraception and a user dependent contraceptive method that does not require daily action. Additionally, in patients taking liver enzyme inducing antiepileptic drugs, DMPA-IM and DMPA-SC are the only non-IUD forms of contraception recommended. With DMPA-IM and DMPA-SC, patients receive substantially higher levels of progestin then what is required to suppress ovulation and therefore the impact of antiepileptic therapy on efficacy is presumed to be minimal. DMPA-IM and DMPA-SC are good contraceptive options for patients taking long term rifampin or rifabutin therapy (i.e., for latent tuberculosis) as there is no evidence that efficacy decreases with such medications. Progestin-only injectables are contraindicated in patients with the presence or history of breast cancer, known or suspected pregnancy, the presence or history of severe liver disease, and unexplained vaginal bleeding. Progestin-only injectables have been shown to have a negative impact on lipoprotein profiles. For this reason, DMPA-IM and DMPA-SC should not be used in patients with poorly controlled hypertension (systolic blood pressure of 160 mm Hg or greater or diastolic blood pressure of 100 mg Hg or greater) or diabetes of more than 20 years duration or evidence of microvascular disease due to fear of increasing cardiovascular risk. Due to concerns for decreased bone mineral density (BMD) with prolonged use, both progestin-only injectables have a United States Food and Drug Administration (US FDA) black box warning against use for more than two consecutive years. Some observational studies suggest progestin-only injectables increase fracture risk while other data indicates decreased BMD is temporary and reversible. In contrast to the US FDA recommendations, the World Health Organization does not recommend restricting duration of progestin-only injectables use due to concerns about BMD. Given the concern for decreased BMD with DMPA-IM and DMPA-SC use, this form of contraception may not be appropriate for patients on chronic steroid therapy, with a history of non-traumatic fractures, or with risk factors for decreased BMD.

Prior to initiating progestin-only injectables, patients should be provided anticipatory guidance including expected return to fertility after discontinuation, possible changes in menstruation, and changes in weight. For patients using the DMPA-IM injections, return to fertility averages between 9 and 10 months after discontinuation. For DMPA-SC injections, return to fertility was noted to be a median of 30 weeks after discontinuation. For patients who desire immediate return to ovulation following discontinuation of contraception, the DMPA-IM and DMPA-SC may not be appropriate contraceptive options. Most patients experience changes in menstrual bleeding patterns (i.e., prolonged or irregular bleeding, lighter or heavier bleeding, or amenorrhea) in the first year of progestin-only injectable use. Patients should be counseled that changes in bleeding are expected and that the irregularity of bleeding usually improves with time. After 1 year of either DMPA-IM or DMPA-SC use 40–50% of patients experience amenorrhea and after 5 years of use 80% experience amenorrhea. For this reason, DMPA-IM and DMPA-SC may be appropriate for patients on anticoagulants or menorrhagia as they protect against anemia due to menstrual bleeding. In terms of weight gain, some studies comparing non-hormonal methods of contraception or no contraception to the progestin-only injectables suggest a slight increase in weight of less than 4.5 pounds in the DMPA-IM and DMPA-SC groups. Blood or laboratory testing, blood pressure monitoring, pelvic examination, breast examination, and cervical cancer screening outside of recommended routine care are not required prior to initiation of DMPA-IM or DMPA-SC injections. Patients should be informed that both contraceptive methods can be administered 2 weeks early or up to 4 weeks late from the scheduled due date; however, all efforts should be made to stay on schedule with injections.

Progestin-only injectables may be a suitable contraceptive option for our patient in the clinical case. When counseling our patient about this method, the healthcare provider should emphasize the difference in efficacy of progestin-only injectables with typical versus perfect use. Additionally, the healthcare provider should discuss possible changes in menstruation including amenorrhea, the delay in return to fertility following discontinuation, and the US FDA black box warning against use for more than 2 years due to concerns for decreased bone mineral density so our patient can make an informed decision when selecting a contraceptive method (Fig. 12.6).

Progestin-Only Injectables Quick Facts

Advantages
Efficacy: >99% with perfect use and 94% with typical use
Discrete form of contraception
User dependent but does not require daily action
Can induce amenorrhea and subsequently protect against
anemia due to menorrhagia

Disadvantages
Does not protect against STIs
User dependent
Delayed return to fertility after discontinuation
US FDA black box warning against use for more than 2 years
due to decreased BMD

Contraindications
Active or history of breast cancer
Known or suspected pregnancy
Presence or history of severe liver
disease
Unexplained vaginal bleeding
Poorly controlled hypertension (systolic
blood pressure ≥ 160 mmHg or diastolic
blood pressure ≥ 100 mmHg)
Long standing diabetes mellitus defined
as more than 20 years or diabetes
mellitus with evidence of microvascular
disease

Fig. 12.6 Progestin-only injectables quick facts

12.6.2 *Progestin-Only Pills*

Progestin-only pills (POPs) also known as the "minipill" are a user dependent form of contraception that prevent pregnancy primarily by thickening cervical mucus and secondarily by inhibiting ovulation which occurs in about 50% of menstrual cycles. POPs may be started any time in a menstrual cycle as long as pregnancy has been ruled out. If POPs are initiated within 5 days from the onset of menstrual bleeding, no additional contraception is required. When POPs are initiated more than 5 days from the onset of menstrual bleeding, patients should be advised to use an additional form of contraception or abstain from sexual intercourse for two full days as POPs require 48 hours to provide a contraceptive effect. As serum steroid levels drop close to baseline 24 hours after administration, it is crucial that patients take POPs at the same time each day. Healthcare providers should counsel patients that with perfect use, POPs provide greater than 99% efficacy but with typical use, 9 out of 100 patients will become pregnant within the first year of using POPs.

POPs can be used in patients with many types of medical conditions. POPs, like all forms of progestin-only contraception, are an acceptable form of contraception for patients taking anticoagulant therapy. Patients with a history of or at risk of venous thromboembolism, myocardial infarction, or stroke can use POPs. POPs can generally be used without contraindication in patients with obesity, hypertension, diabetes mellitus (regardless of duration or presence of microvascular disease), cervical intraepithelial neoplasia, anemia, thrombogenic mutations, cervical cancer, STIs, or human immunodeficiency virus (HIV). In patients with SLE with negative antiphospholipid antibodies and absence of other cardiovascular disease risk factors (i.e., smoking, diabetes mellitus, older age, hypercholesterolemia, and hypertension), POPs can be used but additional follow-up may be necessary. POPs should not be used in patients with current or history of breast cancer or liver disease. POPs should be avoided in patients who have undergone bariatric surgery that has resulted in compromised absorption of oral medications (biliopancreatic diversion or Roux-en-Y gastric bypass) due to the risk of decreased efficacy. Patients who have undergone restrictive types of bariatric surgery (laparoscopic sleeve gastrectomy, laparoscopic adjustable gastric band, or vertical banded gastroplasty) that do not impact oral medication absorption can take POPs without concern for decreased efficacy. Additionally, POPs should be avoided in patients taking medications that affect hepatic enzymes (i.e., antiretroviral therapy, rifampin, antiepileptic therapy, etc.) due to risk of contraception failure with altered metabolism of progestin.

Prior to initiating POPs, patients do not require screening for dyslipidemia, liver disease, cervical cancer outside of regular screening recommendations, or breast disease via clinical breast examination. Patients should be counseled that POPs have not been shown to affect blood pressure or cardiovascular risk. Patients should be informed that a missed dose is defined as POP ingestion more than 3 hours from when the POP should have been taken. If a patient misses a dose, they should take the missed dose as soon as possible in addition to their normal daily POP even if that means taking two pills on the same day. Additionally, patients must use back-up contraception or avoid sexual intercourse until POPs are taken on time for a full 48 hours. If a patient has unprotected sexual intercourse during a period of missed POPs, emergency contraception should be considered. Anticipatory guidance should also include instructions to follow the recommendations for missed pills in the event of severe vomiting or diarrhea within 3 hours of taking a POP due to theoretical concerns for decreased efficacy.

POPs should be included in the discussion of medically appropriate contraceptive options for our patient in the clinical case with emphasis on the user dependent nature of POPs and difference in effectiveness between typical and perfect use. Any patient that chooses POPs for contraception requires additional counseling about missed doses. If our patient selects POPs for her contraceptive method, she should then be informed that a missed dose is defined as being more than 3 hours from when the POP should have been taken. She should also be advised that if she misses a dose, she must use back-up contraception or avoid sexual intercourse until POPs are taken on time for a full 48 hours (Fig. 12.7).

12.6.3 Combination Hormonal Contraception

Combination hormonal contraception (CHC) is a user dependent form of contraception that exists in three formulations: pill, transdermal patch, and vaginal ring and can be started any time during the menstrual cycle as long as pregnancy has been ruled out. If CHC is started within the first 5 days of the menstrual cycle with day

Progestin-Only Pills Quick Facts

Advantages Efficacy: >99% with perfect use and 91% with typical use **Disadvantages** Does not protect against STIs User dependent requiring daily action **Contraindications** Active or history of breast cancer Presence or history of liver disease Previous bariatric surgery that resulted in compromised absorption of medications Medications that affect hepatic enzymes *Close follow up may be necessary	**Appropriate for the following Medical Conditions** History or at risk of VTE, MI, or stroke Obesity Diabetes mellitus for any duration with or without microvascular disease Cervical intraepithelial neoplasia Anemia Thrombogenic mutations Cervical cancer Current STI HIV SLE with negative antiphospholipid antibodies and absence of other cardiovascular disease risk factors*

Fig. 12.7 Progestin-only pills quick facts

one being the first day of menstrual bleeding, no additional contraceptive protection is needed. If CHC is started more than 5 days after the start of menstrual bleeding, the patient should be advised to use additional contraceptive protection or abstain from sexual intercourse for the next 7 days. CHC is typically used for 21–24 consecutive days followed by four to seven hormone free days with either no use or placebo pills. With typical use of all forms of CHC, 9 out of 100 patients will become pregnant within the first year. With perfect use of all types of CHC, the efficacy increases to greater than 99%. Like with other user dependent forms of contraception, healthcare providers should emphasize the difference in efficacy with perfect versus typical use and encourage patients to strive for perfect use to decrease the risk of pregnancy.

Combination hormonal contraception is contraindicated in patients with certain medical conditions and/or taking certain medications. Given the limited data regarding transdermal patch and vaginal ring use, it is recommended that clinicians apply the same contraindications for pill use to all forms of CHC. The following discussion will review contraindications for all forms of CHC.

Estrogen increases hepatic production of serum globulins involved in coagulation such as factor VII, factor X, and fibrinogen. Increased production of serum globulins by estrogen found in CHC leads to increased risk of VTE. While all forms of CHC increase the risk of VTE, it should be noted that the risk of VTE in CHC users is only half as high as the risk of VTE in pregnancy. Patients with risk factors for VTE should be counseled about non-hormonal or progestin-only contraceptive methods. Patients are considered to have unacceptable risk for VTE with CHC use if they have any of the following: smoking at age 35 years or older, history of deep venous thrombosis or pulmonary embolism, plans for major surgery with anticipated prolonged immobilization, inflammatory bowel disease with active or extensive disease, immobilization, corticosteroid use, vitamin deficiencies or fluid depletion, familial thrombophilia (prothrombin G20210A mutation, factor V Leiden, protein C, protein S, or antithrombin deficiency), antiphospholipid syndrome, SLE with positive or unknown antiphospholipid antibodies, or acute or prior superficial venous thrombosis. Patients with such risk factors should be counseled about non-hormonal or progestin-only contraceptive methods.

Patients with SLE or migraine headaches require further evaluation to determine appropriateness of CHC use. When considering contraceptive options for patients with SLE, the healthcare provider should first test for antiphospholipid antibodies including lupus anticoagulant, anticardiolipin antibody, and anti-beta2-glycoprotein antibody. In patients with SLE and positive antiphospholipid antibodies, CHC is contraindicated. In patients with SLE and negative antiphospholipid antibodies with no risk factors for cardiovascular disease (i.e., older age, tobacco use, hypertension, hypercholesterolemia, and diabetes), CHC is an appropriate contraceptive method. Patients should be counseled that the use of CHC does not appear to impact SLE disease activity. In patients with migraine headaches, the healthcare provider needs to first determine whether the migraine headaches are with or without aura. In patients who have migraine headaches without aura, CHC can be used as long as the patient has no risk factors for stroke. In patients with migraine headaches with aura, CHC is not recommended due to an increased risk of stroke with estrogen use.

Patients with risk factors for cardiovascular disease such as older age, obesity, hypertension, and diabetes should be evaluated carefully prior to initiation of CHC. There are no contraindications to CHC use based on age alone. In patients aged 40 years and older who are otherwise healthy, non-smoking, with a normal body mass index, and no cardiovascular risk factors, CHC can be used until age 50–55 years. In perimenopausal patients, the use of CHC has been shown to positively impact bone mineral density and decrease vasomotor symptoms of perimenopause. In patients who are obese but otherwise healthy, CHC can be used without concerns for a significant decrease in efficacy. Patients that undergo bariatric surgery with Roux-en-Y bypass or biliopancreatic diversion should not use oral CHC due to decreased absorption of oral medications but can use non-oral forms of CHC without restriction. In patients who have undergone vertical banded gastroplasty, laparoscopic adjustable gastric band, or laparoscopic sleeve gastrectomy, any form of CHC can be used. Patients with elevated blood pressure must be risk stratified to determine appropriateness of CHC use. In patients with blood pressure <140/90 mm Hg, any form of hormonal contraception including CHC can be used. In patients with systolic blood pressures of 140–159 mm Hg or diastolic blood pressures of 90–99 mm Hg, CHC should generally not be used. Nonetheless, in situations where no other contraceptive method is appropriate or acceptable to the patient and blood pressures range from 140–159/90–99 mm Hg, CHC can be used after discussing the risks of cardiovascular disease with the patient. In patients with systolic blood pressure of 160 mm Hg or greater or diastolic blood pressure of 100 mg Hg or greater or with known vascular disease, CHC should not be used. There is limited data on how to counsel patients on antihypertensive therapy with well controlled blood pressure. The theoretical risks of CHC use in this patient population are deemed to outweigh advantages and patients should, therefore, be counseled about progestin-only or non-hormonal contraceptive methods that are considered safer options. Low dose CHC pills have been shown to slightly increase blood pressure when compared to the use of the copper IUD. For this reason, it is recommended patients have blood pressure checked at follow-up visits after starting CHC. If blood pressure is increased at follow-up visits and there is no alternative explanation for the rise in blood pressure, healthcare providers should consider stopping the CHC. Compared to CHC, progestin-only pills do not have a significant effect on blood pressure or cardiovascular disease risk and are an appropriate option for patients with hypertension who wish to be on a pill form of contraception. There is no data to suggest that CHC affects carbohydrate metabolism and therefore, CHC is unlikely to worsen diabetes. Based on available data, no methods of contraception including CHC are contraindicated in patients with uncomplicated diabetes mellitus with or without insulin use. However, in patients with diabetes of more than 20 years duration and/ or with evidence of microvascular disease including retinopathy, nephropathy, or neuropathy, all forms of CHC are contraindicated. In patients with known ischemic heart disease, history of stroke, or complicated valvular heart disease with pulmonary hypertension, risk for atrial fibrillation, and/or a history of subacute bacterial endocarditis, CHC is contraindicated.

In patients with current or prior breast cancer, active gestational trophoblastic disease, and certain types of liver disease, CHC use is inappropriate. In patients with known BRCA1 or BRCA2 mutations or a family history of breast cancer who have not personally been diagnosed with breast cancer, any form of hormonal contraception including CHC can be used. Furthermore, the use of CHC has been shown to have a protective effect against both endometrial and ovarian cancer with longer durations of therapy corresponding to increased risk reduction. For this reason, CHC use may be beneficial in patients with BRCA1 or BRCA2 mutations. To date, multiple studies have demonstrated that CHC pills are not associated with a significant increase in breast cancer risk. In patients with a personal history of breast cancer, CHC should not be used and instead patients should be offered non-hormonal contraception such as the copper IUD. Patients with gynecologic cancer usually undergo treatment that results in sterility. However, in patients awaiting treatment or with preserved fertility after treatment, CHC can be used without restriction. Hormonal contraception is appropriate for patients with a history of gestational trophoblastic disease if certain criteria are met. CHC can be used in patients with a history of gestational trophoblastic disease who have undergone suction curettage and either have decreasing or undetectable hCG levels or have elevated hCG levels but no active disease is present or suspected. In patients with severe decompensated cirrhosis, hepatocellular adenoma, or malignant hepatoma, CHC is contraindicated.

Prior to discussing appropriate contraceptive options with a patient, the clinician should perform a thorough medication and herbal supplement review as certain medications and herbal supplements can alter CHC metabolism and efficacy. Medications such as antimycobacterial and antiepileptic therapies that induce liver enzymes decrease the efficacy of CHC by lowering serum steroid levels. In patients taking hepatic enzyme inducing therapies, CHC is not appropriate due to the increased risk of contraceptive failure. While antimycobacterial drugs such as rifampin and rifabutin are known to affect CHC metabolism, all other broad-spectrum antibiotics, antifungals, and antiparasitic therapies have not been shown to impact CHC efficacy and can be used while patients are taking CHC for contraception. Patients taking antiretroviral therapy can use CHC without concern for decreased efficacy as long as they are not taking fosamprenavir. Providers should be aware that estrogen has been shown to impact the metabolism of lamotrigine therapy. In patients on lamotrigine who start CHC therapy, lamotrigine levels are likely to decrease during CHC use and increase during hormone free intervals. For patients taking lamotrigine, discussion with the patient's neurologist or psychiatrist is recommended prior to initiating CHC. The use of St. John's wort, an herbal supplement used to treat depression, can impact the efficacy of CHC by increasing hepatic enzyme metabolism. For this reason, clinicians should inquire about supplement use and recommend against CHC use in patients using St. John's wort.

General counseling should be provided to all patients prior to initiating CHC. Patients should be informed that if CHC is used accidentally during pregnancy, there is no known harm to the patient, the course of the pregnancy, or the fetus. Although CHC use is contraindicated in patients with familial thrombophilia, there is no evidence to support routine screening of asymptomatic patients for familial thrombophilia prior to initiating CHC. Patients may inquire about CHC's effect on mood. Healthcare providers should assure patients that depressive symptoms have not been shown to be impacted by the use of any type of hormonal contraception, including CHC. Additionally, patients on selective serotonin reuptake inhibitors (SSRIs) or serotonin and norepinephrine reuptake inhibitors (SNRIs) do not need to worry about medication interactions with CHC as there is no evidence to suggest impact of SSRIs or SNRIs on the metabolism of CHC.

For patients utilizing the patch or vaginal ring, proper technique and basic anticipatory guidance should be provided. For patients who chose to use the patch, counseling should include information about how to properly place the patch and potential side effects. Combined hormonal patches are utilized by applying one patch weekly for the first 3 weeks of the menstrual cycle followed by one patch free week. Patients should be instructed to apply the patch to a clean, dry, intact, and non-irritated location on the upper outer arm, abdomen, back, or buttocks that will not be constricted or significantly rubbed by clothing. Additionally, the healthcare provider should emphasize that no creams, lotions, powders, or oils should be used at the site of application as this may lead to issues with patch adherence. When using the patch, patients can exercise, swim, shower, bathe, and go in hot tubs without issue as long as the patch has proper adherence. To ensure proper adherence, the patient should be instructed to check the patch daily to confirm correct attachment is maintained. Patients should be informed that the patch can cause irritation at the site of application and that some patients may experience headache, breast discomfort, and dysmenorrhea with use. Patients who elect to use the vaginal ring should be instructed to place the vaginal ring inside the vaginal canal for 3 weeks. After 3 weeks, the vaginal ring should be removed for a 1-week ring-free interval prior to placing the next vaginal ring. Patients should be advised that the main side effect of the vaginal ring is headache which occurs in 7% of users. Other less common side effects include nausea, leucorrhea, coital problems, weight gain, and device expulsion.

CHC is an effective user dependent contraceptive option that is appropriate for many patients. However, given the increased risk for VTE and cardiovascular disease as well as interactions with other medications, healthcare providers should

Combined Hormonal Contraception Quick Facts

<u>Advantages</u>
Efficacy: >99% with perfect use and 91% with typical use
Protective effect against endometrial and ovarian cancer

<u>Disadvantages</u>
Does not protect against STIs
User dependent
Increased risk of VTE
Increases blood pressure
Cannot be used with medications or herbal supplements that affect liver enzyme function
Affects the metabolism of lamotrigine

<u>Appropriate for the following Medical Conditions</u>
SLE with negative antiphospholipid antibodies and no risk factors for cardiovascular disease
Migraine headache without aura and no risk factors for stroke
Age 40 years and older provided the patient is otherwise healthy, non-smoking, with a normal BMI, and no cardiovascular risk factors
Obesity but otherwise healthy with no cardiovascular risk factors
Patients with blood pressure <140/90 mm Hg
Uncomplicated diabetes mellitus with or without insulin use
Patients with BRCA1 or BRCA2 mutations or a family history of breast cancer who have not personally been diagnosed with breast cancer
Gynecologic cancer while awaiting treatment or with preserved fertility after treatment
History of gestational trophoblastic disease[*]

<u>Contraindications</u>
Smoking at age 35 years or older
History of deep venous thrombosis or pulmonary embolism
Plans for major surgery with anticipated prolonged immobilization
Inflammatory bowel disease with active or extensive disease
Immobilization
Corticosteroid use
Vitamin deficiencies or fluid depletion
Familial thrombophilia
Antiphospholipid syndrome
SLE with positive or unknown antiphospholipid antibodies
Acute or prior superficial venous thrombosis
Migraine headache with aura
Bariatric surgery that impacts absorption of medications[**]
Systolic blood pressure of 140-159 mm Hg[***]
Diastolic blood pressure of 90-99 mm Hg[***]
Systolic blood pressure ≥160 mm Hg or diastolic blood pressure ≥ 100 mm Hg
Known vascular disease
Diabetes mellitus for more than 20 years duration and/or with microvascular complications
Ischemic heart disease
History of stroke
Complicated valvular heart disease
Current or history of breast cancer
Active gestational trophoblastic disease
Severe decompensated cirrhosis
Hepatocellular adenoma
Malignant hepatoma

[*]After suction curettage and with decreasing or undetectable hCG levels or elevated hCG levels but no active disease is present or suspected
[**]Contraindication to pill form of CHC only. Can use non-oral forms of CHC such as patches or vaginal rings.
[***]If no other contraceptive method is acceptable to the patient, CHC can be used after discussing the risks of cardiovascular disease

Fig. 12.8 Combined hormonal contraception quick facts

ensure their patient has no medical contraindications to CHC use prior to discussing CHC as a contraceptive option. In the clinical case, our patient has a history of migraine with aura which is a contraindication to CHC use due to increased risk of stroke. Our patient should be advised that CHC is not appropriate and alternative contraceptive options should be discussed (Fig. 12.8).

12.6.4 *Barrier Contraception*

Barrier contraception is a broad category of user dependent non-hormonal contraception that includes not only external and internal condoms but also diaphragms and cervical caps. For the purposes of this chapter, we will use barrier contraception to refer to only external formerly known as male and internal formerly known as female condoms as the other forms of barrier contraception are not widely used. External and internal condoms are the only form of contraception that protect against STIs. When used correctly, the external and internal condom can protect against HIV and herpes simplex virus. The exception to the protection against STIs is the use of the non-latex lambskin external condom. The external condom comes in two different forms: latex and non-latex. The latex external condom is the most effective at preventing pregnancy and protecting against STIs. The latex condom should not be used in patients who are sensitive or allergic to latex as these individuals may experience allergic contact dermatitis, irritation, or even anaphylactic symptoms when exposed to latex containing products. Additionally, the latex condom can only be used with water-based lubricants like lubricating jellies (i.e., K-Y Jelly). The use of oil-based lubricants can damage latex condoms and therefore, decrease efficacy. The non-latex external condom is made of either polyisoprene, polyurethane, or lamb intestine commonly referred to as lambskin. The polyisoprene external condom is made from a synthetic version of the sap of the hevea tree and is as strong as latex. The advantages of the polyisoprene external condom include increased stretch which lends to less slippage or breakage compared to other types of external condoms. The disadvantage of the polyisoprene external condom is increased thickness which decreases heat transfer between partners which results in decreased sensitivity. The polyurethane condom is derived from a type of plastic that does not stretch well. This results in an increased risk of slippage and reported higher breakage rates compared to other types of external condoms. The benefits of the polyurethane external condom include being thinner than most other external condoms which allows for increased transmission of heat and enhanced sensitivity during sexual intercourse, having little to no smell, and ability to be used with oil-based lubricants. The lambskin external condom is made from lamb intestines which allows for good transmission of heat and enhanced sensitivity between partners. The major disadvantage of the lambskin external condom is it lacks protection against STIs and is therefore, only effective as a method of contraception. The internal condom consists of two flexible rings, one that is inserted into the vagina and one that remains outside the vagina. The internal condom can be inserted up to 8 hours prior to sexual intercourse to provide hormonal free contraception. The main disadvantages of the internal condom include discomfort, feeling the two rings during intercourse, and difficulties with proper placement.

The efficacy of barrier contraception (internal and external condoms) varies significantly with typical use versus perfect use. With typical use, the external condom is 82% effective in preventing pregnancy. However, only 2 in 100 patients will become pregnant within the first year with perfect use of the external condom.

Barrier Contraception Quick Facts

General Information
Internal Condom Efficacy: 95% with perfect use and 79% with typical use
External Condom Efficacy: 98% with perfect use and 82% with typical use
Non-hormonal
Protect against STIs[*]
No absolute contraindications to use

Internal Condom
Discomfort before and during intercourse
Difficulties with proper placement

Latex External Condom
Cannot be used with oil-based lubricants
Contraindicated in patients with a latex sensitivity or allergy

Polyisoprene External Condom
Increased stretch lends to less slippage or breakage
Increased thickness lends to decreased heat transfer and sensitivity during sexual intercourse

Polyurethane External Condom
Thinner which lends to increased heat transfer and sensitivity during sexual intercourse
Little to no smell
Can be used with oil-based lubricants
Poor stretch lends to increased risk of slippage and breakage

Lambskin External Condom
Good transmission of heat and enhanced sensitivity during sexual intercourse
No protection against STIs – only provides contraception

[*]Except the external non-latex lambskin condom

Fig. 12.9 Barrier contraception quick facts

Patients who use the internal condom with perfect use experience pregnancy at a rate of 5 in 100 patients within the first year of use. With typical use of the female condom 21 in 100 patients will become pregnant within the first year of use. Healthcare providers should recognize the user dependent nature of this contraceptive method and ensure patients can perform proper technique when using either the external or internal condoms in order to strive for perfect use.

Given the low efficacy rates with typical use, barrier contraception may not be the best option for our patient in the clinical case. That being said, the use of barrier contraception should be discussed as a possible option given it is a hormone free contraceptive method that can protect against STIs without absolute medical contraindications to use. If our patient elects to use barrier contraception, the healthcare provider should ensure she knows proper technique, avoids oil-based lubricants if using latex condoms, and is aware that the lambskin condom does not protect against STIs (Fig. 12.9).

12.6.5 *Fertility Awareness*

Fertility awareness is a user dependent hormone free method of contraception that centers on correctly recognizing the fertile days, typically between days 8 and 19 of the menstrual cycle. Patients may use changes in cervical secretions or body temperature in addition to calendar days to monitor their menstrual cycles for periods

Fertility Awareness Quick Facts

Advantages	**Disadvantages**
Non-hormonal	User dependent
No medical conditions with	Efficacy: 76%
absolute contraindication to use	Does not protect against STIs

Fig. 12.10 Fertility awareness quick facts

of fertility. During fertile days patients who practice fertility awareness will abstain from sexual intercourse or use internal or external condoms to avoid pregnancy. With typical use, 24 of 100 patients will become pregnant within the first year of using fertility awareness, the lowest efficacy of all the contraceptive methods discussed in this chapter. Apart from the low efficacy rate, the disadvantages of this method of contraception include no protection against STIs and difficulty of use in patients with irregular menstrual cycles. Additionally, patients who take lithium, tricyclic antidepressants, anti-anxiety medications, and certain antibiotics and anti-inflammatory drugs that impact fertility signs or cycle regularity may be at increased risk of pregnancy using this contraceptive method. The advantage of fertility awareness is there are no medical conditions with absolute contraindications to its use.

A brief overview of this method should be included in comprehensive contraception counseling with our patient in the clinical case. However, the healthcare provider should emphasize the low efficacy rate of fertility awareness and spend time discussing more efficacious options with our patient (Fig. 12.10).

12.6.6 Conclusion

All contraceptive options are medically appropriate for our patient in the clinical case with the exception of CHC. After discussing the various contraceptive options, healthcare providers should be prepared for patients to ask for a recommendation. In our patient case, the most efficacious user independent reversible options should be recommended first which would be the LARC methods.

Contraception is an important component of care for patients with child bearing potential that can be offered in the primary care setting. In order to provide appropriate counseling, primary care providers should be well versed in the efficacy, benefits, and risks including contraindications of the various contraceptive methods available. When discussing contraceptive options with patients, clinicians must avoid expressing their own biases and preferences unless solicited. Patients with child bearing potential should be encouraged to elect the contraceptive method that is not just medically appropriate but also aligns most with their values and preferences.

Suggested Reading

1. Colquitt CW, Martin TS. Contraceptive methods: a review of nonbarrier and barrier products. J Pharm Pract. 2017;30(1):130–5.
2. Curtis KM, Tepper NK, Jatlaoui TC, Berry-Bibee E, Horton LG, Zapata LB, et al. US medical eligibility criteria for contraceptive use, 2016. Morb Mortal Wkly Rep Recomm Rep. 2016;65(3):1–103.
3. Jacobstein R, Polis CB. Progestin-only contraception: injectables and implants. Best Pract Res Clin Obstet Gynaecol. 2014;28(6):795–806.
4. American College of Obstetricians and Gynecologists. ACOG practice bulletin no. 208: benefits and risks of sterilization. Obstet Gynecol. 2019;133(3):e194–207.
5. Curtis KM, Peipert JF. Long-acting reversible contraception. N Engl J Med. 2017;376(5):461–8.
6. American College of Obstetricians and Gynecologists. ACOG Practice Bulletin No. 206: use of hormonal contraception in women with coexisting medical conditions. Obstet Gynecol. 2019;2:128–50.
7. Madden T, Blumenthal P. Contraceptive vaginal ring. Clin Obstet Gynecol. 2007;50(4):878–85.
8. Galzote RM, Rafie S, Teal R, Mody SK. Transdermal delivery of combined hormonal contraception: a review of the current literature. Int J Women's Health. 2017;9:315.
9. Trussell J, Guthrie K. Choosing a contraceptive: efficacy, safety, and personal considerations. In: Hatcher RA, Trussell J, Nelson AL, Cates W, Stewart FH, Kowal D, editors. Contraceptive technology. 19th revised ed. New York: Ardent Media, Inc; 2007. p. 19–47.

Chapter 13
Non-Ob Treatment of the Pregnant Patient

Madison Malone and Molly Heublein

Ms. K is a 36-year-old woman with a history of depression who presents to your clinic for routine follow-up. She mentions she is thinking about becoming pregnant soon.

Pre-conception counseling

The goal of pre-conception counseling is to optimize pre-pregnancy health and minimize modifiable risk factors for complications. Pre-pregnancy care may improve reproductive outcomes and should be a routine part of medical care for any person with the potential to become pregnant, inclusive of all gender identities and presentations. Counseling should occur multiple times over the reproductive lifespan of a patient, regardless of whether a patient is using contraception or planning for pregnancy, and adapt to a patient's changing health status and reproductive goals. In the primary care setting, it may be appropriate to incorporate elements of pre-conception counseling to the annual physical, as these encounters have similar goals of establishing healthy habits, reviewing management of chronic diseases, and screening for health-related behaviors. Using a question such as "Are you thinking of becoming pregnant this year?" may be helpful in beginning your discussion. Using open-ended questions can help tailor the discussion regarding birth control options, pre-pregnancy counseling, and abortion counseling to a particular patient. For patients who take a known teratogenic medication for a chronic medical condition, or for patients with newly diagnosed, poorly controlled conditions (i.e., new diabetes with elevated blood sugar), pre-conception counseling is an especially important forum for discussing the risks of pregnancy prior to medication alteration or disease control.

In conducting pre-pregnancy counseling, a helpful approach can be to ask a series of questions to guide the patient-interview and recommendations:

M. Malone (✉)· M. Heublein
Department of Medicine, University of California San Francisco, San Francisco, USA
e-mail: madisone.malone@ucsf.edu; Molly.Heublin@ucsf.edu

M. Mahmoudi (ed.), *Common Cases in Women's Primary Care Clinics*,
https://doi.org/10.1007/978-3-031-48569-5_13

1. *How do the patient's medical conditions impact pregnancy?*
2. *How does pregnancy impact the patients' medical conditions?*
3. *What medications might need to be changed or started?*

Universal counseling recommendations

While certain aspects of counseling may be highly individualized, many recommendations are broadly applicable and reinforce a healthy lifestyle such as regular moderate-intensity exercise (30 minutes per day, 5 days per week) and eating a well-balanced diet. Patients attempting pregnancy or currently pregnant should be counseled to avoid foods high in mercury such as bigeye tuna, king mackerel, marlin, orange roughy, shark, swordfish, tilefish, and white albacore tuna. Physicians should use the history and physical exam to assess for risk of pre-existing nutritional deficiencies and test for deficiencies as appropriate. Risk factors include low BMI, history of gastric bypass, and gastrointestinal disorders, among others.

Providers should review medication lists thoroughly, including use of the over-the-counter medications and supplements. The FDA and ACOG, as well as several other independent organizations, have established guidelines regarding the safety of various medications during pregnancy. Medications with known teratogenic effects should be stopped. All patients should be started on folic acid supplementation during the pre-conception period, ideally 3 months prior to conception, to reduce the risk of fetal neural tube defects. For patients at average risk, 400mcg per day of folic acid is acceptable. For patients at higher-than-average risk, such as those with seizure disorders or prior pregnancy with a neural tube defect, 4 mg of folic acid daily is recommended. Patients should be encouraged to take a daily prenatal vitamin—most prenatal vitamins contain adequate folic acid and vitamin use is associated with decreased risk of miscarriage. Prenatal vitamins should include at least the minimum quantities of recommended micronutrients for pregnant people (Table 13.1).

A review of a patient's family and medical history may also be helpful in offering pre-conception genetic testing for patients at risk. In general, at-risk populations

Table 13.1 Recommended prenatal vitamins

Nutrient	Recommended daily amount	Need in pregnancy
Calcium	1000 mg	Fetal bone and teeth development
Choline	450 mg	Fetal brain development
Folic acid (vitamin B9)	400 mcg	Fetal brain and spinal cord development
Iron	27 mg	Facilitates increased maternal blood volume
Iodine	220 mcg	Fetal brain development
Vitamin A	770 mcg	Fetal skin, bone, and eye development
Vitamin B12	2.6 mcg	Facilitates increased maternal blood volume and aids in fetal nervous system development
Vitamin C	85 mg	Fetal gum, teeth, and bone development
Vitamin D	600 IU	Fetal skin, bone, and eye development

include patients with Ashkenazi Jewish, French-Canadian, or Cajun decent. All patients considering pregnancy should be offered carrier screening for cystic fibrosis.

Patients should be routinely screened for hepatitis B and C prior to conception, and routine STI testing should be obtained per current guidelines. Routine cancer screening such as cervical cancer screening should be up to date. Review of current immunization status is also critical. Prior to conception, patients should be offered a yearly influenza vaccine, HPV vaccination (not currently recommended during pregnancy), and at least one lifetime Tdap vaccine. The CDC recommends delaying pregnancy after rubella or varicella vaccination at least 1 month before trying to conceive.

Couples should also take steps to prevent infections known to cause fetal birth defects, especially Zika virus. CDC guidelines recommend that male partners traveling to areas with high Zika prevalence should delay attempting pregnancy with a partner for at least 3 months. Female partners should avoid pregnancy for a minimum of 2 months.

Her current medications include sertraline 150 mg daily and acetaminophen as needed.

Chronic disease optimization

Chronic disease management is especially important in pre-conception counseling, as improving control of pre-existing chronic conditions may reduce fetal and maternal complications during pregnancy. Care should be given to consider both how pre-existing conditions may impact pregnancy and how pregnancy may impact pre-existing conditions.

Pre-existing diabetes prior to pregnancy, or pregestational diabetes, is a known risk factor for congenital anomalies. Poor blood sugar control during pregnancy may increase fetal risk of macrosomia and birth complications related to large gestational size. Achieving an A1c < 6.5% prior to conception may reduce these risks. Metformin is a commonly used medication in reproductive-age patients, whether for PCOS or diabetes, and is safe to continue in pregnancy. However, for patients with poorly controlled diabetes on metformin alone, insulin should be initiated.

Pre-existing hypertension, also called chronic hypertension, should also be well controlled with a goal of normotension (SBP < 130, DBP < 80) to reduce risk of vasculopathy, intrauterine growth restriction, and preeclampsia. Patients may need cross-titration of medications given the known teratogenic effects of some antihypertensive medications (i.e., ACE inhibitors and ARBs). Nifedipine, labetalol, and hydralazine are typical drugs of choice.

Untreated thyroid disease, particularly hypothyroidism, poses risks even early in pregnancy including spontaneous abortion, preterm birth, placental abruption, preeclampsia, and fetal death. It is recommended to screen for hypothyroidism in patients with symptoms or risk factors, rather than as part of routine lab testing. Patients with known and treated hypothyroidism should consult with an endocrinologist or a maternal/fetal medicine specialist regarding management of thyroid medications during pregnancy, as thyroid hormone requirements may increase

30–50%. Additionally, thyroid function tests should be interpreted using trimester-specific reference ranges.

Maintaining a BMI within the normal range prior to conception may reduce fetal and maternal complications during pregnancy. Both low and high BMI are associated with complications. In addition to obesity-related complications in non-pregnant patients such as increased risk of thromboembolic events, hypertension, diabetes, stroke, and heart disease, obese pregnant patients are at additional risk of miscarriage, preterm delivery, and cesarean delivery. Patients with low BMI are at increased risk for infants with low birth weights.

Psychiatric disease, possibly the most common chronic condition affecting young reproductive-age patients, should also be optimized prior to conception. It is estimated that 10–16% of pregnant women meet criteria for depression and up to 70% have depressive symptoms.

Management of psychotropic medications during pregnancy is challenging for multiple reasons. Pregnant patients are routinely left out of clinical trials, and over-all risk of most medications during pregnancy is therefore unknown. Studies exploring these topics are additionally limited by "confounding by indication." Further, researchers are unable to include pregnant patients in most randomized control trials due to ethical concerns. However, there is also substantial risk involved in discontinuing these medications. Untreated maternal depression is associated with adverse outcomes including low birth weight, poor fetal growth, and postnatal complications. Therefore, discussions regarding medication changes should include detailed risk/benefit discussions with each individual patient. SSRIs and a few other psychotropics are commonly prescribed by primary care physicians and will therefore be the focus of this discussion (Table 13.2).

Briefly regarding other psychotropic classes, all antipsychotic medications are FDA class C with exception of clozapine (Clozaril) which is class B. Typical (first generation) antipsychotics have a larger reproductive safety profile, and no significant teratogenic effects have been associated with use of chlorpromazine (Thorazine), haloperidol (Haldol), or perphenazine (Trilafon) during pregnancy. All benzodiazepines are class D or X; alprazolam (Xanax), chlordiazepoxide (Librium), and diazepam have been associated with neonatal lethargy, poor respiratory effort, feeding difficulties, and hypothermia if benzodiazepine use occurred shortly before delivery. However, use of benzodiazepines during pregnancy is generally not considered teratogenic. Mood stabilizers including carbamazepine, valproic acid, lithium, and lamotrigine are all class C and D. Given the complex nature of these medications and the diseases they treat, management of these medications during pregnancy should involve a psychiatrist when possible.

Screening for substance use

Screening for substance use, including caffeine, tobacco, alcohol, and other substances is an important aspect of pre-conception counseling and should be discussed routinely. Moderate caffeine consumption (<200 mg per day, approximately 2 cups of coffee) is unlikely to pose increased risk during pregnancy. In contrast, current recommendations advise against any tobacco or alcohol use given established risks of these substances. Tobacco use is associated with numerous fetal and maternal

Table 13.2 Psychotropic medication safety during pregnancy

Psychotropic medication	Summary of evidence	FDA	ACOG recommendations
SSRIs	Use of SSRIs late in pregnancy may be associated with mild transient neonatal symptoms including central nervous symptom, motor, respiratory, or gastrointestinal signs and neonatal pulmonary hypertension		
Sertraline (Zoloft)	Based on animal and human studies, sertraline is not thought to increase risk of congenital anomalies. Inconsistent results regarding risk of neonatal pulmonary hypertension	C	Individualized counseling recommended
Citalopram (Celexa) Escitalopram (Lexapro)	Risk of transient neonatal symptoms	C	
Fluoxetine (Prozac)	Based on animal and human studies, fluoxetine is not thought to increase risk of congenital anomalies. Inconsistent results regarding fetal heart defects, neonatal pulmonary hypertension Long-term studies suggest exposure does not adversely affect neurodevelopmental outcomes	C	
Fluvoxamine	Based on animal and human studies, fluvoxamine is not thought to increase risk of congenital anomalies. No specific reports of neonatal pulmonary hypertension	C	
Paroxetine (Paxil)	Inconsistent association with fetal cardiovascular anomalies	D	Discontinuation prior to conception; consider fetal echocardiography if exposure occurs during early pregnancy
Other antidepressants			
Amitriptyline	Interference of embryo development in animal studies. Human studies have not found increased rates of birth defects	C	Most tricyclics are considered safe during pregnancy and lactation (with exception of doxepin)
Nortriptyline	No increased rate of birth defects in human studies	C	
Buspirone (Buspar)	Animal studies have not shown increased rates of congenital anomalies; however, there are no controlled human data	B	
Bupropion (Wellbutrin)	Animal studies have not shown increased rates of congenital anomalies. Human studies have had inconsistent results regarding risk of cardiac defects	B	
Duloxetine	Based on animal and human studies, duloxetine is not thought to increase risk of congenital anomalies	C	

(continued)

Table 13.2 (continued)

Psychotropic medication	Summary of evidence	FDA	ACOG recommendations
Venlafaxine	Not thought to increase risk of congenital anomalies. Inconsistent associations between exposure and malformations in human studies	C	
Mirtazapine	Based on animal and human studies, mirtazapine is not thought to increase risk of congenital anomalies	C	
Trazodone	Based on animal and (limited) human studies in pregnancy, trazodone is not thought to increase risk of congenital anomalies	C	

SSRI = selective serotonin reuptake inhibitor
FDA classification: *A* = controlled studies show no risk; *B* = no evidence of risk in humans; *C* = risk cannot be ruled out; *D* = positive evidence of risk; *X* = contraindicated in pregnancy
Summary of evidence per Reprotox database

complications including increased fetal mortality and even childhood asthma and obesity. Alcohol use during pregnancy can cause fetal effects at any stage of pregnancy. In severe cases, alcohol exposure can cause fetal alcohol spectrum disorders and even cause lifelong cognitive impairment. While there is no safe level of alcohol use during pregnancy, it is generally considered that heavier alcohol use poses most risk. Cannabis is the most-used substance in pregnancy though its risk profile may be similar to that of tobacco. Current guidelines recommend discontinuation of cannabis use in pregnant patients, even if cannabis was used pre-pregnancy for medicinal purposes.

She has an allergy listed in her chart as "rash to penicillin."

Approach to reported penicillin allergy in people with reproductive potential

Reported penicillin allergy is known to be associated with increased morbidity in pregnant people, including increased risk of cesarean delivery and increase in total length of hospitalization. This is likely due to delayed or alternative treatment for pregnant people with known group B strep colonization, a known risk factor for neonatal sepsis. However, only a small proportion of people with a reported allergy have a true allergy to penicillin. Therefore, all people planning to become pregnant should be referred for penicillin allergy testing, before or during pregnancy.

Upon her next visit to clinic, she is 6 weeks pregnant. She has not yet had her first visit with her OB/Gyn, however is experiencing several bothersome symptoms and asks how best to manage them.

Evaluation and treatment of common conditions in early pregnancy

Early in pregnancy, prior to a patient's first Ob/Gyn appointment, it is common for people to present to their primary care doctor for help with managing both pregnancy-related symptoms and other common complaints unrelated to pregnancy.

Nausea and vomiting

Nausea is a common symptom during early pregnancy that can often be managed with lifestyle modifications and over-the-counter medications. However, nausea occurring before 4 weeks estimated gestation or onset after 12 weeks should be investigated further for possible pathologic causes such as molar pregnancy. In severe cases, nausea and vomiting may progress to hyperemesis gravidarum, sometimes requiring hospital admission for IV anti-emetics, IV fluids, and enteral tube feeding. Early treatment can prevent progression and complications such as poor fetal weight gain and malnutrition.

Assessment of the patient should include evaluation of volume status including vital signs and orthostatic blood pressure measurements. On exam, it may be helpful to assess moisture of mucus membranes and skin turgor as part of your volume examination. If there is evidence of severe dehydration, referral to the emergency department is often necessary.

Universal recommendations for treatment include lifestyle modifications such as eating frequent, small meals and substituting foods with potent taste or smell with more bland foods. For mild symptoms, daily pyridoxine (vitamin B6) is first line. Over-the-counter antihistamines such as doxylamine and diphenhydramine are safe and effective though can often cause significant drowsiness, limiting their usefulness during the day. Natural ginger can often be helpful, in the form of tea, gum, or capsules. For refractory symptoms, metoclopramide is recommended. Ondansetron can also be used, but cautious use is recommended during the first trimester.

Constipation

Evaluation for constipation should include an assessment of hydration and exercise habits. Patients with a history of constipation may have worsened symptoms during pregnancy. Lifestyle recommendations are first line and include increasing hydration, daily exercise, and increasing natural dietary fiber. For mild symptoms, osmotic laxatives are preferred, such as Metamucil, docusate, or milk of magnesia. For refractory symptoms, stimulant laxatives such as senna or bisacodyl are often effective.

Headaches

As in any patient, red flag symptoms for headaches include neurologic changes, fevers, thunderclap onset, associated hypertension, or non-responsiveness to medications. In later pregnancy (after 20 weeks gestation) headaches can be a sign of preeclampsia and need urgent intervention. However, for mild headaches without red flag symptoms, numerous safe treatment options are available. Ensure adequate hydration and sleep and investigate provoking factors. For stress-associated headaches, relaxation techniques can be useful. For mild symptoms, magnesium oxide 400 mg, Tylenol, and small caffeinated beverages are first line. Metoclopramide and amitriptyline are safe second line options. NSAIDs should generally be avoided, especially in the third trimester.

Over-the-counter medications

Over-the-counter medications are commonly used by pregnant and non-pregnant patients for a variety of mild symptoms. Knowledge of which medications are safe during pregnancy is a critical part of pre-conception and pregnancy counseling (Table 13.3)

Table 13.3 Safety of common over-the-counter medications during pregnancy

Class	FDA pregnancy risk classification by trimester
Pain reliever	
Acetaminophen (Tylenol)	B/B/B
Aspirin	D/D/D
NSAIDs (ibuprofen/Advil, naproxen/Aleve, Motrin)	B/B/D
Antihistamines	
Pseudoephedrine (Pseudoephed)	B
Guaifenesin	C
Dextromethorphan	C
Diphenhydramine (Benadryl)	B
Loratadine (Claritin)	B
Fexofenadine (Allegra)	C
Antidiarrheals	
Bismuth subsalicylate (Pepto Bismol)	C/C/D
Loperamide (Imodium)	B/B/B
Atropine/diphenoxylate (Lomotil)	C/C/C
Antacids	
Aluminum hydroxide/magnesium hydroxide (Maalox)	B
Calcium carbonate (Tums)	C
Simethicone (Mylanta)	C
Famotidine (Pepcid)	B
Anti-emetics	
Meclizine (Antivert)	B

FDA classification: *A* = controlled studies show no risk; *B* = no evidence of risk in humans; *C* = risk cannot be ruled out; *D* = positive evidence of risk; *X* = contraindicated in pregnancy

Ms. K has an uncomplicated pregnancy and delivers a healthy full-term baby. She returns to the clinic at 6 months post-partum after discharging from her OB's clinic for a routine exam.

Post-partum visit

Obstetricians will typically conclude their care of the post-partum patient between 6 and 12 weeks post-partum. Therefore, it is important for primary care physicians to be aware of how a patient's pregnancy may continue to affect them in the months after delivery.

The post-partum visit should be similar to an annual visit, including an overall assessment of the patient's physical, psychological, and social well-being. Begin with open-ended questions to tailor the discussion to your patient.

Review medications with the patient carefully and ensure ongoing adherence to daily prenatal vitamins for the duration breastfeeding. Obtain a detailed understanding of complications that arose during pregnancy. In the setting of extreme physiologic changes that occur during pregnancy, any complications or conditions that arose during the pregnancy may give insight to previously undiagnosed medical conditions and the patient's risk for developing future conditions. For patients who developed gestational hypertension, preeclampsia, or gestational diabetes, they should be counseled that these conditions increase their lifetime risk of cardiometabolic disease. It is also important to discuss future pregnancy planning to tailor discussions regarding contraception management. Patients should be advised that pregnancy can still occur while breastfeeding.

In addition to a thorough physical exam, your evaluation should include assessment of blood pressure, A1c, and, only if significant anemia occurred during pregnancy, complete blood counts. If these are normal, patients can return to routine hypertension and diabetes screening.

Post-partum depression and anxiety are common, especially in patients with a history of psychiatric illness. Screening for post-partum depression with PHQ-9 or the Edinburg Postnatal Depression Scale is a critical part of the post-partum assessment and should be repeated at each visit for at least 1 year post-partum. The peripartum and post-partum periods are also high-risk times for interpersonal violence, and an assessment of a patients' safety and risk for interpersonal or domestic violence is essential.

13.1 Conclusion

Pre-conception care is a fundamental part of primary care, and preparing for pregnancy can greatly improve both maternal and fetal health. At each annual visit, physicians are encouraged to incorporate pre-conception counseling for patients with reproductive potential. Use of open-ended questions about plans for pregnancy or pregnancy prevention can guide counseling. During pre-conception counseling, consider: How will pregnancy impact medical conditions and how will medical conditions impact pregnancy? Review each patient's current health status and encourage good lifestyle habits such as healthy diet and exercise. Control of diabetes, hypertension, thyroid disease, and obesity prior to pregnancy leads to better maternal and fetal outcomes. Stop or attempt to reduce alcohol consumption, drug use, and cannabis use, even if used for medicinal purposes. A thorough review of current medications to assess for safety in pregnancy is critical. For medications that have little data regarding safety during pregnancy, a detailed risk/benefit discussion about continuation or discontinuation should occur; this applies to many psychiatric medications. In counseling, include education regarding the safety of over-the-counter medications and supplements. All patients should be started on a prenatal vitamin and folate supplementation, ideally prior to conception. Primary care physicians should be equipped to help patients manage common symptoms that occur early in pregnancy prior to the first obstetrics visit, especially first trimester nausea and vomiting. After pregnancy, providers should review complications which occurred during pregnancy that may confer later-life risk for cardiovascular disease.

Routine screening for post-partum depression, anxiety, and interpersonal violence is critical.

Suggested Reading

1. Armstrong C. ACOG guidelines on psychiatric medication use during pregnancy and lactation. Am Fam Physician. 2008;78(6):772.
2. Black RA, Hill DA. Over-the-counter medications in pregnancy. Am Fam Physician. 2003;67(12):2517–24.
3. Chen, X, Williams PN, Watto MF, Garbitelli B. #305 obstetrics for internist. [Internet] The curbsiders internal medicine podcast; 2021 Nov 5 [cited 2023 April 18]. Available from: https://thecurbsiders.com/episode-list
4. Desai SH, Kaplan MS, Chen Q, Macy EM. Morbidity in pregnant women associated with unverified penicillin allergies, antibiotic use, and group B streptococcus infections. Perm J. 2017;6(21):16–080.
5. Gregory DS, Wu V, Tuladhar P. The pregnant patient: managing common acute medical problems. Am Fam Physician. 2018;98(9):595–602.
6. American College of Obstetricians and Gynecologists. Nutrition during pregnancy. ACOG frequently asked questions No. 001. 2022 March.
7. American College of Obstetricians and Gynecologists. Optimizing postpartum care. ACOG Committee Opinion No. 736. Obstet Gynecol. 2018;131:e140–50.
8. American College of Obstetricians and Gynecologists. Prepregnancy counseling. ACOG Committee Opinion No. 762. Obstet Gynecol. 2019;133:e78–89.
9. Reprotox [Internet]. Apple valley (MN): The reproductive toxicology center, [cited 2023 April 18]. Available from: https://reprotox.org

Chapter 14
Menopause

Sondos Al Sad

14.1 Case Presentation

Ms. RO is a Somali widower noted to be 61 years old in her medical chart. Presenting with hot flashes and irregular menses for the past 6 months, she reports two heavy periods lasting 11 days compared to her 6-day periods. She reported her periods were regular until the last couple of years, they changed from every 26 days to every 33–35 days. She is G6P6006, all uncomplicated vaginal births. She reported mild urge incontinence recently, she states, "It is typical for moms to leak." She is not currently sexually active. When asked about menstruating to this age, she noted that her true age is 57 years, but her date of birth was modified for immigration purposes. She does not know much about the menstrual history of females in her family but denies any problems with cancers or reproductions in first- or second-degree relatives. Her biggest concern is prolonged menstrual bleeding as it is interfering with her religious rituals. Her BMI is 32.4, blood pressure is 119/82.

14.2 Introduction

Menopause is the permanent cessation of menses resulting from the loss of ovarian follicular function. It can occur naturally due to aging or induced due to iatrogenic or pathological reasons. The average age for menopause is around 52 years of age. All women who survive past midlife are destined to experience menopause but each in their own unique way depending on their life course and determinants of health.

S. Al Sad (✉)
Family and Community Medicine, Women's Health Primary Care, San Francisco, USA
e-mail: Sondos.Alsad@ucsf.edu

© The Author(s), under exclusive license to Springer Nature
Switzerland AG 2024
M. Mahmoudi (ed.), *Common Cases in Women's Primary Care Clinics*,
https://doi.org/10.1007/978-3-031-48569-5_14

Table 14.1 Menopause terminology

Term	Definition
Natural menopause	Spontaneous cessation of menses for 12 months after 40 years of age
Induced menopause	Menopause is caused by bilateral oophorectomy or secondary to chemotherapy or radiation therapy, with subsequent ovarian damage
Premature menopause	Menopause occurs before age 40 (induced or spontaneous)
Primary ovarian insufficiency (POI) (*previously known as premature ovarian failure*)	A continuum of impaired ovarian function (intermittent to permanent) usually with extended periods of amenorrhea in women younger than age 40
Perimenopause (*replacing the term climacteric*)	It begins with the onset of intermenstrual cycle irregularities (± 7 days) and/or other menopause-related symptoms and extends beyond the FMP to include the 12 months after menopause, thus lasting 1 year longer than the menopause transition. They are the most symptomatic years
Menopause transition	The span of time that begins with the onset of intermenstrual cycle irregularities (± 7 days) and/or other menopause-related symptoms and extends through menopause (the FMP)
Final menopause period (FMP)	The menstrual period is followed by 12 consecutive months of amenorrhea
Postmenopausal	No menses for 12 consecutive months
Genitourinary syndrome of menopause (replaced atrophic vaginitis/vaginal atrophy)	A constellation of symptoms impacting vulvovaginal tissues and pelvic floor.

Women are living longer with a life expectancy of mid-eighties with more than 50 million women worldwide reaching menopause annually.

While menopause is a natural event that impacts almost half of the population worldwide, it is a noteworthy signal of a new phase in life, and a priceless opportunity to reassess health status and goals. An insightful understanding of the physiologic changes, evidence-based management of menopause symptoms, and disease risk reduction are essential in providing optimal healthcare (see Table 14.1).

14.3 Physiology of Menopause

The menstrual cycle is orchestrated through a sophisticated interplay of the hypothalamic-pituitary-ovarian axis (Fig. 14.1). Loss of ovarian follicles with aging leads to the menopause transition and eventually to the cessation of menses. Follicular loss begins in utero; women are born with 1 to 2 million follicles. By the menopause transition, a few hundred to a few thousand follicles remain.

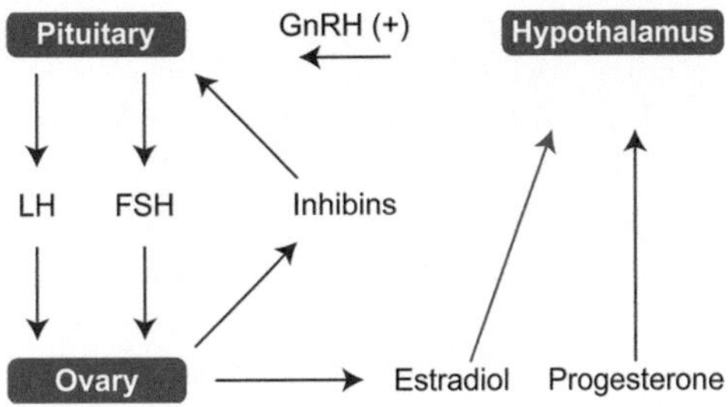

Fig. 14.1 Hypothalamic-pituitary-ovarian axis (*GnRH* Gonadotropin-releasing hormone, *LH* Luteinizing hormone, *FSH* Follicular stimulating hormone)

14.3.1 Endocrine Characteristics of Menopausal Transition (Perimenopause)

Ovarian

Major ovarian hormones are steroids (estradiol and progesterone) and peptides (inhibins and activins). Estradiol and inhibins are secretory products of the predominant ovarian cells (granulosa cells) and progesterone is produced by the corpus luteum.

Estradiol is primarily produced by predominant follicles and as the ovarian follicular function decreases its circulating levels decrease. Estrone is derived primarily from the metabolism of estradiol and from peripheral aromatization of androstenedione to estrone in adipose tissue and muscle. Estrone predominates menopausal transition as estradiol levels decline. Estrogens have three receptors (α, β, and G-protein coupled receptors) present in the ovaries, nervous system, breasts, cardiovascular system, bone, soft tissue, and many others.

Inhibin A and inhibin B are major ovarian peptides involved in pituitary feedback. Inhibin A is secreted in parallel with estradiol and progesterone and fluctuates during the menstrual cycle being at its highest peak during the luteal phase. Inhibin B levels fluctuate during a cycle exhibiting a midcycle peak and lowest concentrations during the luteal phase. Inhibin B and FSH form a closed-loop negative feedback system during the follicular phase, with the levels of inhibin B fine-tuning pituitary FSH regulation. Thus, both ovarian estradiol and inhibins contribute to the pituitary-ovarian axis.

Circulating androgens are produced by the ovaries, the adrenal glands, and through peripheral conversion of circulating androstenedione and dehydroepiandrosterone (DHEA) to testosterone. A decrease in testosterone levels is found to be transient and they normalize after menopause. The menopause transition is associated with a drop in the sex hormone-binding globulin (SHBG) levels. Reduced SHBG levels alter the ratio of testosterone to SHBG (i.e., free androgen index). The free androgen index rises maximally during the 2 years before the FMP.

Anti-Mullerian hormone (AMH) has been identified as a marker of ovarian reserve. It is exclusively produced by the granulosa cells of preantral and small ovarian follicles and reflects the transition of resting primordial follicles to growing follicles. AMH levels have been used primarily to assess ovarian reserve in women seeking fertility assessment. Interestingly, AMH levels have shown an age-related continual decline to undetectable levels 5 years prior to menopause. Also, the FSH-inhibin B ratio has been reported to be inversely correlated with AMH, and measuring both might be useful to characterize menopause status. More standardized assays and data from populations outside fertility testing are needed to expand the AMH role in the characterization of menopause.

Antral follicle count, as determined by ultrasound evaluation of the ovary, is of limited use in primary care settings.

Ovarian aging manifestations (see Fig. 14.2):

- Ovaries decrease in size (e.g., not easily visualized on an ultrasound).
- Substantial decrease in the number of follicles.
- Decrease in the ovarian production of inhibin and AMH.
- Remaining follicles respond poorly to elevated FSH and LH.

Pituitary

Relevant pituitary hormones are follicle-stimulating hormone (FSH) and—to a lesser extent—luteinizing hormone (LH). Low estradiol signals the pituitary gland to increase FSH levels, which represents a commonly measured clinical sign in early reproductive aging. LH falls less dramatically compared to FSH and is of no known clinical significance as a biomarker for menopause, thus far. The postmenopausal loss of gonadal feedback alters the forms of LH and FSH secreted, resulting in slower clearance and prolonged half-life.

In the postmenopausal phase, there is a steady age-related decline in serum levels of LH and FSH independent of the loss of ovarian hormonal feedback. This indicates that the dynamics of hypothalamic gonadotropin-releasing hormone (GnRH) secretion are altered. The amount of GnRH secreted is increased in postmenopausal women, although accompanied by a decrease in GnRH pulse frequency. The decline of LH and FSH in the presence of increased GnRH secretion results from an age-related diminished pituitary response to GnRH.

Fig. 14.2 Hormonal changes during the menopause transition

⬇ Circulating estrogens

⬇ Ratio of estrogen to androgen

⬇ Sex hormone-binding globulin secretion

⬆ Peripheral aromatization of DHEA to estrone

⇄ Reversal of estradiol (E_2) to estrone (E_1) ratio

⬌ No significant change in testosterone levels

While circadian rhythmicity of the pituitary hormones adrenocorticotropic hormone (ACTH) and thyroid-stimulating hormone (TSH) remains intact, gonadotropin secretion in postmenopausal women does not follow a circadian rhythm.

Adrenals

Adrenal glucocorticoid secretion follows a circadian pattern of secretion, with peak values in the morning and a nadir in the late afternoon. Cortisol and ACTH levels rise with increasing age, and serum concentrations at all ages are higher in women than in men. Blunting of the cortisol circadian rhythm is characteristic of aging in both sexes. A year following the onset of the late menopause transition stage, cortisol levels were reported to rise significantly, coinciding with an increase in DHEAS, urinary metabolites of estrogen, and FSH. Women with an increase in cortisol were found to have significantly more severe hot flashes. Cortisol levels stabilized around the time of the FMP.

As research evolves, we are learning more about estrogen receptors, the steroidal nature of hormonal therapy, the role of the thermoregulatory neuroendocrine system, and potential treatments to specifically address these changes to decrease morbidity and improve quality of life.

14.4 Clinical Implications

14.4.1 Presentation

Menopause is the marker for ovarian follicular retirement and menstrual changes are the hallmark of the menopausal transition. It is a retrospective diagnosis after 12 months from the final menopause period (FMP). Most follicular loss occurs from atresia versus ovulation (<500 follicles ovulated over a lifetime) and proceeds as a continuum but not at a constant rate. During the transition to menopause and beyond, women experience many physical changes, most of which are normal consequences of ovarian and somatic aging. However, some of the changes associated with menopausal transition could be signs of underlying illnesses or warning for an increased risk of aging-related morbidities.

Classic Symptoms
- Change in menstrual cycle pattern (during perimenopause).
- Vasomotor symptoms (hot flashes and night sweats).
- Vulvovaginal symptoms (e.g., vaginal dryness, dyspareunia, and urinary symptoms).
- Sleep disturbances.

Other Symptoms Associated with Menopause

- Cognitive concerns (memory, concentration).
- Psychological symptoms (depression, anxiety, moodiness).

Body Changes Reported with Menopause Transition

- Weight changes are mostly related to lifestyle rather than hormonal changes. However, menopause may be related to adipose distribution more toward androgenic (midsection adiposity) rather than gynecoid.
- Tooth loss after menopause has been associated with osteoporosis, as for each 1% annual decrease in whole-body bone mineral density (BMD), the risk for tooth loss quadruples.
- A decline in skin collagen to 30% in the first five postmenopausal years with a steady 2% yearly decline over the following decades.
- Increase in the ratio of androgen to estrogen during the menopause transition may influence hair changes leading to female pattern hair loss or unwanted hair growth (e.g., chin hair).

14.4.2 Evaluation

Due to the wide age range (40–58 years) for natural menopause, chronologic age is a poor indicator of the menopausal transition. The Stages of Reproductive Workshop (STRAW) provided a standardized definition of reproductive aging based on menstrual cycle bleeding criteria and follicle-stimulating hormone (FSH) levels to promote consistency in reporting, research, and clinical terminology. A decade later, the STRAW+10 workshop incorporated new criteria to the staging related to FSH, antral follicle count (AFC), Anti-Mullerian hormone (AMH), inhibin B, and estradiol level changes (Fig. 14.3). Staging provided by STRAW is not applicable to women with menstrual disorders.

Menopause is primarily a clinical diagnosis and diagnostic workup more likely to be utilized in the setting of early menopause, menopause transition, and the syndromes of menopause (see Table 14.2).

We should tailor our diagnostic workup to the patient's presentation and may include:

- Detailed clinical history including menstrual cycle or pattern changes, menarche, parity, perinatal complications, sleep patterns, gynecologic history, and some clinics use instruments for menopause symptoms such as the Utian Quality of

Stage	-5	-4	-3b	-3a	-2	-1	+1a	+1b	+1c	+2
Terminology	REPRODUCTIVE				MENOPAUSAL TRANSITION		POSTMENOPAUSE			
	Early	Peak	Late		Early	Late	Early			Late
					PERIMENOPAUSE					
Duration		Variable			Variable	1-3 years	2 years (1+1)		3-6 years	
Principal criteria										
Menstrual Cycle	Variable to Regular	Regular	Regular	Subtle Changes in Flow/Length	Variable Length Persistent >= 7-day difference in length of consecutive cycles	Interval of amenorrhea of >=60 days				
Supportive criteria										
Endocrine FSH			Low	Variable	Variable	>25IU/L*	Variable	Stabilizes		
AMH			Low	Low	Low	Low	Low	Very Low		
Inhibin B			Low	Low	Low	Low	Low	Very Low		
Antral Follicle Count (limited use)			Low	Low	Low	Low	Very Low	Very Low		
Descriptive Characteristics										
Symptoms						Vasomotor symptoms Likely	Vasomotor symptoms Most Likely**			Increasing symptoms of GSM

FMP: final menopause period, GSM: Genitourinary syndrome of menopause
*Approximate expected level based on assays using current international pituitary
** 10-15% of women have persistent vasomotor symptoms

Fig. 14.3 Staging reproductive aging workshop +10 (STRAW+10)

Life Scale (UQOL) or Menopause-Specific Quality of Life Questionnaire (MSQoL), past medical history of thyroid disorders, reproductive cancers, hepatobiliary disease, clotting disorders, cardiovascular disease, osteoporosis, or mental illness. Current and past sexual activity, alcohol, tobacco use, dietary regimen, and level of physical activity are important in painting a holistic management plan and appropriate screenings.

- Physical examination should include blood pressure, weight, body mass index (BMI), cardiovascular, breast, and pelvic examination.
- Laboratory tests are mostly to rule out secondary causes of presenting symptoms such as thyroid panel, complete blood count, blood diatheses studies, liver function test, and biometric screening for risk stratification as in fasting blood sugar or hemoglobin A1C and lipid panel. Little evidence to support checking vitamin and mineral levels such as vitamin B12, vitamin D, and magnesium depending on the reported dietary regimen and risk of osteoporosis.
- Further evaluation should include preventive screening for breast cancer, colon cancer, and osteoporosis for informed clinical management. A transvaginal ultrasound is indicated to rule out a pelvic pathology (e.g., fibroids, polyps, or adenomyosis)

Table 14.2 Differential diagnosis of early menopausal symptoms (younger than 40 years)

Causes	Evaluation	Differential diagnosis
Genetic disorders		
• **X chromosome disorders (monosomy, trisomy, or translocations, deletions)** • **Specific genetic disorders** • **Mutations involving enzymes important for reproduction** – **Galactosemia** – **17α-hydroxylase deficiency** – **Aromatase deficiency** *Associated autoimmune disorders* • **Autoimmune polyendocrine syndromes** – **Hypothyroidism** – **Adrenal insufficiency** – **Hypoparathyroidism** – **Type 1 DM** • **Dry eye syndrome** • **Myasthenia gravis** • **Rheumatoid arthritis** • **Systemic lupus erythematosus** • **Congenital thymic aplasia** *Miscellaneous disorders* – **Metabolic syndromes** – **Infections (mumps, HIV)** *Iatrogenic causes* – **Pelvic radiation** – **Chemotherapy (alkylating agents)** *Surgical menopause* – **Oophorectomy** – **Ovarian cystectomy** – **Consequence of hysterectomy or uterine artery embolization**	• Clinical history and physical examination • Family history of early menopause • LH, FSH, estradiol, and prolactin levels • If FSH is initially elevated, repeat FSH and estradiol levels on at least 2 occasions, usually 1 month apart • TSH and thyroid peroxidase antibodies • Fasting blood glucose • Serum calcium and phosphorus concentrations • Pelvic ultrasound • *Not indicated* – Progesterone withdrawal test – Ovarian antibodies – Ovarian biopsy Refer (endocrine or genetics) • Karyotype (consider molecular cytogenetic studies of the X chromosome) • FMR1 gene premutation testing • Adrenal antibodies (evaluate adrenal reserve with ACTH testing if positive)	*Low FSH conditions* • Pregnancy • Hypothalamic amenorrhea – Secondary to constitutional disorder • Uncontrolled DM • Celiac disease – Extremes of lifestyle • Exercise • Caloric restriction • Perceived stress – Lesions of the hypothalamus/pituitary – GnRH agonist/ antagonist therapy • Hyperprolactinemia • Hypothyroidism and hyperthyroidism • PCOS *Elevated FSH condition* • POI

DM Diabetes mellitus, *HIV* Human immunodeficiency virus, *LH* Luteinizing hormone, *FSH* Follicle-stimulating hormone, *FMR1* Fragile X messenger ribonucleoprotein 1, *ACTH* Adrenocorticotropic hormone, *GnRH* Gonadotropin-releasing hormone, *PCOS* Polycystic ovarian syndrome, *POI* Premature ovarian insufficiency

14.4.3 Our Case

Ms. RO showed interest in learning more about menopause and if her symptoms mean she has heart problems. We had a lengthy discussion about perimenopausal changes including vasomotor symptoms and lifestyle changes. She speaks good

English but prefers health education resources in Somali. She understood that her abnormal uterine bleeding requires further evaluation and agreed to get some labs done, schedule a transvaginal ultrasound, and return for an endometrial biopsy procedure in the clinic. I was able to locate resources in Somali about menopause on Medline Plus. Her labs came back in 2 days with borderline elevated LDL (129), suboptimal HDL (42), high FSH (129), postmenopausal estradiol levels (10), low vitamin D, suboptimal vitamin B12 (she eats a regular diet, no pork or alcohol. Sources of meat are mainly goat and lamb. Few vegetables besides cooked stew) and other labs are within normal limits (CBC, CMP, TSH). Her transvaginal ultrasound showed a retroverted uterus of 10.2 cm fundal height with endometrial thickening of 9 mm (thick for age). She has not done pap tests before or a mammogram.

14.4.4   Clinical Issues

Subfecundity and Fertility

Delaying conception in industrialized countries is on the rise posing biopsychosocial challenges for women desiring pregnancy at later ages. By mid-thirties functional ovarian reserve decreases dramatically, and spontaneous miscarriages may occur in half of the pregnancies by mid-40 s. Several complications may present during advanced maternal gestation. Hence, for women desiring pregnancy past 35 years of age, a timely evaluation and referral to a fertility specialist are warranted.

Conversely, spontaneous pregnancy is still possible up to 1 year after menopause so discussing contraception during the menopause transition is substantial.

Abnormal Uterine Bleeding

Due to anovulatory cycles, all forms of abnormal uterine bleeding (AUB) may occur. Refer to Chap. 6 for the evaluation and management of menstrual disorders. Postmenopausal bleeding is unique to menopause clinics and warrants further evaluation for histological and structural etiologies with endometrial biopsy and transvaginal ultrasound, respectively (see Chap. 3).

A differential of postmenopausal bleeding:

- Vulvar (e.g., lesions)
- Urethral (e.g., caruncles)
- Cervix (e.g., friable tissue, polyps, neoplasia)
- Vaginal (e.g., lesions, GSM)
- Uterine (e.g., fibroids, polyps, malignancy)
- Hormonal therapy (e.g., Tamoxifen)
- Rule out anal/rectal sources of bleeding.

Vasomotor Symptoms of Menopause

Three in four perimenopausal women in the United States (US) report vasomotor symptoms (VMS). Vasomotor symptoms (known as hot flashes or flushes) are recurrent, transient episodes of flushing accompanied by a sensation of warmth to intense heat on the upper body and face/head (reports of whole-body sweats as well) (Fig. 14.4). VMS is highly occurring during perimenopause and the first two postmenopausal years. Up to 15% of postmenopausal women report severe VMS and persistent symptoms past late menopause. VMS does significantly impact the quality of life, and career performance, and may be associated with increased metabolic syndrome and cardiovascular disease.

Contributing factors to VMS:

- Warm environment, hot drinks, spicy food, stress, higher BMI, cigarette smoking, alcohol intake
- Drugs: Selective estrogen receptor modulators (SERMs), selective serotonin reuptake inhibitors (SSRIs), aromatase inhibitors (AIs)
- Disease conditions include thyroid disease, infection, leukemia, pancreatic tumors, autoimmune disorders, and anxiety.
- Serum estrogen levels are not predictive of hot flash frequency or severity.

Genitourinary Syndrome of Menopause

Unlike VMS, genitourinary syndrome of menopause (GSM) progresses over time. It encompasses vulvovaginal changes associated with perimenopause. GSM is more favorable than vaginal atrophy in menopause practices and research. It occurs due to loss of estrogen in the vulvovaginal tissues, inflammation and tissue changes in the vaginal microbiome, and an increased vaginal pH from an acidic environment to an alkaline one. GSM may manifest as vaginal dryness, vulvovaginal itching or irritation, dyspareunia (mostly superficial), urinary frequency, urinary incontinence, and postmenopausal bleeding. (Refer to Chaps. 5, 8, and 17 for differential diagnostic workup based on presenting symptoms.)

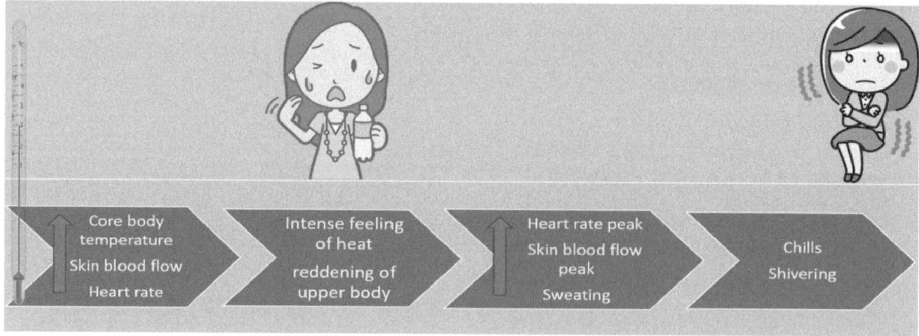

Fig. 14.4 Anatomy of a hot flash

Sleep Disturbances

Women report sleep disturbances more than men at all ages. Sleep disturbance is more prevalent in perimenopausal, postmenopausal, and surgically menopausal women than in premenopausal women. There is an independent relationship between menopausal stages and sleep disturbance beyond the effects of aging and other confounders. Sociocultural factors affect the levels of sleep disturbance at various menopausal stages. Sleep disturbances are associated with fatigue, irritability, chronic illnesses, and mood disorders.

For focused management, it is important to rule out and address potential other causes (e.g., sleep apnea, pain, excessive alcohol intake, or medications). Clinical decision-making depends on the type of sleep disturbance (acute or chronic, primary, or secondary to other conditions), the context of the sleep problem (distressing vasomotor symptoms or life stress), and the severity of daytime consequences.

Sexual Health

The aforementioned changes negatively impact sexual health in women transitioning through midlife. Decreased fertility may discourage those thinking of sex as a tool for procreation only, VMS and sleep disturbances may contribute to fatigability and less availability for sexual encounters, GSM may impede vaginal intercourse due to vaginal dryness and pain, and prolonged AUB affects vaginal intimacy. Biological menopause is one component of many in a woman's sexual function. Alleviating menopausal symptoms can enhance the sexual well-being of women and narrow the differential for female sexual disorders.

Neuropsychological Health

Declines in estrogen perimenopause are associated with declines in cognitive functioning and an increased risk of depressive symptoms. Some studies suggest that these changes are transient and may improve postmenopausal. Nonetheless, perimenopausal depression is increasingly recognized as a new subtype of depressive disorder with specific clinical characteristics.

These neuropsychological changes may be related to social stressors during midlife such as an empty nest, caregiver burden for elders and children simultaneously "sandwich generation," infertility, sleep disturbance, chronic illnesses, loss of a partner, and stress at work or family. Women with a history of premenstrual syndrome or dysphoria, sexual dysfunction, physical inactivity, or hot flashes are more vulnerable to depressive symptoms. Early recognition of factors associated with cognitive and mood changes around menopause can improve outcomes and change the course through early intervention and timely counseling.

Metabolic Changes

Changes in lipid profile, the higher lifetime risk of diabetes, weight fluctuation, and physical inactivity during perimenopause contribute to increased incidence of cardiovascular disease (CVD) in women. CVD presents differently in women and has increased drastically in females younger than 55 years of age. Premature and early onset menopause has been linked to a higher risk of CVD; however, this varies by social determinants of health (e.g., ethnicity or cultural background) and is confounded by the effects of aging. (Refer to Chap. 11 for more details.)

Osteoporosis

Postmenopausal women are at substantial risk of developing osteoporosis and identifying those at risk during the menopause transition can significantly improve quality of life and prevent detrimental health outcomes. More on osteoporosis in Chap. 16.

14.5 Our Case

Ms. RO returned to the clinic to discuss pathology results and share updates on her lifestyle changes. She reports walking 30 minutes a day 4–5 days a week, eating salad with dinner every day, and adding 1–2 raw vegetables to her breakfast. She also reports that she does ritual fasting (13 hours with no food or drinks from dawn to dusk) on Thursdays when she is not menstruating. Her last menstrual period was 6 weeks ago with no spotting. Her hot flashes are worse when she is stressed out and happen 2–3 times a week. She is not currently interested in mammograms or medications. Her endometrial biopsy came back normal as well as her pap and HPV testing. She is open to having a hormonal IUD if her bleeding resumes or persists. She reports that drinking moringa leaf extract and sage herbal tea helps with her symptoms. She is open to seeing a nutritional counselor for her high LDL and supplementing with vitamin D.

14.6 Management

14.6.1 Lifestyle Prescription

Reassurance is of immense importance when women present with changes suggestive of the menopause transition. Providers can be initiative-taking and screen for changes in patients in their mid-thirties and encourage women to become more aware of their cycles and perimenstrual changes.

Emphasize the value of healthy lifestyle changes through a sustainable and gradual pace and schedule regular follow-ups as necessary to support women during their midlife transition.

Patient's prescription:

- Perimenopausal diet should be predominantly plant-based diet to decrease cancer risk with healthy fatty acids to provide substrates for steroidal hormones.
- Maintain a healthy weight which should be tailored to ethnicity and other social determinants of health rather than an absolute BMI range.
- Obtain adequate calcium and vitamin D:

  - For calcium: 1200 mg/d from food (preferably) and/or supplement
  - For vitamin D: recommended dietary allowance is 600 IU/d until age 70 and 800 IU/d after age 70

- Daily appropriate exercise, not close to bedtime.
- Avoid alcohol consumption.
- Avoid smoking in all forms.
- Institute measure to mitigate fall risks at all costs including supportive footwear.
- Sleep hygiene measures (use cool, dark, quiet room, use the bedroom only for sleep and sexual activities, use lightweight sleepwear, avoid heavy evening meals, alcohol, caffeine, and nicotine, use mindfulness and relaxation techniques, and maintain a regular sleep schedule even on weekends)
- Reduce sexual discomfort and increase sensitivity with moisturizers, lubricants, and vibrators.
- Stress management through self-care activities and self-advocacy in work environments.

Provider's contribution:

- Address patient's concerns including quality of life matters not only morbidities (sexual health, skincare, pelvic hygiene, and self-care).
- Recognize sexual orientation and cultural background in your counseling.
- Optimal management of chronic metabolic disease (blood pressure and glycemic regulation).
- Rule out secondary causes and manage them accordingly.
- Maintain preventive screenings per guidelines.
- Consider an interdisciplinary approach with early interventions such as referral to cognitive behavioral therapy for sleep disturbances, pelvic floor therapy for GSM or urinary incontinence, sex therapy for sexual health concerns, or psychotherapy for depressive symptoms.

14.6.2 Pharmacological Therapy

Medications should be considered for menopausal symptoms impacting the quality of life or predisposing women to disease risk (e.g., osteoporosis or depression). Early intervention during the menopause transition or within 10 years from menopause was found to reduce the risk of osteoporosis and mitigate the incidence of depression. Choice of therapy can be guided by coexisting morbidities, pharmacogenetics, adverse reactions to medications, and most importantly patient preferences.

Menopausal Hormonal Therapy

Menopausal hormonal therapy (MHT) has evolved over the past decades. Recent evidence changes showed favorable health outcomes with MHT intervention in early menopause and menopause transition. A follow-up analysis of Women's Health Initiative (WHI), randomized clinical trials such as KEEPS (Kronos Early Estrogen Prevention Study), and ELITE (Early versus Late Intervention Trial with Estradiol) studies demonstrated favorable safety profile of MHT and lower trends of all-cause mortality among younger women with estrogen alone (Table 14.3).

Oral contraceptives (OCPs) offer a viable option for symptomatic perimenopause and contraception as they can suppress vasomotor symptoms, restore predictable bleeding, decrease dysmenorrhea, enhance BMD, and lower the risk of endometrial and ovarian cancer. OCPs have higher doses of hormones compared to

Table 14.3 Menopausal hormonal therapy types

Formulations	Indication(s)	Contraindication(s)
Estrogen therapy (ET) (women with no uterus)	Premature menopause (POI) Moderate-severe VMS Osteoporosis prevention	Absolute: Active cancer diagnosis, active CVD, current VTE. MI, pregnancy Relative: History of cancer, VTE, liver disease, high triglycerides
Estrogen progesterone therapy (EPT) (women with an intact uterus)	Same as above Sleep disturbances may benefit from progesterone	Same as above, more so with increased risk of breast cancer
Selective estrogen-receptor modulators (SERM) (Osphena, Duavee)	Same indications as above for women with breast tenderness, increased density, or uterine bleeding with EPT	
Vaginal estrogen (Estrace) Vaginal DHEAs (Intrarosa)	GSM treatment	Unexplained vaginal bleeding
Oral contraceptives (OCP) higher doses than MHT Higher risk of VTE	Symptomatic perimenopause and contraception	Relative: Active smoking hypertension, diabetes, obesity, and other comorbidities
Bioidentical hormonal therapy (compounded hormonal therapy)	Not recommended due to lack of FDA testing. They are not tested for efficacy, safety, batch standardization, or purity	

POI Primary ovarian insufficiency, *VTE* venous thromboembolism, *MI* myocardial infarction

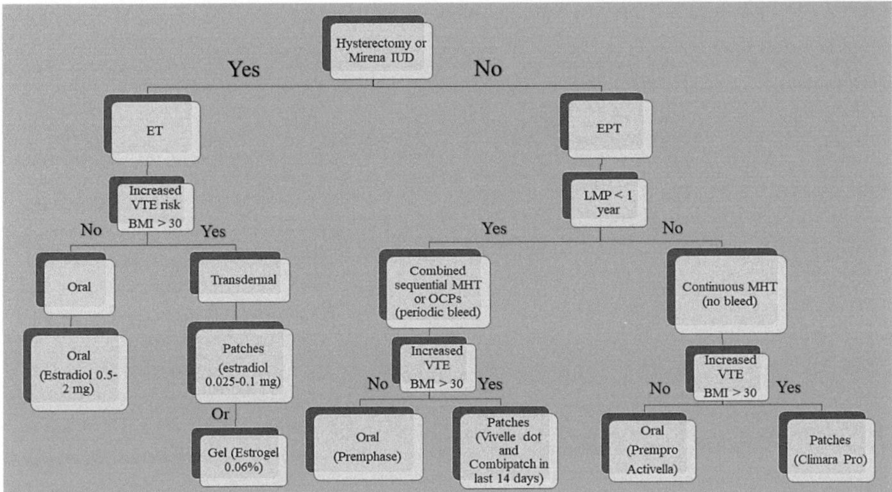

Fig. 14.5 A simplified guide to menopausal hormonal therapy. (*IUD* Intrauterine device, *ET* Estrogen therapy, *EPT* Estrogen progesterone therapy, *LMP* Last menstrual period, *VTE* Venous thromboembolism, *MHT* Menopausal hormonal therapy)

MHT hence a higher VTE risk. Choosing OCPs versus MHT better be approached with shared decision-making and individualized approach. Consider stopping OCPs around 50 years of age and transitioning to MHT if menopausal symptoms persist.

Bioidentical hormones have molecules that are identical to our body's hormones. Non-bioidentical like Premarin or medroxyprogesterone (MPA) act like estrogen and progesterone, respectively, but are different from our body's hormones.

MHT is indicated in moderate to severe menopausal symptoms and premature menopause. Clinical indications supported with quality evidence are VMS, GSM, and osteoporosis prevention. There is limited evidence of its benefits for cognition, skin changes, or weight fluctuations. It is important to set your patient's expectations to current evidence-based indications and choose MHT based on individual needs. Most contraindications are relative according to the growing body of menopause research (see Fig. 14.5).

Extending MHT long-term is acceptable for women who request it and are informed of pertinent benefits and risks, prevention of osteoporosis-related fractures if more tolerated than alternate therapies, and there are no contraindications with up-to-date cancer screenings. After 3 years of EPT discontinuation, the rate of cardiovascular events, fractures, and colon cancer was the same as in the placebo group, and a notable increase in the rate of all cancers and mortality from breast cancer. After 3 years of ET discontinuation, no increase in CVD, DVT, stroke, hip fracture, colorectal cancer, or total mortality, and the decrease in breast cancer persisted. There is a 50% chance of vasomotor symptoms recurring with MHT cessation whether tapered or abruptly discontinued (see Table 14.4). Testosterone is not recommended for menopausal symptoms treatment or libido enhancement.

Table 14.4 Risk–benefit profile of menopausal hormonal therapy

Outcome/symptom	Formulation	Benefit	Risk	Probable benefit or risk
Vasomotor symptoms	Estrogen (E)	Yes		
	estrogen + progestogen (E + P)	Yes		
Osteoporosis	E	Yes		
	E + P			
Coronary heart disease	E	Yes	Yes	Decreased risk in women <60, within 10 y of menopause Increased risk in women many years past menopause
	E + P	Neutral	Neutral	
Stroke	E		Yes	
	E + P		Yes	
Type 2 diabetes	E	Yes		
	E + P	Yes		
Venous thromboembolism	E		Yes	
	E + P		Yes	
All-cause mortality	E	Neutral	Neutral	Trends toward decreased risk when started early in menopause and neutral or increased risk when started later in menopause
	E + P			
Breast cancer	E	Yes	Yes	
	E + P			
Endometrial cancer	E	Yes		
	E + P			
Colon cancer	E	Neutral		
	E + P	Yes		
Fractures	E	Yes		
	E + P	Yes		

E + P: Estrogen + Progesterone

Menopausal Non-Hormonal Therapy

Women with contraindications to MHT or not interested in hormonal therapy may benefit from a non-hormonal prescription. Start at the lowest dose and titrate to therapeutic effect and counsel for proper tapering for patients who are likely to self-manage.

- Non-hormonal lubricants and topical gels
- Antidepressant

  - SSRIs: FDA-approved low-dose paroxetine. Citalopram and escitalopram showed significant improvement in randomized controlled trials (RCTs).
  - SNRIs: Venlafaxine has shown improvement in RCTs and desvenlafaxine has favorable weight and sexual side effects with parallel symptom relief to other SNRIs.

- Hypnotic
  - Eszopiclone
- Anticonvulsant
  - Gabapentin has shown improvement in hot flashes and sleep disturbances.
- Antihypertensive
  - Clonidine

14.6.3 Alternative and Complementary Therapy

More than half of women self-medicate their menopausal symptoms and over 60% of them feel uninformed about alternative and complementary treatment options. There is limited research on most complementary options available to women which leads to commercialized health, delay in the use of effective therapy, and use of inappropriate therapies.

A metanalysis showed promising therapeutic effects with Black Cohosh with or without St. John's wort. North American Menopause Society (NAMS) does not recommend over-the-counter supplements, vitamins, herbal therapies, relaxation techniques, and chiropractic interventions for menopausal symptoms. Yoga, regular exercise, and acupuncture do not have sufficient evidence in alleviating menopausal symptoms, but they may have other health benefits.

The Study of Women's Health Across the Nation (SWAN) found that women experience perimenopause differently across ethnic groups hence an inquisitive open dialogue tempered with compassion is encouraged for an informed decision-making process. One in ten USA residents is foreign-born with 15% speaking a second language at home and more than a third of adult women are of multi-ethnic backgrounds. These diversified courses of menopause should be reflected in the resources and research designs offered to improve health outcomes around menopause and women's midlife wellness.

14.7 Summary

Menopause is a terrific opportunity for women to set a fresh outlook on their health and celebrate living to that point. Providers can seize this opportunity through counseling and emphasizing the importance of healthy lifestyle changes, disease risk reduction, and preventive screening. Reassurance and health education remain the mainstay therapy for longevity and wellness. NAMS does not recommend compounded hormonal therapy due to a lack of safety profile data. Menopausal hormonal therapy is safe to prescribe long-term to informed patients with significant symptoms and no absolute contraindications. Non-hormonal treatment options for menopausal symptoms are great alternatives, especially in the setting of coexisting mood disorders or sleep disturbances. Complementary and alternative medicine does not have much evidence to support its prescriptions. Further diversified research with global representation is warranted.

Suggested Reading

1. Medina L, Sabo S, Vespa J. Living longer: historical and projected life expectancy in the United States, 1960 to 2060. Suitland: US Department of Commerce, US Census Bureau; 2020.
2. Chakraborty B, Byemerwa J, Krebs T, Lim F, Chang CY, McDonnell DP. Estrogen receptor signaling in the immune system. Endocr Rev. 2023;44(1):117–41.
3. Ciocca DR, Vargas Roig LM. Estrogen receptors in human nontarget tissues: biological and clinical implications. Endocr Rev. 1995;16(1):35–62.
4. North American Menopause Society. Menopause practice: a Clinician's guide. Mayfield Heights: North American Menopause Society; 2014.
5. Utian WH, Janata JW, Kingsberg SA, Schluchter M, Hamilton JC. The Utian quality of life (UQOL) scale: development and validation of an instrument to quantify quality of life through and beyond menopause. Menopause. 2018;25(11):1224–31.
6. Hilditch JR, Lewis J, Peter A, van Maris B, Ross A, Franssen E, et al. A menopause-specific quality of life questionnaire: development and psychometric properties. Maturitas. 2008;61(1–2):107–21.
7. Tuomikoski P, Savolainen-Peltonen H. Vasomotor symptoms and metabolic syndrome. Maturitas. 2017;97:61–5.
8. Xu Q, Lang CP. Examining the relationship between subjective sleep disturbance and menopause: a systematic review and meta-analysis. Menopause. 2014;21(12):1301–18.
9. Basson R. Women's sexual dysfunction: revised and expanded definitions. CMAJ. 2005;172(10):1327–33.
10. Worsley R, Davis SR, Gavrilidis E, Gibbs Z, Lee S, Burger H, Kulkarni J. Hormonal therapies for new onset and relapsed depression during perimenopause. Maturitas. 2012;73(2):127–33.
11. de Kruif M, Spijker AT, Molendijk ML. Depression during the perimenopause: a meta-analysis. J Affect Disord. 2016;206:174–80.
12. El Khoudary SR. Age at menopause onset and risk of cardiovascular disease around the world. Maturitas. 2020;141:33–8.
13. Mehta J, Kling JM, Manson JE. Risks, benefits, and treatment modalities of menopausal hormone therapy: current concepts. Front Endocrinol. 2021;12:564781.
14. Castelo-Branco C, Gambacciani M, Cano A, Minkin MJ, Rachoń D, Ruan X, et al. Review & meta-analysis: isopropanolic black cohosh extract iCR for menopausal symptoms–an update on the evidence. Climacteric. 2021;24(2):109–19.

Chapter 15
Eating Disorders in Women's Health Primary Care Practice

Melinda Wang, Elizabeth Saunders, Erin C. Accurso, and Judith Walsh-Cassidy

15.1 Introduction

Eating disorders are common among women of reproductive age and are associated with significant morbidity and mortality, but identification and diagnosis can be challenging. Approximately 95% of individuals with anorexia nervosa are women with a prevalence of 0.5–1% among adolescent girls; about 10% of women between 16 and 25 years old may have evidence of subclinical anorexia nervosa. Bulimia nervosa has a prevalence of 3–10% among adolescents and college-aged women and a 1–1.5% prevalence among women of reproductive age. The estimated prevalence of binge eating disorder is approximately 2–3% of the general population, approximately 30% of women who are pursuing weight management strategies, and approximately 50% of women with severe obesity. It is estimated about 33% of women with insulin dependent diabetes mellitus have an underlying eating disorder or disturbance. Other eating disorders such as night eating syndrome are also more prevalent among individuals with elevated BMI and those seeking bariatric surgery.

Primary care providers play an important role in the identification and management of eating disorders among women, with studies estimating that at least half of individuals with eating disorders are identified by primary care providers. Awareness of risk factors and presentations of eating disorders and screening methods are important tools in the primary care provider's armamentarium. However, eating disorders are not often included in educational curricula among primary care providers. Individuals with mild eating disorders may be managed solely by their primary care providers, while management of moderate to severe eating disorder cases requires closer multidisciplinary collaboration between mental health providers,

M. Wang (✉) · E. Saunders · E. C. Accurso · J. Walsh-Cassidy
University of California, San Francisco, USA
e-mail: melinda.wang3@ucsf.edu; elizabeth.saunders@ucsf.edu; erin.accurso@ucsf.edu; judith.walsh@ucsf.edu

M. Mahmoudi (ed.), *Common Cases in Women's Primary Care Clinics*, https://doi.org/10.1007/978-3-031-48569-5_15

medical providers, and often dietitians. As psychiatric disorders, eating disorders generally require mental health treatment, although the format and intensity of treatment may vary. Concurrent medical management is essential to provide medical interventions as needed to ensure medical stability of the patient. Nutritional assessment and counseling also play an important role in nutritional rehabilitation, particularly for patients with malnutrition. This chapter seeks to explore the diagnosis and management of eating disorders, focusing on the role of primary care providers within the integrated management team.

15.2 Case 1

Ms. Jones is a 30-year-old woman with history of obesity, major depressive disorder, and generalized anxiety who presents to primary care for concerns of infertility. She was previously on hormonal oral contraception since the age of 16 for menorrhagia and menstrual cramps but stopped taking her oral contraceptives 1 year ago to attempt to conceive with her partner. She takes escitalopram for depression and denies taking any other prescription medications, but she admits to using diet pills she found over the internet to assist with weight loss. She drinks alcohol socially and has smoked five cigarettes per day since she was in high school. She does not use any recreational drugs. She was previously on a dance team while in high school. While she no longer dances, she has been participating in rock climbing in her local gym and also does daily aerobic exercises at the gym. She is concerned that her weight may be the reason she is having difficulty with conception. Her family history is notable for major depressive disorder in her mother. She wishes to discuss next steps for evaluation of infertility.

15.3 Discussion

15.3.1 Screening

Screening is an important tool for primary care providers in the identification of eating disorders. It is estimated that only about 10% of individuals with bulimia nervosa are identified, and only 50% of those identified are referred to treatment. Therefore, increased screening and awareness of eating disorders will increase identification of eating disorders in the primary care population.

The National Institutes of Health provides recommendations for signs and symptoms that should lead to further screening and evaluation of eating disorders in the primary care setting. These symptoms include psychological concerns, gastrointestinal symptoms, menstrual irregularities or amenorrhea, and patient concerns about weight. Signs that should be assessed include low body mass index (BMI) and physical signs of starvation or repeated vomiting. In mild cases, there may be more subtle clues to eating disorders.

Additional considerations for specific eating disorders have also been identified. Anorexia nervosa has been associated with participation in activities that place emphasis on body shape including ballet, modeling, and gymnastics. Other concerns associated with anorexia nervosa include amenorrhea, abdominal discomfort, bloating/constipation, and cold intolerance. If individuals present with progressive weight loss or if there are concerns voiced by family members, these should also prompt concern for a possible underlying eating disorder. Individuals should also be asked about a family history of eating disorders, a risk factor for developing an eating disorder. Unsuccessful attempts at weight loss and gastroesophageal reflux disease (GERD) should also raise concerns for possible underlying bulimia nervosa. Elevated BMI and diabetes have also been associated with eating disorders. Clinical suspicion in the presence of these signs and symptoms should prompt a provider to evaluate individuals for eating disorders. Screening questions that can be asked include the following:

1. Do you think you have an eating problem?
2. Do you worry excessively about your weight?

For patients who also have a history of diabetes, the Diabetes Eating Problem Survey can also be used to screen patients for concomitant eating disorder. The questions include "Do you feel like your eating is out of control?" and "Do you take less insulin than you need because of concerns about your eating or weight?"

Although some women may not reach formal diagnostic criteria for anorexia nervosa or bulimia nervosa, they may be classified as having the "female athlete triad." The female athlete triad consists of low energy availability with or without disordered eating, amenorrhea, and osteoporosis due to hypoestrogenism. It is estimated that 15–62% of women athletes may have an underlying eating disorder. The Female Athlete Triad Coalition 2014 consensus guidelines recommend screening individuals annually during sport pre-participation evaluations with triad-specific questions including menstrual history, concerns about weight, eating disorders, and history of low bone density or stress factors starting at the high school or collegiate level. The International Olympic Committee-endorsed Periodic Health Examination also includes eight screening questions for the female athlete triad.

In the case of Ms. Jones, there are certain subtle features in her initial history that should raise suspicion for possible eating disorder and prompt further evaluation. First, she endorses using diet pills for weight loss and participates in aerobic activities that have a focus on body shape such as being part of a dance team in high school and doing daily aerobic exercises on top of rock climbing as an adult. Second, her focus on her weight and elevated BMI places her at risk for possible underlying eating disorder. Given these factors, an underlying eating disorder should be considered in her evaluation.

15.3.2 Eating Disorders

Below we provide details regarding the diagnostic criteria for common eating disorders according to the DSM-V (Table 15.1).

Anorexia Nervosa

Anorexia nervosa is defined as a restriction in intake leading to low body weight that is less than minimally normal or less than 15% of expected. Individuals also have an intense fear of weight gain and participate in persistent behaviors to avoid weight gain despite low body weights. Patients with anorexia nervosa have a significant emphasis on body weight and shape and will lack recognition of the severity of their current low body weight. Severity of anorexia nervosa is defined by BMI. Patients with BMI <17 kg/m^2 are defined as mild, 16–16.99 kg/m^2 are considered moderate, 15–15.99 kg/m^2 are considered severe, and < 15 kg/m^2 are considered extreme. Anorexia nervosa can also be associated with other psychiatric conditions. For example, among patients with anorexia nervosa, patients may also have obsessive compulsive disorder (OCD) (25% prevalence) and dysthymia (50–75% prevalence). Patients may present with depression and anxiety that can often precede the diagnosis of anorexia nervosa.

Table 15.1 DSM-V criteria overview for common eating disorders

Eating Disorder	General Criteria
Anorexia nervosa	• Restriction of energy intake compared to relative requirements leading to significantly low body weight • Intense fear of gaining weight. • Disturbance in perception of one's body weight/shape
Bulimia nervosa	• Recurrent episodes of binge eating (lack of control, discrete period of time) • Recurrent inappropriate compensatory behavior to prevent weight gain • Both binge eating and compensatory behavior for at least 3 months • Focus on body weight/shape
Binge eating disorder	• Recurrent episodes of binge eating • Distress regarding binge eating • At least once per week for 3 months • Not associated with compensatory behavior
Avoidant/restrictive food intake disorder	• Feeding disturbance with significant weight loss, nutritional deficiency, psychosocial functioning impairment, or dependence on supplementary feeding • No other underlying eating disorder or focus on one's body weight/shape • Not explained by social or other medical factors
Other specified feeding and eating disorders	• Symptoms characteristic of eating disorder • Does not meet full criteria

There are two recognized subtypes of anorexia nervosa. The restricting type is defined as weight loss from excessive exercise and calorie restriction without episodes of binging or purging in the 3 months prior to evaluation. If patients subsequently develop bulimia nervosa, they often will develop crossover symptoms within 5 years of the diagnosis of anorexia nervosa. The binge eating/purging subtype is defined as engagement in binging and purging behavior in the 3 months prior to evaluation.

Individuals with anorexia nervosa have a high morbidity and mortality, with a mortality rate of 10–15%. Causes of death include starvation, suicide, and medical complications from their disease process. Factors associated with poor prognosis include severity of disease, presence of vomiting, challenging family dynamics, male gender, chronicity, and lack of response to early treatment. Those who do initially recover often have a protracted recovery period, and while some may recover completely, others may develop chronic anorexia nervosa.

Bulimia Nervosa

Bulimia nervosa is defined as recurrent episodes of binge eating at least once per week over a period of 3 months characterized by overeating within 2 h and a sense of lack of control during these episodes. Patients will subsequently participate in compensatory behaviors to prevent weight gain including self-induced vomiting, laxative, diuretic, or diet pill misuse, fasting, or excessive exercise. Their self-evaluation will also be influenced by their body shape and weight. Severity is defined by number of episodes per week. Patients who participate in compensatory behaviors 1–3 times per week are considered mild, 4–7 times per week are considered moderate, 8–13 times per week are considered severe, and ≥ 14 times per week are considered extreme.

Bulimia nervosa is also associated with mood disorders including depression. About 50% of individuals will recover from bulimia nervosa and about one-quarter of patients will continue to have abnormal eating habits. Mortality rate is increased in patients who are pre-morbid or have paternal elevated BMI.

Binge Eating Disorder

Binge eating disorder often occurs in patients 25–50 years old and is defined as recurrent episodes of binge eating with episodes characterized by three or more of the following: eating more quickly than normal, eating until they are uncomfortably full, eating when not hungry, eating alone due to embarrassment, sense of disgust, depression, or guilt after episodes. Severity of disease is characterized by number of binge eating episodes per week. Patients with 1–3 episodes per week are considered mild, 4–7 times per week are considered moderate, 8–13 times per week are considered severe, and ≥ 14 times per week are considered extreme.

Unlike patients with bulimia nervosa, patients with binge eating disorder do not use compensatory behaviors. Compared to patients with overeating who typically overeat in positive social situations, patients with binge eating disorder typically binge eat alone with subjective distress.

Avoidant/Restrictive Food Intake Disorder

Avoidant/restrictive food intake disorder (ARFID) is defined as aversion to eating due to lack of interest, avoidance of sensory characteristics, or aversion to consequences of eating that lead to significant weight loss, nutritional deficiency, requiring enteral feeding or nutritional supplements, or interference with psychosocial functioning.

Other Specified Feeding and Eating Disorders

Patients who do not meet criteria for the above eating disorders are classified in the other specified feeding and eating disorders (OSFED) category. Atypical anorexia nervosa includes patients who have the characteristics of anorexia nervosa but do not meet current low body weight criteria. This can include people with an elevated BMI. Patients can also have bulimia nervosa and binge eating disorder with low frequency or limited duration. Purging disorder includes patients who participate in purging behaviors but do not participate in binge eating. Night eating syndrome is defined as episodes of excessive food consumption in the evening exacerbated by stress with insomnia and morning anorexia. Further discussion of additional disorders outside the scope of this discussion is described in the DSM-V.

Often times, the initial screening and evaluation for eating disorder can detect the presence of some type of eating disorder but the exact diagnosis is unclear. Referral to a mental health provider is useful to determine a formal diagnosis for an eating disorder and for the initiation of treatment (see below for more management details).

15.3.3 *Evaluation*

Evaluation should be initiated when there is an initial suspicion for an underlying eating disorder or if a patient screens positive for concern for an eating disorder. Initial suspicion should prompt questions in the history including the patient's previous weight and pattern of weight loss, menstrual history, exercise habits, insomnia, alcohol/other drug use, and daytime hyperactivity. Questions regarding the patient's eating habits should include what the patient eats in a day, a history of eating more than they would like (binge eating), and use of laxatives, diuretics, or diet pills. It is also helpful to elicit individuals' attitudes toward their body weight and shape with questions such as how the patient themselves views their body shape/weight. Patients should also be asked about a family history of depression or alcohol abuse and a personal history of rape/sexual assault, childhood abuse, or depression which are known risk factors for development of eating disorders. Questions specific to bulimia nervosa also include whether the patient ever eats in secret and how satisfied they are with their eating habits. The SCOFF questionnaire is also an effective evaluation tool with high sensitivity (100%) and specificity (87.5%) for identification of early stages of both anorexia nervosa and bulimia nervosa and takes less than 2 min to complete. The SCOFF questionnaire questions include the following:

1. Do you ever make yourself **S**ick because you feel uncomfortably full?
2. Do you ever worry you have lost **C**ontrol over how much you eat?
3. Have you recently lost more than **O**ne stone (14 pounds) in a 3-month period?
4. Do you believe yourself to be **F**at when others say you are too thin?
5. Would you say **F**ood dominates your life?

Other screening tests specific for binge eating disorder include the eating attitudes test, a 26-item self-reported inventory to screen for eating disorders, and the questionnaire on eating and weight patterns-revised.

The gold standard assessment for eating disorders consists of the eating disorder examination (EDE) interview and the eating disorder examination-questionnaire (EDE-Q) which are more often used in collaboration with mental health providers when an underlying eating disorder is suspected. These surveys have four sub-scales that include restraint, concerns about eating, concerns about body shape, and concerns about weight. The surveys also include behavioral symptoms including number of bulimic days/episodes, frequency of binge eating, presence of self-induced vomiting, excessive exercise, and misuse of medications including laxatives and diuretics.

When examining the patient, vital signs should be assessed, specifically examining for evidence of hypotension, bradycardia, or orthostasis. Careful examination of dentition for tooth enamel erosion and dental caries, parotid gland for enlargement via palpation behind the masseter muscle anterior to the ear, heart auscultation for new murmurs (such as mitral valve prolapse from disproportionate size between left ventricle and mitral valve), and skin for injuries associated with recurrent self-induced emesis (such as knuckle calluses known as Russell's sign), peripheral edema, yellow skin (from elevated serum beta-carotene levels), and lanugo (fine, soft hair throughout body) can also point to a concern for eating disorder or severity of eating disorder (Fig. 15.1). Laboratory values that should be assessed generally include electrolytes, including magnesium, calcium, and phosphorus, albumin, and cell count. Patients who binge or purge may present with metabolic abnormalities such as hypochloremic metabolic alkalosis. If a patient has amenorrhea, additional evaluation with pregnancy test, FSH, LH, TSH, and prolactin may be helpful. In severe cases, metabolic abnormalities can present with EKG changes as well. If there is concern for hypoestrogenism, a DEXA scan may be useful to assess severity

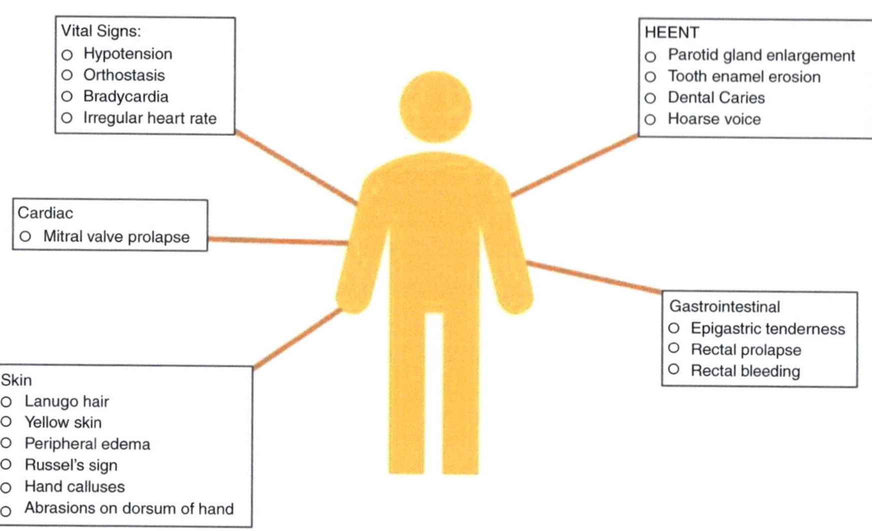

Fig. 15.1 Symptoms on physical exam associated with eating disorders

of bone loss. In patients with concomitant diabetes, other signs include chronically elevated A1c, repeated episodes of diabetic ketoacidosis, or wide daily fluctuations in glucose levels for patients with continuous glucose monitoring. Patients may also have low A1c with eating disorders if they achieve a low A1c with restrictive eating behaviors.

During her visit, Mrs. Jones' vital signs are notable for a body mass index of 31.0 kg/m^2. Her exam is also notable for calluses over her metacarpophalangeal (MCP)joints that she attributes to her rock-climbing gear. Laboratory testing was notable for potassium of 3.3 mmol/l, bicarbonate of 20 mEq/L, chloride of 90 mEq/L. She had normal thyroid stimulating hormone and complete blood count. Mrs. Jones has objective evidence concerning for possible underlying eating disorder. On physical exam and laboratory evaluation, she has evidence of recurrent self-induced vomiting including calluses over her MCP joints (Russel sign), hypokalemia, and hypochloremic metabolic alkalosis. These findings in combination with her increased BMI and concerns about her weight are concerning for possible bulimia nervosa. It would be appropriate to administer the SCOFF questionnaire to further assess for an underlying eating disorder.

15.3.4 Comprehensive Treatment Plan

Upon further evaluation using the SCOFF questionnaire and upon referral to a mental health provider, Mrs. Jones is found to have evidence concerning for bulimia nervosa. She is also referred to a dietitian. Her primary care provider collaborates with these providers to help manage her bulimia nervosa. She engages in cognitive behavioral therapy with her mental health provider in the outpatient setting and trials fluoxetine to help treat her bulimia nervosa.

Management of eating disorders often requires active collaboration within a multidisciplinary team consisting of a patient's primary care provider, a dietitian, and a mental health provider with the ultimate goals of normalizing eating patterns, meeting nutritional needs, and reaching ideal body weight for those who are underweight. The primary care provider should primarily coordinate treatment within the team, identify and manage medical complications associated with the eating disorder, and determine whether a patient requires inpatient hospitalization. If a comprehensive team is not available or if the eating disorder is mild, primary care providers should also manage the patient's eating disorder with routine weight monitoring and food intake monitoring. Primary care providers can also use tools like food diaries and contract setting for weight/food intake in certain patients. A registered dietitian will monitor a patient's nutritional intake, often through use of food diaries, and provide suggestions on how to increase or balance nutrition to support a healthy weight. Mental health providers will often provide individual/family psychotherapy and cognitive behavioral therapy as appropriate for patients with eating disorders. This section will focus on specific treatment modalities for common eating disorders.

Identification of Level of Care

Primary care providers are tasked with determining the appropriate level of care for patients with eating disorders depending on the severity of their disorder. Further determination of level of care may be assessed in conjunction with a mental health provider. The levels of care include hospitalization, inpatient residential treatment program, partial hospitalization (PHP), intensive outpatient programs (IOP), and outpatient treatment (Fig. 15.2).

Patients may meet inpatient hospitalization criteria based on medical stability. Disease severity characterized by rapid weight loss, loss of>30% of their ideal body weight, and a large number of binge/purge episodes may qualify patients for inpatient hospitalization. Severe bulimia nervosa is defined as 8–13 episodes and extreme bulimia nervosa is defined as ≥14 episodes per week. Patients who do not respond to outpatient therapy or are unable to reliably follow-up may benefit from more intensive care such as inpatient hospitalization. Additionally, individuals with severe depression or suicidality or concurrent substance use disorder may benefit from inpatient treatment. Other indications for hospitalization include medical complications secondary to the eating disorder such as arrhythmia/bradycardia,

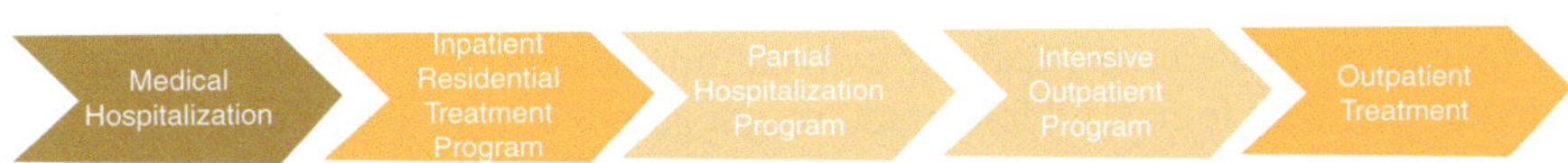

Fig. 15.2 Continuum of level of care for patients with eating disorders

hypotension, hypoglycemia, hypokalemia, hypophosphatemia, or evidence of inadequate cerebral perfusion. Day programs such as partial hospitalization and intensive outpatient programs may be considered depending on patient motivation level and availability of programs. Patients who require withdrawal of laxatives or diuretics may require intensive non-outpatient treatment level of care.

Non-Pharmacological Interventions

Non-pharmacological interventions and behavioral interventions in eating disorders often depend on the type of eating disorder. This section provides recommendations for weight gain strategies and mental health treatments of common types of eating disorders and the behavioral interventions or psychotherapy options for each.

Patients with anorexia nervosa often benefit from identifying a target weight, often defined as within 10% of patient's highest weight before onset of illness or 3–5 pounds above weight where menses is resumed in patients who are not on hormonal contraception or do not have a history of amenorrhea from other causes. Patients should be monitored for gradual weight gain of 0.5–1 pound per week with weekly patient weights. For patients who do not want to know their weight, shared decision making regarding alternative monitoring such as weekly nursing visits or more intensive monitoring should be considered. Providers should also be aware of possible water loading. Water loading is the act of artificially increasing one's weight by increasing one's water intake beyond normal levels of hydration to induce diuresis by cutting down fluid intake prior to weight checks. If there is concern for water loading, urine specific gravity can be monitored.

In anorexia nervosa, patients may benefit from contract setting with all members of the patient's treatment team. The contract can include specific details such as indications for hospitalizations or higher level of care, follow-up, and completion of a food diary. Patients may also discuss with a registered dietitian their portion sizes, intervals between meals, emotions or physical sensations associated with eating. Patients can also participate in goal settings specifically around the addition of foods in their diet, interval between meals, and portion sizes. Cognitive behavioral therapy has also been used in patients with anorexia nervosa and is more effective in patients with high severity anorexia nervosa. Among younger patients, family therapy is often indicated, with individual therapy as an alternative for some adolescents when family therapy is not feasible.

Patients with bulimia nervosa often respond positively to cognitive behavioral therapy, interpersonal therapy, and dialectical behavioral therapy that focus on modification of their behavior and thinking around their binge/purge episodes. Similarly, binge eating disorder also benefits from cognitive behavioral therapy, behavioral weight management, and nutritional guidance. Self-care manuals have also been shown to be effective among patients with bulimia nervosa and binge eating disorder.

In patients with female athlete triad, weight gain is a mainstay of treatment. Goal weight is defined as reaching one or more of the following: reversal of weight loss, return of menstruation, weight gain ≥ 18.5 kg/m^2, or energy expenditure ≥ 2000 kcal per day, often requiring >3000 kcal per day to promote weight restoration. Patients may benefit from referral to nutrition counseling or sport dietician and collaboration with patient's coach. For patients with concomitant eating disorder, management of the underlying eating disorder is important. Weight bearing exercises should also be considered for bone density management although whether high-impact activity leads to increased fractures in this population remains unclear.

In patients with eating disorder and diabetes, providers should be aware of morality language such as "good" or "bad" A1c values or "correcting" blood sugar values. Patients may benefit from coordination between all members of the patient's treatment team including possibly an endocrinologist.

Medical Management and Pharmacotherapy

The medical management and pharmacotherapy options for eating disorders are an adjunct to psychotherapy and behavioral interventions. This section describes specific medications and medical management recommendations to date.

High dose fluoxetine has been approved by the Food and Drug Administration (FDA) for treatment of bulimia nervosa and should be considered first line therapy, although there is evidence that most antidepressants such as tricyclic antidepressants, other serotonin selective reuptake inhibitors (SSRI)/serotonin-norepinephrine reuptake inhibitors (SNRIs), and monoamine oxidase inhibitors (MAOIs) may benefit this disorder. Medications for binge eating disorder include sibutramine, which is contraindicated in patients with cardiovascular disease, topiramate, and orlistat. Bupropion should be avoided due to increased risk of seizures in eating disorders. Of note, there is no strong evidence that antidepressants such as SSRIs are useful in the management of anorexia nervosa.

For patients who have associated fear and anxiety associated with eating, providers can consider the use of anxiolytics before eating. Hormonal contraception may mask resumption of menses which can provide additional challenges in assessing return of healthy weight and remove an important motivational factor associated with weight restoration among patients. In conjunction with evaluation by a dietitian, patients may also benefit from vitamin supplementation including daily multivitamin with iron and calcium and zinc supplementation. Patients can also be treated with metoclopramide for abdominal bloating. Due to risk of refeeding syndrome, fatal electrolyte, and fluid shifts after re-establishing nutrition in malnourished patients, patient's electrolytes should be regularly monitored and patients should be prescribed electrolyte repletion to prevent development of refeeding syndrome.

Complications and Management

Patients particularly with high severity eating disorders have an increased risk of developing medical complications. This section describes complications associated with certain eating disorders and provides management recommendations.

Patients with high severity anorexia nervosa are at risk of developing cardiovascular complications. For example, patients may develop arrhythmias or sudden death due to QT prolongation from certain electrolyte abnormalities. Close monitoring of electrolytes and use of electrocardiogram particularly among patients with known electrolyte abnormalities are necessary. In particular, patients at risk of refeeding syndrome may develop hypokalemia, hypocalcemia, hypomagnesemia, and hypophosphatemia. Patients should therefore receive oral nutritional repletion and electrolyte repletion as needed. Patients with severe electrolyte abnormalities may require inpatient hospitalization. Other hormonal abnormalities that may develop include thyroid abnormalities, high cortisol levels, and neurogenic diabetes insipidus. Patients may also develop gastrointestinal complications including gastroparesis, constipation, and refeeding pancreatitis; dermatologic complications such as dry skin, carotenodermia, lanugo, and starvation-associated pruritis; and hematologic complications such as pancytopenia. They may also have difficulty with temperature regulation. These symptoms can be treated with symptomatic management and often improve with management of the underlying eating disorder.

Those who engage in purging, particularly in bulimia nervosa, may also develop complications associated with recurrent forced emesis. In particular, patients may develop dental erosion from gastric acid, which often will worsen with teeth brushing after episodes. Patients may develop parotid gland hypertrophy and esophageal symptoms including GERD, and in severe cases, esophageal rupture due to recurrent vomiting. Pulmonary symptoms such as aspiration pneumonitis and pneumomediastinum may also develop. Laboratory abnormalities including hypokalemia, hypoglycemia, hypochloremic metabolic alkalosis from recurrent vomiting, and metabolic acidosis from misuse of laxatives can also develop. Patients can also develop constipation from laxative abuse, chronic diarrhea, and post-binge pancreatitis. Cardiovascular complications including arrhythmias from electrolyte imbalance, mitral valve prolapse from weight loss, and hypertension due to misuse of diet pills can also develop. Patients who have type I diabetes have an increased risk of microvascular complications, particularly if they have poor glycemic control occasionally due to underdosing their insulin to promote weight loss.

Gynecological Health

Menstrual irregularities and secondary amenorrhea can occur with eating disorders even with normal BMI and should be evaluated on a routine basis. About 30% of women with anorexia nervosa develop delays in normal menstruation and fertility after their weight returns to normal. Conversely, in bulimia nervosa, fertility issues occur at a similar rate as in the regular patient population. Due to menstrual irregularities or amenorrhea, unplanned pregnancies can occur as patients may have inadequate contraception use and misconceptions regarding their ability to conceive. Discussing expectations regarding menstruation and fertility is important in patients with eating disorders.

It is possible that Mrs. Jones' secondary amenorrhea is associated with her long term CHC use; however, given her underlying bulimia nervosa, it would be reasonable to consider eating disorder as a possible contribution to her amenorrhea. Of note, she should be reassured that rates of infertility among patients with eating disorders are similar to those in the general population and should therefore undergo routine infertility evaluation and management.

Bone Health

Due to hypothalamic hypogonadism that leads to a hypoestrogenic state in patients with severe disease, patients may develop osteoporosis with increased risk of fracture and often will not develop withdrawal bleeding after a progesterone challenge. Patients with the female athlete triad are also at increased risk of stress fractures. As discussed above, DEXA scan may be useful in evaluation if there is concern for hypoestrogenism in women with eating disorders. For patients with Z-score lower than expected for age (≤ -2.0) and high fracture risk, patients should be counseled regarding their risk of clinical fractures and the importance of slow weight gain to goal weight as primary management. Patients should also be treated with calcium and vitamin D supplementation. There is minimal evidence surrounding the use of oral contraceptives to reduce the risk of bone loss. There are also limited data on the use of hormone therapy, bisphosphonates such as alendronate, or teriparatide in premenopausal women, and these medications should be considered on a case-by-case basis based on clinical context.

Pregnancy and Eating Disorders

As previously discussed, pregnancy can occur in patients with eating disorders, particularly due to menstrual irregularities and misconceptions about ability to conceive. If an eating disorder is diagnosed prior to pregnancy, patients should be educated regarding risks of pregnancy and recommended to postpone pregnancy until after they have recovered from their eating disorder. If a patient with an underlying eating disorder has a positive pregnancy test, early referral to specialized care and expectation management are crucial. Prior studies have shown that those with bulimia nervosa also are at higher likelihood of having a history of miscarriage.

Patients should be referred to a high-risk pregnancy obstetrician in addition to their outpatient care team including their dietitian and mental health provider. They should be provided guidance regarding the importance of nutrition for the fetus' health. Pregnant people with anorexia nervosa, for example, may have babies that are small for gestational age, microcephaly, intrauterine growth restriction, and premature labor. Pregnant people with eating disorders should also engage in early discussions regarding expected body shape changes/weight changes, cravings, and hyperemesis gravidarum. Body shape and weight changes during pregnancy can increase anxiety and further complicate the management of eating disorders. Some patients may develop recurrence of or worsening of an underlying disorder due to these changes. Conversely, other patients may improve their underlying eating disorder for fear of harming the fetus. Patients should have regular follow-up in the prenatal period. Patients should be counseled regarding the use of laxatives, appetite suppressants, and diuretics, which can be unsafe during pregnancy.

In the postpartum period, people with eating disorders should be monitored closely. Women with eating disorders are at higher risk of developing postpartum depression with one-third of women developing postpartum depression. They may also develop anemia and problems with episiotomy repair due to malnutrition. There is also an increased risk of relapse in the postpartum period or an increase in binge eating in patients with eating disorders. Postpartum women with eating disorders may also develop challenges with breastfeeding and therefore benefit from increased breastfeeding support. They should be monitored closely in the postpartum period for weight, eating patterns, binge/purge episodes, and misuse of diet pills, laxatives, diuretics, or other medications to assist with weight loss.

15.4 Conclusion

Eating disorders such as anorexia nervosa have high risk of morbidity and mortality. Primary care providers play a crucial role in the diagnosis and management of eating disorders. The presentation of women with eating disorders may be variable and primary care providers should be aware of the various types of patients who may be at risk for development of eating disorders. Once clinically suspected, providers should perform careful screening and evaluation. The management of eating disorders once diagnosed requires close coordination of care in a multidisciplinary team including the primary care provider, a mental health provider, and a nutritionist. For patients who are pregnant, involvement of a high-risk obstetrician will also be necessary. Primary care providers should not only evaluate the appropriate level of care patients require but also monitor patients closely for the development of medical complications of eating disorders. Successful management of patients with eating disorders often requires psychiatric care with adjunctive medications. Close follow-up at all stages of care is crucial among patients with eating disorders. The current detection rates of eating disorders are estimated to be low. Providers may be more likely to identify and comfortably manage eating disorders with increased awareness of eating disorders among primary care providers.

Suggested Reading

1. Ward VB. Eating disorders in pregnancy. BMJ. 2008;336(7635):93–6.
2. Berg KC, Peterson CB, Frazier P, Crow SJ. Psychometric evaluation of the eating disorder examination and eating disorder examination-questionnaire: a systematic review of the literature. Int J Eat Disord. 2012;45(3):428–38.
3. Walsh JM, Wheat ME, Freund K. Detection, evaluation, and treatment of eating disorders. J Gen Intern Med. 2000;15(8):577–90.
4. Sim LA, McAlpine DE, Grothe KB, Himes SM, Cockerill RG, Clark MM, editors. Identification and treatment of eating disorders in the primary care setting. Mayo Clinic Proceedings; 2010, Elsevier.
5. Sangvai D. Eating disorders in the primary care setting. Prim Care. 2016;43(2):301–12.
6. Rome ES, Ammerman S. Medical complications of eating disorders: an update. J Adolesc Health. 2003;33(6):418–26.
7. Pritts SD, Susman J. Diagnosis of eating disorders in primary care. Am Fam Physician. 2003;67(2):297–304.
8. Mond JM, Myers TC, Crosby RD, Hay PJ, Mitchell JE. Bulimic eating disorders in primary care: hidden morbidity still? J Clin Psychol Med Settings. 2010;17(1):56–63.
9. Lemly DC, Dreier MJ, Birnbaum S, Eddy KT, Thomas JJ. Caring for adults with eating disorders in primary care. Primary Care Comp CNS Disorder. 2022;24(1):39060.
10. Klein DA, Sylvester J, Schvey NA. Eating disorders in primary care: diagnosis and management. Am Fam Physician. 2021;103(1):22–32.
11. Keski-Rahkonen A, Raevuori A, Hoek HW. Epidemiology of eating disorders: an update. Ann Rev Eating Disorder. 2018:66–76.
12. Gurney VW, Halmi KA. An eating disorder curriculum for primary care providers. Int J Eat Disord. 2001;30(2):209–12.
13. Allen S, Dalton WT. Treatment of eating disorders in primary care: a systematic review. J Health Psychol. 2011;16(8):1165–76.
14. Association AD. Position of the American dietetic association: nutrition intervention in the treatment of anorexia nervosa, bulimia nervosa, and eating disorders not otherwise specified (EDNOS). J Am Diet Assoc. 2001;101(7):810–9.
15. De Souza MJ, Nattiv A, Joy E, Misra M, Williams NI, Mallinson RJ, et al. Female athlete triad coalition consensus statement on treatment and return to play of the female athlete triad: 1st international conference held in San Francisco, California, May 2012 and 2nd international conference held in Indianapolis, Indiana, May 2013. Br J Sports Med. 2014;48(4):289.

Chapter 16
Osteoporosis

Christina Lalani and Atul Lalani

16.1 Introduction

16.1.1 Pathophysiology and Presentation

Although all adults achieve their peak bone mass by their mid-twenties, there are important differences in the evolution of bone mass in males and females [1]. In males, there is a progressive decline in bone mass after achievement of peak bone mass. However, in females, bone mass typically plateaus until menopause, after which there is a period of accelerated bone loss. Healthy bone undergoes continuous remodeling, which includes cycles of bone resorption and bone formation. However, bone mass can become decreased in the setting of low peak bone mass, increased bone resorption, or decreased bone formation [1]. Osteoporosis is a metabolic bone disease that results in disruption of the normal structure of the bone leading to consequential bone fragility and a higher predisposition to fractures. According to the CDC, the prevalence of osteoporosis in the USA is 12.6% (2017–2018), which has increased in recent years.

Osteoporosis is an asymptomatic disease process until patients develop a fracture, and even then, fractures are often incidentally identified on imaging that is completed for other indications [2]. The most common site of fracture in osteoporosis is a vertebral compression fracture which can present with pain in the acute setting but can present asymptomatically with evidence of height loss or kyphosis on

C. Lalani (✉)
Beth Israel Deaconess Medical Center, Boston, MA, USA

A. Lalani
East Valley Endocrinology, Scottsdale, AZ, USA

© The Author(s), under exclusive license to Springer Nature Switzerland AG 2024

M. Mahmoudi (ed.), *Common Cases in Women's Primary Care Clinics*, https://doi.org/10.1007/978-3-031-48569-5_16

"

exam in the chronic setting [2]. When patients present with an acute vertebral compression fracture, they classically report the onset of acute back pain without significant trauma. The pain can be variable in quality but is most often well-localized to the mid spine. Although the pain should resolve within 4–6 weeks on average, slower healing fractures can result in a more prolonged duration of pain. Other common sites of fracture include hip fractures and Colles fractures (distal radial fractures).

16.2 Case Presentation

16.2.1 Initial Presentation

Ms. Johnson is a 67-year-old female with a history of hypertension, hyperlipidemia, GERD, and non-insulin dependent diabetes who presents to her primary care clinic for an annual visit. Her medications include losartan 50 mg daily, rosuvastatin 20 mg daily, omeprazole 40 mg daily, and metformin 500 mg daily. She has no known drug allergies. For her social history, she lives in an apartment with her husband and is independent in all activities of daily living. She ambulates independently and manages her own medications. She reports current tobacco use and has smoked ½ pack per day of cigarettes since age 20. She consumes 1–2 glasses of wine per day. She eats a balanced diet of foods primarily prepared at home but does not do any exercise currently. She has a family history of heart attack in her father at age 70 and hip fracture in her mother at age 72. At the clinic visit today, she is overall feeling well and denies any specific concerns. Her review of symptoms is negative for headaches, chest pain, shortness of breath, pre-syncope, syncope, weight loss/gain, night sweats, fevers, chills palpitations, nausea/vomiting, diarrhea, cold intolerance, and heat intolerance. Based on this patient's age, her primary care doctor, Dr. Roberts, orders a bone density scan for screening for osteoporosis.

16.2.2 Initial Testing and Management

Ms. Johnson undergoes a DEXA scan with the following results: T-score for femoral neck: −2.6, T-score for proximal femur: −2.3, and T-score for lumbar spine: −2.0. She returns to Dr. Roberts' office to discuss her test results. Dr. Roberts shares with the patient that her DEXA scan results are consistent with a diagnosis of osteoporosis. He tells her that guidelines recommend the initiation of treatment for her new diagnosis to reduce the risk of fracture in the setting of her weakened bones.

As a first step, Dr. Roberts orders additional laboratory testing including a biochemical profile, 25-hydroxy vitamin D, and complete blood count. The results of the patient's laboratory testing are outlined in Fig. 16.1. Her laboratory results are overall unremarkable except for her 25-hydroxy vitamin D level of 18 ng/mL, which

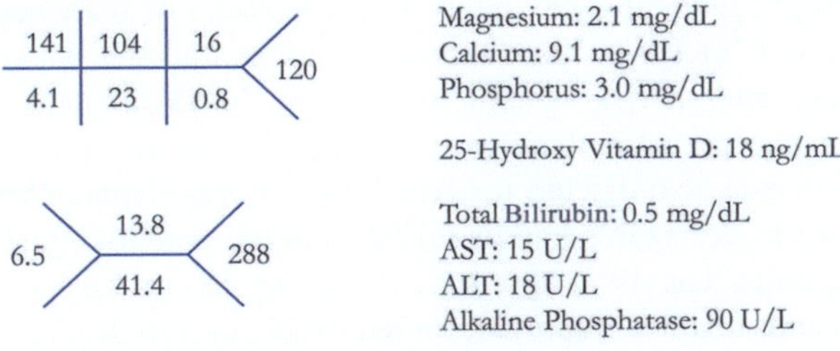

Fig. 16.1 Baseline laboratory results

is consistent with vitamin D insufficiency. Based on the patient's medical history and current presentation, there are no concerns for other causes of secondary osteoporosis. She is started on 1000 international units daily of vitamin D3 with a plan to repeat her laboratory testing in 3 months to assess for improvement.

In the meanwhile, she follows up with Dr. Roberts to discuss other non-pharmacological treatments for osteoporosis. Her doctor completes an assessment of her daily calcium intake and finds that Ms. Johnson is consuming more than 1200 mg of calcium per day. He determines that she does not need to start a calcium supplement at this time. He also begins to assess Ms. Johnson's current exercise tolerance and physical activity. Ms. Johnson shares that she generally does not set aside time for exercise but is active around her house with household tasks and cooking. She does have a flight of stairs in her home, which she is able to climb without any difficulty. Her doctor discusses multiple options for slowly incorporating more physical activity and Ms. Johnson ultimately decides that she is going to work on going for a 30 minute walk after dinner three times a week. Dr. Roberts emphasizes that it is more important that she does at least 150 min of physical activity per week than it is that she does high intensity activity. Increasing weight-bearing exercise of any kind is beneficial for her health from an osteoporosis perspective. The final aspect of lifestyle management that her primary care doctor discusses is the patient's tobacco use. Although she is initially hesitant about cutting down her smoking, Ms. Johnson ultimately decides that she is open to trying nicotine patches to help with slowly decreasing her tobacco intake.

16.2.3 Follow-Up and Initiation of Pharmacological Therapy

Ms. Johnson follows up in clinic 3 months after starting vitamin D supplementation. She obtains repeat labs that show a 25-hydroxy vitamin D level of 25 ng/mL, which is within normal limits. At this visit, Dr. Roberts discusses multiple different options for pharmacological therapy. Since Ms. Johnson does not have severe osteoporosis (T-score of ≤ -3 or T-score of ≤ -2.5 with a fragility fracture), the first-line treatment for her osteoporosis is a bisphosphonate. Dr. Roberts discusses the potential side effects that are specific to oral bisphosphonates including gastrointestinal reflux, esophagitis, and ulcers. Dr. Roberts also shares that both oral and IV bisphosphonates can cause the side effect of osteonecrosis of the jaw or atypical femur fractures. Ms. Johnson mentions that she is overdue for a dental extraction and after a risk–benefit discussion, the decision is made to defer initiation of bisphosphonate therapy until after her dental extraction. Dr. Roberts and Ms. Johnson also discuss the feasibility of oral bisphosphonate treatment in the setting of Ms. Johnson's known GERD and the potential gastrointestinal side effects. She decides that she is agreeable to trialing an oral bisphosphonate for now. She understands that it is important for her to stay upright for 30–60 min after taking the medication and is confident that she will be able to do this consistently. After completion of her dental work, Ms. Johnson is eventually initiated on alendronate 70 mg weekly.

Unfortunately, after 4 weeks of therapy, she contacts Dr. Roberts' office due to concerns about worsening acid reflux in the setting of taking alendronate. After discussing different options for alternative therapy, the decision is ultimately made to switch to IV bisphosphonate therapy with initiation of IV zoledronic acid. Ms. Johnson understands that she may have 1–3 days of flu-like symptoms after receiving her injection of IV zoledronic acid, but she will not have ongoing gastrointestinal symptoms. She is started on 5 mg IV zoledronic acid every 12 months.

16.2.4 Monitoring After Initiation of Therapy

After 2 years of therapy, Ms. Johnson returns to clinic for follow-up. Dr. Roberts elects to obtain a repeat DEXA scan to assess how Ms. Johnson's bone density has evolved since the initiation of IV zoledronic acid. She completes a repeat DEXA scan with the following results: T-score for femoral neck: −2.7, T-score for proximal femur: −2.3, and T-score for lumbar spine: −1.9. Since Ms. Johnson is tolerating IV zoledronic acid well and her bone density T-scores are similar to her prior scan, Dr. Roberts elects to continue IV zoledronic acid for now and repeat a bone density scan in 1 year.

16.2.5 Transition of Therapy

Unfortunately, in the interim, Ms. Johnson has a ground level fall after which she has a left wrist fracture. She returns to clinic for follow-up. Dr. Roberts discusses his concerns about Ms. Johnson having a fracture despite treatment with an IV bisphosphonate. He checks in on Ms. Roberts' adherence with calcium and vitamin D and she reports that she has been taking vitamin D supplementation and continues to have high calcium intake with her diet. He rechecks Ms. Johnson's vitamin D level and calcium level and both are within normal limits. Her laboratory results do not show concern for a secondary cause of osteoporosis. He also confirms that she has not missed any doses of IV bisphosphonates and has presented for her annual injection. Dr. Roberts discusses potential options for alternative therapy given her fragility fracture while on treatment with an IV bisphosphonate. He recommends initiation of teriparatide for 2 years. Ms. Johnson does not have any contraindications to receiving teriparatide including primary or secondary hyperparathyroidism, hypercalcemic disorders, or an increased risk of osteosarcoma. He shares that this will require a daily injection into the thigh or abdominal wall. Although Ms. Johnson is hesitant about a daily injection, she shares that her husband will be able to help with these injections and is open to trialing teriparatide.

Dr. Roberts discusses the potential side effects of teriparatide. He shares that with the first few doses, Ms. Johnson may have orthostatic hypotension or tachycardia. He encourages her to lie down when she takes her first few doses. Other potential side effects include nausea, hypercalcemia, calciphylaxis, and hypercalciuria. Dr. Roberts elects to monitor Ms. Johnson's calcium every 3 months to ensure that she does not develop hypercalcemia.

16.2.6   Follow-Up on Teriparatide

After 1 year of therapy, Dr. Roberts elects to obtain a repeat DEXA scan to reassess Ms. Johnson's bone density on teriparatide. She completes a repeat DEXA scan with the following results: T-score for femoral neck: −2.3, T-score for proximal femur: −1.9, and T-score for lumbar spine: −1.5. Given her improving bone density, Dr. Roberts elects to continue teriparatide for an additional year. After completion of 2 years of teriparatide, she is transitioned back to IV zoledronic acid.

16.3   Discussion

16.3.1   Definition and Diagnosis

The diagnosis of osteoporosis is typically made using a dual-energy X-ray absorptiometry (DEXA) scan, also called a bone density scan. A DEXA scan uses small amounts of radiation to evaluate the density of a patient's lumbar vertebrae, femur, and sometimes forearm. According to the World Health Organization, osteoporosis is defined as having a bone mineral density in the femur neck region, proximal femur, or lumbar spine that is at least 2.5 standard deviations below the average bone mineral density of a young adult female (Table 16.1).

Table 16.1 Interpretation of bone density T-score

T-score on bone density scan	Classification
−1.0 to +1.0	Normal bone density
−1.0 to −2.5	Osteopenia
≤ −2.5	Osteoporosis

This criterion should only be applied to postmenopausal women and men older than 50 years old. The presence of a fragility fracture, a fracture that results from a fall from standing height or less, is also diagnostic of osteoporosis, especially in bones such as the spine, hip, wrist, humerus, rib, and pelvis. A clinical diagnosis of osteoporosis can also be made if an individual's 10-year probability of a major osteoporotic fracture (meaning a fracture of the spine, hip, shoulder, or forearm) is at least 20% or the 10-year probability of a hip fracture is at least 3%. The most frequently used tool to assess an individual's risk of fracture is the Fracture Risk Assessment Tool (FRAX), which models fracture risk based on an individual's femoral neck bone mineral density and additional clinical risk factors [3]. The relevant risk factors included in the calculation tool include age, sex, weight, height, previous fracture, history of fractured hip in parent, current smoking, current glucocorticoid use, history of rheumatoid arthritis, secondary osteoporosis, and consumption of more than 3 alcoholic drinks per day [3].

Other potential causes of bone fracture and reduced bone mineral density beyond osteoporosis include osteomalacia, malignancy, Paget disease, and hyperparathyroidism. It is also important to consider physical abuse in the differential diagnosis when patients present with fractures in atypical locations or have fractures that are out of proportion to the degree of bone mineral density loss.

When patients are found to have osteoporosis, in addition to completing a bone density scan, the initial evaluation should include a calcium, phosphate, creatinine, liver function tests, 25-hydroxy vitamin D, and complete blood count. Additional testing can be considered depending on the patient's history and the concern for secondary causes of osteoporosis. For example, screening for multiple myeloma would be reasonable in a patient who presents with anemia and weight loss as well as concern for bone mineral density loss.

16.3.2　Screening for Osteoporosis

The guidelines for screening for osteoporosis with a bone density scan are variable dependent on the country and availability of resources for both screening and intervention. In the USA, most society guidelines recommend screening for osteoporosis with a bone density scan for all women over 65 [4]. This guideline is influenced by the findings of multiple studies that show a reduction in fractures with the implementation of population screening [5]. Screening can also be considered in younger postmenopausal female patients with higher clinical risk for fractures including previous fracture, glucocorticoid therapy, parental history of hip fracture, low body weight, cigarette smoking, excessive alcohol consumption, rheumatoid arthritis, or concern for secondary causes of osteoporosis. There are no standardized guidelines on screening for osteoporosis in premenopausal individuals, but it is reasonable to consider screening in women with a history of fragility fracture or known secondary causes of osteoporosis. The list of secondary causes of osteoporosis is extensive but includes conditions like gastrointestinal malabsorption, vitamin D or calcium deficiency, hyperparathyroidism, hyperthyroidism, Cushing's syndrome, hypogonadism, alcoholism, renal disease, liver disease, and several different medications [6].

There is some variability in the guidelines on screening for osteoporosis in males. According to the National Osteoporosis Foundation, International Society for Clinical Densitometry, and Endocrine Society, all men older than 70 years old should undergo screening for osteoporosis with a bone density scan. However, since osteoporosis is less frequently seen in men, there are fewer clinical trials evaluating the management of osteoporosis in men and there is less data on whether there is a benefit to routine screening in this population. As a result, the United States Preventive Services Task Force does not make a recommendation on screening in males.

As an example of the variability in guidelines between various societies, according to the Association of Clinical Endocrinologists, screening with bone density of the lumbar spine and proximal femur should be completed in the following categories of individuals: all women 65 years and older, any adult with fracture not caused by severe trauma, and younger postmenopausal women with risk factors for fracture. In contrast, the National Osteoporosis Foundation also recommends screening in all men older than 70, women in the menopausal transition with clinical risk factors for fracture, men who are age 50–69 with clinical risk factors for fracture, and adults who have medical conditions or take medications associated with low bone mass or bone loss. There are no definitive guidelines on the need for repeat screening and the frequency for surveillance imaging in patients who are not diagnosed with osteoporosis on initial evaluation.

16.3.3 Management of Osteoporosis

All patients with osteoporosis should be counseled on lifestyle modification including smoking cessation, limiting alcohol intake, and completing regular weight-bearing exercise. It is recommended that individuals with osteoporosis exercise for at least 30 minutes three times a week. Patients should also consume at least 1000–1200 mg of calcium per day and 600–1000 international units of vitamin D per day.

Prior studies have primarily shown a benefit for the use of additional pharmacologic therapies in postmenopausal osteoporosis. In the USA, pharmacologic therapy is recommended for postmenopausal females who meet the criteria for diagnosis of osteoporosis as above. This differs from the criteria for intervention in other countries. For example, the United Kingdom National Osteoporosis Guideline group recommends intervention based on an age-dependent intervention threshold. Initiation of medical therapy should only be done after normalization of calcium and achievement of a 25-hydroxy vitamin D level of at least 20 ng/mL. This entails pursuing work-up and management of hypocalcemia or hypercalcemia prior to initiation of medical therapy.

In premenopausal females, additional pharmacologic therapy is typically only considered in individuals with fracture, active bone loss, and/or ongoing secondary causes of osteoporosis and bone loss. The FDA has approved the use of bisphosphonates and teriparatide in premenopausal women who are receiving glucocorticoids. However, since there is limited safety data on the use of pharmacological therapy for osteoporosis in premenopausal women, the overall duration of treatment should be minimized to whatever extent possible. In cases of secondary osteoporosis, treatment should be focused on management of the underlying cause, when possible. For example, estrogen is the appropriate therapy in women with hypogonadism and osteoporosis.

Bisphosphonates

Bisphosphonates are typically the first-line therapy for postmenopausal female patients with osteoporosis and oral bisphosphonates are preferred to IV bisphosphonates from a cost-effectiveness perspective when they can be tolerated. The first-line oral bisphosphonates include alendronate or risedronate because they have efficacy in reducing vertebral and hip fractures in addition to improving bone mineral density. Contraindications for oral bisphosphonates include esophageal disorders, inability to remain upright after administration, or surgical anastomoses in the gastrointestinal tract. In these patients, the preferred treatment is IV zoledronic acid. Bisphosphonates should not be used at all in patients with an eGFR <30 mL/minute without consultation with a metabolic bone disease expert. Other options for individuals who are unable to tolerate IV bisphosphonates include denosumab and anabolic agents. The most notable adverse event associated with the use of bisphosphonates is osteonecrosis of the jaw. To minimize the risk of this event, if patients are planned for dental surgery, initiation of a bisphosphonate should often be deferred until after the patient has healed from the surgery.

Denosumab

Denosumab is an alternative to bisphosphonates for postmenopausal women who have contraindications to bisphosphonates or are unable to tolerate them. It is also a reasonable option in individuals at a high risk of fracture and individuals with chronic kidney disease. There is some concern about increased risk of vertebral fracture after discontinuing denosumab, which could suggest a need for indefinite treatment.

Anabolic Agents

Anabolic agents that can be used in osteoporosis include teriparatide, abaloparatide, and romosozumab. Anabolic agents can be prescribed as an alternative to bisphosphonates for patients who are postmenopausal with severe osteoporosis (T-score of ≤ -3 or T-score of ≤ -2.5 with a fragility fracture). While some experts recommend use of anabolic agents first line in the management of severe osteoporosis, others prefer to use bisphosphonates as first line due to the cost of anabolic therapy, subcutaneous administration, and lack of long-term safety data. Although they are not first line for the treatment of osteoporosis more generally, anabolic agents can also be considered in patients who are unable to tolerate either IV or oral bisphosphonates. Treatment with an anabolic agent is limited to 12–24 months, depending on which agent is selected, and patients are typically treated with an anti-resorptive agent, such as a bisphosphonate, after discontinuation.

Selective Estrogen Receptor Modulators

Selective estrogen receptor modulators (SERMs) such as raloxifene have less anti-resorptive effects than bisphosphonates. As a result, these are typically indicated for patients who are unable to take bisphosphonates or denosumab or who have an increased risk of invasive breast cancer. SERMs should not be used in premenopausal women since they can worsen bone loss by blocking the action of estrogen on bone.

16.3.4   Monitoring After Treatment

Although there is no standardization across guidelines, it is reasonable to repeat a DEXA scan 1–2 years after initiation of therapy to assess for stability or improvement in bone density [4]. After this, monitoring can occur every 2 years unless there is a change in therapy or concern for ongoing bone loss. Of note, the American College of Physicians does not recommend monitoring during therapy since treatment can reduce fracture risk even without an improvement in bone density. If monitoring is done, there is some controversy on the interpretation of a decrease in bone density. While some would argue that this suggests a treatment failure and a need to transition to an alternative agent, others would argue that small decreases do not necessarily suggest treatment failure and repeat imaging should be done after 1–2 years to follow-up. Patients who continue to have fractures after at least 1 year of treatment with a bisphosphonate should be transitioned to an anabolic agent.

Ms. Johnson's initial case presentation and the evolution in her treatment course highlight examples of several possible pathways for the treatment of osteoporosis. At her initial presentation to Dr. Roberts' clinic, Ms. Johnson merits screening for osteoporosis as she is a postmenopausal female who is older than 65 years old. This screening should be completed by a primary care physician. If Ms. Johnson were younger than 65 years old and premenopausal, there would not be a standardized recommendation for the appropriate timeline for screening for osteoporosis. If Ms. Johnson had a history of fragility fracture or a history that raised concern for the risk of secondary causes of osteoporosis, it could be reasonable to consider the initiation of screening with a bone density scan even prior to age 65. In this case, it would be important to have a risk–benefit discussion with the patient to discuss the most appropriate path forward.

Ms. Johnson is diagnosed with osteoporosis based on her bone density T-score in her femoral neck of −2.6. This suggests that her bone density in her femoral neck is 2.6 standard deviations below that of the average young healthy female. Although her bone density in the proximal femur (T-score: −2.3) and in the lumbar spine (T-score: −2.0) would not meet criteria for osteoporosis, diagnosis only requires a T-score less than 2.5 in one of the three measured regions.

After Ms. Johnson is diagnosed with osteoporosis, Dr. Roberts very appropriately obtains a thorough medical history and orders appropriate laboratory testing to gain a deeper understanding of her risk factors for secondary osteoporosis. Prior to initiating medical therapy for osteoporosis, it is important to rule out reversible causes of osteoporosis and treat those appropriately. In Ms. Johnson's case, her vitamin D should be repleted prior to starting other treatment for osteoporosis. Another key component of the management of osteoporosis is the optimization of lifestyle factors. The incorporation of physical activity and modification of reversible lifestyle factors will often require frequent follow-up and consistent motivational interviewing to ultimately achieve sustainable change.

Ms. Johnson's initial therapy is an oral bisphosphonate, which is the first-line treatment for osteoporosis. When she is unable to tolerate the oral bisphosphonate, Dr. Roberts elects to offer an IV bisphosphonate as an alternative. At this time, it would also be reasonable to consider other treatment options such as denosumab or an anabolic agent. Although there is no standardized guideline on when or how often to monitor bone density after the initiation of therapy, Dr. Roberts elects to repeat a DEXA scan after 1 year. If Ms. Johnson's bone density had not improved or worsened after 1 year of therapy, there would be two different options for next steps. He could either continue bisphosphonate therapy and continue to monitor bone density in 1–2 years or he could transition the patient to an alternative agent. The occurrence of a fragility fracture is an appropriate indication to transition Ms. Johnson's treatment to an anabolic agent. Most providers will resume a bisphosphonate agent after completion of 1–2 years of treatment with an anabolic agent.

16.4   Conclusion

Osteoporosis is a metabolic bone disease that is increasingly present in individuals, especially women, with increasing age. It is important to evaluate the risk of osteoporosis and indications for screening for osteoporosis in all patients in the primary care setting. In addition to other high-risk individuals, all female patients over age 65 should be screened. Although there are several treatment options for osteoporosis, the first-line treatment for most patients is the initiation of an oral bisphosphonate. Other treatment options can be considered in the setting of bisphosphonate intolerance or failure of therapy. The duration of treatment depends on the patient's response to therapy.

Suggested Reading

1. International Osteoporosis Foundation | IOF Compendium of Osteoporosis. International Osteoporosis Foundation; n.d. Retrieved November 16, 2022, from https://www.osteoporosis.foundation/sites/iofbonehealth/files/2020-01/IOF-Compendium-of-Osteoporosis-web-V02.pdf
2. Sozen T, Ozisik L, Calik Basaran N. An overview and management of osteoporosis. Eur J Rheumatol. 2017;4(1):46–56. https://doi.org/10.5152/eurjrheum.2016.048.
3. Welcome to FRAX®. FRAX Fracture Risk Assessment Tool. Retrieved November 16, 2022, from https://www.sheffield.ac.uk/FRAX/
4. LeBoff MS, Greenspan SL, Insogna KL, Lewiecki EM, Saag KG, Singer AJ, Siris ES. The clinician's guide to prevention and treatment of osteoporosis. Osteoporos Int. 2022;33(10):2049–102. https://doi.org/10.1007/s00198-021-05900-y.
5. Merlijn T, Swart KMA, van der Horst HE, Netelenbos JC, Elders PJM. Fracture prevention by screening for high fracture risk: a systematic review and meta-analysis. Osteoporos Int. 2019;31(2):251–7. https://doi.org/10.1007/s00198-019-05226-w.
6. DeLange Hudec SM, Camacho PM. Secondary causes of osteoporosis. Endocr Pract. 2013;19(1):120–8. https://doi.org/10.4158/ep12059.ra.

Part III
Common Infections in Women

Chapter 17
Urinary Tract Infection

Stephanie Zuo and Megan Bradley

17.1 Introduction

Urinary tract infections (UTIs) are one of the most common bacterial infections and occur much more frequently in women compared to men in part due to the shorter female urethra. Generally, episodes of acute cystitis and pyelonephritis occurring in healthy, non-pregnant women who do not have abnormalities of the urinary tract are classified as uncomplicated UTIs, while all other UTIs are considered complicated. Repeated episodes of infection can qualify a patient for recurrent UTIs, for which the diagnosis, prevention, and management are discussed in this chapter. Asymptomatic bacteriuria occurs more frequently in older women and is another important condition that should be understood as we seek to promote antibiotic stewardship. Lastly, management of UTIs in pregnancy is discussed.

17.1.1 Case

A 31-year-old nulliparous woman presents to her gynecologist as well as urinary urgency and frequency with burning on urination for the past 2 weeks. She reports that the symptoms are accompanied with lower abdominal pressure and discomfort, and she has had to urinate every 30 min to an hour. Her urine has recently become cloudy and foul-smelling. She reports a transient low-grade fever that resolved. She denies back pain, nausea/vomiting, hematuria, or vaginal discharge.

S. Zuo (✉) · M. Bradley
Department of Obstetrics, Gynecology, and Reproductive Sciences, University of Pittsburgh Medical Center, Pittsburgh, PA, USA
e-mail: zuos@upmc.edu; bradleym4@upmc.edu

M. Mahmoudi (ed.), *Common Cases in Women's Primary Care Clinics*,
https://doi.org/10.1007/978-3-031-48569-5_17

She reports similar symptoms 10 years ago when she was in college. She is sexually active with one partner and uses condoms. She has no significant past medical or surgical history.

It appears your patient likely has a UTI. How is this defined and how will you next evaluate this patient?

17.2 Definitions

UTIs can be classified into lower UTIs (i.e. infection of the bladder or lower urinary tract) and upper UTIs (i.e. infection of the kidney or upper urinary tract). For this chapter, the focus will be on the diagnosis and management of lower UTIs.

An uncomplicated UTI is defined as a UTI that affects an individual who is otherwise healthy and does not have any structural or functional urinary tract abnormalities, is not pregnant, and has not been recently instrumented (for example, with cystoscopy or urinary catheterization, including long-term indwelling catheters). By definition, complicated UTIs encompass all other UTIs. This includes women who have urologic abnormalities, are immunocompromised, or are pregnant. Recurrent UTIs are defined as two or more UTIs in 6 months or three or more UTIs in 12 months. Finally, asymptomatic bacteriuria is defined as the presence of bacteria in an uncontaminated urine specimen collected from a patient who has no urinary symptoms or signs of a UTI.

17.2.1 Continuation of Case

You decide to first perform a physical exam. On exam, the patient is afebrile with normal vital signs. She is well-appearing and has mild suprapubic tenderness. She does not have costovertebral tenderness, vaginal discharge, or any other significant physical exam findings. You suspect she has an uncomplicated UTI.

17.3 Uncomplicated Urinary Tract Infections

The most common symptom of suspected uncomplicated UTI in women presenting for care is dysuria. Other UTI symptoms include increased urgency, urinary frequency, and suprapubic discomfort. Occasionally, mild incontinence and hematuria can occur during UTIs. Flank pain, fever, and nausea/vomiting should raise concern for pyelonephritis.

The top risk factors for uncomplicated UTI in premenopausal women include sexual intercourse, use of spermicides, and history of UTI. There may be a genetic component of patient susceptibility to UTI since history of maternal UTI and young age at first UTI have been identified as risk factors. Notably, behaviors such as post-coital voiding patterns, frequency of urination, wiping patterns, douching, and use of hot tubs have not shown a significant association with UTIs. For postmenopausal women, an important risk factor to consider for uncomplicated UTI is vaginal atrophy.

Given similarities in presentation with sexually transmitted urethritis or vaginitis, the primary care physician should take care to consider this in the differential diagnosis of a women with UTI symptoms. If symptoms of vaginal discharge or irritation are present, the likelihood of a UTI is decreased, and a pelvic examination should be performed and appropriate testing pursued.

17.3.1 Continuation of Case

What are your next steps for diagnostic testing?

UTIs are diagnosed using both urinary symptoms and a positive urine culture, which is typically considered to be at least 1000 colony-forming units (CFU)/mL of a known uropathogen in the setting of urinary tract symptoms. In healthy women without a history of recurrent UTI who have a specific combination of symptoms (dysuria and urinary frequency without vaginal discharge or irritation), the probability of UTI is more than 90%. For these patients, additional testing is not necessary to make a diagnosis of UTI. Virtual/telephone-based provider-guided presumptive therapy is reasonable. It should be noted that in less definitive patient presentations and in older women, urinary symptoms do not always coincide with bacteriuria. In fact, over 20% of women who report typical UTI symptoms have negative urine cultures. Older women are more likely to experience lower urinary tract symptoms related to overactive bladder without having a UTI.

Use of point-of-care urinalysis or urine dipstick testing can be helpful in women with suggestive but not diagnostic features of a UTI, but these tests cannot definitively diagnose or rule out infection. Nitrites, which are produced by gram-negative bacteria, are most indicative of a possible UTI, followed by leukocyte esterase, which corresponds to white blood cells in the urine (also known as pyuria) and blood (usually microscopic hematuria). Having a combined presence of both nitrites and leukocyte esterase or blood increases the positive predictive value for a urinary tract infection to 92%. Providers should recognize the risk of false-positive results on urine dipstick testing due to poor collection techniques and vaginal contamination of voided samples.

Urine culture is the standard for diagnosis of UTI, but it is typically not necessary in the diagnosis of uncomplicated cystitis due to the accuracy in diagnosis by patient symptom report alone and the time required for culture results. For women with complicated or recurrent UTI or in women with a history of initial drug failure, multi-drug resistant organisms, or multiple drug allergies, a urine culture should be collected. The advantage of urine culture is that treatment can be tailored to the isolated uropathogen as well as its antibiotic susceptibility, which prevents overtreatment and inappropriate use of antibiotics. Notably, urine cultures should be interpreted in clinical context. Certain organisms, even at high concentrations (for example, lactobacillus) are typically considered contaminants in women with uncomplicated cystitis, while women with acute symptoms highly suspicious of UTI with low (for example, 1000 CFU/mL) concentrations of uropathogens often have true bacteriuria and should be treated appropriately. The most common uropathogen in uncomplicated UTIs is *Escherichia coli*, which makes up 75% of cases.

17.3.2 Continuation of Case

You perform a point-of-care urinalysis to assess for possible UTI. It results with nitrites, moderate leukocyte esterase, and trace blood. You then send a urine sample for urine culture. The patient desires to be treated empirically prior to receiving her finalized urine culture results. Which antibiotic do you choose?

The preferred treatment for uncomplicated UTIs is outpatient oral antibiotic therapy. Choice of antibiotic regimen should consider medical history, history of drug reactions, other recent infections or positive urine cultures, and local patterns of antibiotic resistance. The Infectious Diseases Society of America published clinical practice guidelines in 2010 for premenopausal, non-pregnant women with no known urologic abnormalities or comorbidities experiencing acute uncomplicated UTI. Antibiotic regimens are listed in Table 17.1. Nitrofurantoin, trimethoprim-sulfamethoxazole (TMP-SMX), and fosfomycin are recommended as first-line antibiotic therapy. For these antibiotics, clinical efficacy is high.

Nitrofurantoin concentrates in the lower urinary tract but is bacteriostatic and has minimal tissue penetration. Therefore, it should be avoided in cases with a possibility of pyelonephritis. It is overall well-tolerated and is highly effective against *E. coli* and other gram-negative uropathogens, in spite of rising resistance levels. Although previously contraindicated in patients with renal impairment, nitrofurantoin has been shown to be safe in patients with a creatinine clearance as low as 30 mL/min. For those with lower creatinine clearances, there is a decrease in efficacy due to inadequate urine levels of the drug, but no increase in toxicity. There is a rare chance of pulmonary toxicity that may be either cytotoxic or immune-mediated in nature which may occur with chronic nitrofurantoin therapy (e.g. for long-term UTI prophylaxis).

The combination of trimethoprim and sulfamethoxazole in TMP-SMX works synergistically against a wide range of organisms. It is inexpensive and well-tolerated, but there is concern about growing resistance to the antibiotic since the mid-1990s. In a large national study of urine antimicrobial resistance in the USA, 22.2% of *E. coli* isolates were resistant to TMP-SMX from urine samples collected in 2012. As per ISDA recommendations, TMP-SMX should not be empirically prescribed in communities with greater than 20% resistance.

Fosfomycin tromethamine is the stable salt form of fosfomycin, which has activity against both gram-positive and gram-negative organisms. It becomes highly

Table 17.1 Antibiotic regimens for acute cystitis

	Dose	Side effects	Estimated clinical efficacy	Comments
First-line antibiotics				
Nitrofurantoin monohydrate/macrocrystals	100 mg BID x 5 days	*Common*: nausea, headache, flatulence, diarrhea *Rare*: pulmonary fibrosis, hepatitis, pancreatitis	90–95%	Avoid if suspicious for pyelonephritis; FDA pregnancy category B
Trimethoprim/sulfamethoxazole	160/800 mg (1 DS tablet) BID × 3 days	*Common*: nausea, vomiting, rash, photosensitivity *Rare*: Stevens-Johnson syndrome, toxic epidermal necrolysis, hepatitis	86–100%	Avoid if prevalence of local resistance >20%, adjustment of dosage needed in cases of renal impairment; FDA pregnancy category C
Fosfomycin trometamol	3 g single dose packet (may be repeated 72 h later)	*Common*: nausea, diarrhea, headache *Rare*: dizziness, rash, abdominal pain, elevated liver enzymes	63–91%	Most laboratories do not test for resistance, may be useful for multi-drug resistant pathogens but may have inferior efficacy; FDA pregnancy category B
Second-line antibiotics				
Beta-lactams	Dose varies; typically 3- to 7-day regimen	*Common*: nausea, diarrhea, rash *Rare*: encephalopathy	85–98%	Avoid empiric use of penicillins due to poor efficacy; FDA pregnancy category B
Fluoroquinolones	Dose varies; typically 3-day regimen	*Common*: nausea, headache, dizziness, insomnia *Rare*: peripheral neuropathy, tendinopathy, tendon rupture, QT interval prolongation, hepatotoxicity	79–98%	Higher risk of tendon rupture in older or immunosuppressed patients, increased resistance limits usefulness, when possible reserve use for pyelonephritis; FDA pregnancy category C

concentrated in the urine after a single dose. Fosfomycin appears to be somewhat less efficacious compared to other short-term antibiotic regimens, which may be due to high interindividual variability in concentrations of fosfomycin in the urine. Despite this, it is still recommended as a first-line antibiotic given low rates of adverse effects. Most microbiology laboratories do not routinely report susceptibility data for fosfomycin, but generally, fosfomycin is active against many multi-drug resistant uropathogens. It remains a first-line drug in these cases, although resistance among Klebsiella species is growing and treatment regimens of two or three doses may be required.

In circumstances when first-line agents are not appropriate, reasonable alternatives include fluoroquinolones and beta-lactams. Generally, beta-lactams have greater rates of adverse events and are less efficacious compared to the first-line agents. Although frequently prescribed for uncomplicated UTIs, fluoroquinolones face increasing resistance and concerns about safety, with a U.S. Food and Drug Administration black box warning of a heightened risk for tendinitis and tendon rupture.

Women are sometimes interested in trying non-antibiotic therapies first in the management of uncomplicated UTIs. Given the overall benign nature of cystitis, it is reasonable for clinicians to delay antibiotic therapy in healthy women while awaiting urine cultures, especially in the case of a patient with multiple drug intolerances or concern for alternative sources of her symptoms. However, there is limited data on the role of non-antibiotic therapies, such as cranberry extract products, anti-inflammatory medications, and increased fluid intake, for the management of uncomplicated UTIs.

If symptoms resolve, no further follow-up is needed after treatment of uncomplicated UTIs.

17.3.3 Continuation of Case

You decide to prescribe a 5-day course of nitrofurantoin for UTI treatment. You give the patient precautions to notify the office if she does not experience resolution of her symptoms or if she experiences fever or costovertebral angle tenderness, as this would raise concerns for development of a complicated UTI.

17.4 Complicated Urinary Tract Infections

Complicated UTIs are more difficult to treat than uncomplicated infections and therefore require different management strategies. There are multiple factors that can cause a UTI to be categorized as complicated, including host factors (e.g. poorly controlled diabetes, immunosuppression, impaired renal function), anatomic abnormalities (e.g. bladder outlet obstruction, fistula), functional problems of the bladder (e.g. incomplete voiding because of dysfunction of the bladder detrusor muscle), and when urinary devices are present (e.g. indwelling bladder catheters). UTIs that occur in pregnant patients and patients who have had a renal transplant or history of spinal cord injury also qualify as complicated. Additionally, UTIs that fail to resolve on first-line therapy should be considered a complicated UTI.

Severe complicated UTIs can present with systemic symptoms concerning for urosepsis. Clinical judgment is needed to determine if resuscitation and observation in the emergency department and/or hospitalization for inpatient supervision are necessary in these patients. Over 620,000 hospital admissions per year are due to complicated UTI in the USA, most of which are non-catheter related. Pre-treatment urine cultures are important in patients with suspected complicated UTIs since multi-drug resistant uropathogens are more likely in this population. Initial antibiotic regimens for treatment should be broad-spectrum and may be based on previous urine culture results and local resistance patterns. Once susceptibilities from pre-treatment urine cultures result, antibiotic therapy should be tailored as appropriate. Longer durations of antibiotics (i.e. 7–14 days) are required to adequately treat complicated UTIs.

17.4.1 Continuation of Case

Three months later, you receive a call from the patient. She reports experiencing bothersome urinary frequency and urgency once again and would like to be treated as soon as possible.

17.5 Recurrent Urinary Tract Infections

Recurrent UTIs are defined as having at least two culture-proven episodes in the past 6 months or at least three culture-proven episodes in the past year. This may be due to bacterial relapse or reinfection. Bacterial relapse, also known as bacterial persistence, occurs when symptoms return within 2 weeks of treatment due to the same offending organism, usually as a result of failure of initial therapy. Bacterial reinfection is recurrent infection with a different organism, with the same organism more than 2 weeks after treatment, or after a sterile intervening culture.

Twenty percent of women who experience their first UTI will experience a recurrence within 3–4 months. The incidence of recurrent UTIs is highest among women ages 18–34 and 55–64. In premenopausal women, risk factors for recurrent UTIs are similar to that of sporadic infection and include frequent intercourse, spermicide use, and history of UTI prior to the age of 15. For postmenopausal women, a decrease in circulating estrogen causes an increase in vaginal pH, resulting in dramatic changes in the urogenital microbiome. This allows uropathogens, typically from the rectum, to colonize the vagina and distal urethra. Similar to acute UTI, *E. coli* is the most common uropathogen for recurrent UTI. However, in postmenopausal women, other uropathogens, including *Klebsiella pneumoniae* and *Enterococcus faecalis*, compose up to 35% of recurrent UTIs.

Evaluation and management of recurrent UTIs should be performed by a specialist (i.e. urology, urogynecology). Typical evaluation includes a physical examination, including a focused neurologic and a pelvic examination. Bladder emptying should be assessed either by urethral catheterization or using ultrasonography (bladder scan). Typically, radiographic imaging and cystourethroscopy are not necessary, but can be considered.

Unlike management of uncomplicated UTI, patients with recurrent UTI should always have a urine culture with sensitivity collected prior to initiation of treatment. This is due to the higher chance of antibiotic resistance in this patient population.

17.5.1 Continuation of Case

You send a urine culture and empirically prescribe her a course of TMP-SMX. You also review her risk factors for recurrent UTI. You recommend she consider a non-antibiotic prophylactic strategy for the prevention of UTIs in the future. What options are available to the patient?

The mainstay for management of recurrent UTI is prevention, with a goal of avoiding and/or suppressing future infections. The most common antibiotic and non-antibiotic preventative therapies are discussed in this section. Generally, for postmenopausal women, local estrogen therapy is the recommended first step, given robust evidence on its effectiveness, followed by antibiotic prophylaxis for patients who continue to have persistent UTIs.

17.5.2 Non-antibiotic Prophylaxis

Due to the risk of antimicrobial resistance with antibiotic prophylaxis, there is a rising interest in the use of non-antibiotic therapies for recurrent UTI prophylaxis (Table 17.2).

Behavioral changes are a suitable first-line option that patients can use to reduce UTI frequency with minimal effort, although effectiveness appears to be limited and certain interventions may have no significant effect. These include cessation of spermicide use, increasing hydration to 1.5 L daily, wiping front to back, voiding after sexual intercourse, and avoiding delayed voiding

Of the non-antibiotic prophylactic options, vaginal estrogen therapy is the most efficacious in reducing UTIs. Local estrogen therapy increases *Lactobacillus*, decreases vaginal pH, and improves vaginal tissue quality, which reduces the chance for vaginal colonization by uropathogens. In one landmark study, the occurrence of UTIs for women using intravaginal estrogen cream went from 5.9 to 0.5 episodes per year. Vaginal estrogen therapy comes in multiple forms including creams, tablets, and rings. There is minimal systemic absorption of vaginal estrogen, but in patients with a history of breast or endometrial cancer or who have had a history of venous thromboembolism, risks and benefits should be carefully weighed. Unlike vaginal estrogen, systemic oral estrogens have not been shown to be effective in reducing UTI frequency.

Table 17.2 Non-antibiotic prophylaxis for recurrent urinary tract infections

	Strength of evidence	Mechanism of action	Comments
Vaginal estrogen therapy	Moderate	Decreases vaginal pH to allow for dominance of *Lactobacillus*, which prevents colonization of vagina and distal urethra with uropathogenic organisms	Various formulations include cream, ring, and tablet Oral estrogens do not decrease UTIs
Methenamine hippurate	Low	Converts to formaldehyde in acidic urine, creating an antiseptic environment	Dose is 1 g twice a day and can be taken with vitamin C tablets to increase acidity of urine and maximize methenamine therapeutic efficacy
D-mannose	Low	Sugar which competitively binds to type 1 pili of enteric bacteria to prevent adherence to urothelium	Dose is 2 g daily and noted to have fewer side effects than daily nitrofurantoin prophylactic dosing
Cranberry extract	Low/very low	Proanthocyanidins (PACs) prevent adhesion of bacteria to urothelium	36 mg PACs or more provide optimal antibacterial effect (currently available in medication form under trade name, Ellura)
Lactobacillus probiotic supplements	Very low	Increase *Lactobacillus* populations in the vagina	Both oral capsules and suppositories have been studied without evidence of benefit

Methenamine hippurate converts to formaldehyde from hexamine, which acts as a bacteriostatic agent and acidifies the urine. In a recent randomized trial, methenamine hippurate was as effective as trimethoprim in preventing UTIs over 1 year, although rates were noted to be high among the treatment groups. Previous studies have found that methenamine hippurate may be effective in preventing UTIs in patients without renal tract abnormalities, but was not found to be effective in patients with neurogenic bladder or those with renal tract abnormalities. Long-term use of methenamine has been found to be safe with minimal side effects and no evidence of development of drug resistance.

D-mannose binds to the type 1 pili of bacteria to prevent adhesion to the urothelium and may also act as an immune modulator. A recent meta-analysis showed that d-mannose may have similar effectiveness as antibiotic prophylaxis in preventing UTIs. Studies on D-mannose found minimal adverse side effects and good compliance, although data remains limited.

Cranberry extract is well-known in popular media for preventing UTIs. Cranberries contain proanthocyanidins (PACs) which inhibit the adherence of fimbriated E. coli to the bladder mucosa. The recommended amount of PACs in supplements should be 36 mg or greater. This may be difficult to measure in cranberry juices or powders or inaccurate in natural tablets or capsules. Although there is moderate heterogeneity in the data, a 2012 Cochrane review found that cranberry products do not significantly reduce the risk of repeat UTI compared to placebo or no treatment. However, newer data suggests that cranberry may reduce the risk of UTI by 26% and that there may be a role for cranberry products in certain individuals or cases, especially in combination with other non-antibiotic prophylactic therapies.

Lastly, both oral and vaginal lactobacilli probiotics have been examined for the prevention of UTIs, but due to lack of data and mixed results, current guidelines are unable to support their use. Although prior studies found improvement in UTI frequency with use of vaginal *lactobacillus*, a more recent meta-analysis showed no significant effect for the use of probiotics in UTI prevention. Ultimately, more research is needed to determine whether *lactobacillus* probiotics are a useful option for UTI prophylaxis.

17.5.3 Antibiotic Prophylaxis

Antibiotic prophylaxis is very effective at reducing symptomatic UTI with a 92–99% rate of effectiveness. They may be taken continuously or post-coitally. Antibiotic options with dosages for continuous prophylaxis are shown in Table 17.3. Historically, the duration of continuous prophylaxis ranged from 6 to 12 months, but we generally recommend an initial 3–6-month trial with cessation of antibiotics if UTIs cease. Continuous antibiotic therapy increases the chance of multi-drug resistance, which is why they are not the first-line preventative therapy for recurrent UTIs. Other common side effects are vaginal and oral candidiasis and gastrointestinal symptoms.

In select women who experience recurrent UTIs after sexual activity, postcoital prophylaxis using a one-time dose of antibiotics either before or after intercourse can be offered. Treatment effectiveness is 85% while also allowing for less antibiotic burden compared to continuous dosing.

Intravesical instillations of antibiotics, such as gentamicin, have been studied in women with recurrent UTIs, particularly those with neurogenic bladders requiring

Table 17.3 Continuous antibiotic prophylaxis dosing

Nitrofurantoin monohydrate/macrocrystals	50 mg daily, 100 mg daily
Trimethoprim	100 mg daily
Trimethoprim/sulfamethoxazole	40/200 mg daily
Cephalexin	125 mg daily, 250 mg daily
Fosfomycin trometamol	3 g every 10 days

All UTI antibiotic prophylaxis should be reviewed after 3–6 months and considerations should be made to deprescribe, if possible.

intermittent self-catheterization or indwelling catheters. Patients typically respond well with a 71–88% success rate in reducing symptomatic UTIs at least up to 6 months after completion of intravesical antibiotic therapy. There is no agreed upon regimen for frequency of instillations (ranging from nightly to once a week) and length of therapy (ranging from 2 weeks to 3 months). Although side effects of intravesical antibiotic therapy are not well-documented, most reported adverse events were minor, including allergy, suprapubic discomfort, UTI, and diarrhea.

17.6 Asymptomatic Bacteriuria

17.6.1 Continuation of Case

At her next visit, the patient brings in a urine culture result showing 100,000 CFU/ mL E. coli. She states that she wanted to make sure her UTI had been treated appropriately, so she requested a test be sent at her local urgent care center. At the time, she did not have any urinary symptoms. You are concerned she has asymptomatic bacteriuria. What are your next steps?

Asymptomatic bacteriuria is defined as the presence of one or more species of bacteria in the urine at a concentration of $\geq 10^5$ CFU/mL, irrespective of the presence of pyuria, in the absence of signs of symptoms of a UTI. The prevalence of asymptomatic bacteriuria ranges from 1.0% to 5.0% in premenopausal women and 2.8–8.6% in healthy postmenopausal women. In women with diabetes and women over the age of 70, it can be as high as 10.8-16%. Asymptomatic bacteriuria is also common in people with spinal cord injuries, urologic abnormalities, renal transplant, or impaired voiding, as well as in older, institutionalized populations.

In the past, pyuria was considered to be a useful indicator in discriminating acute UTI from asymptomatic bacteriuria. However, studies in older adults have found that pyuria and urinary inflammatory markers are not helpful to distinguish between infection and asymptomatic bacteriuria and should not be used to guide management. The symptom of dysuria is a preferred discriminating factor for the diagnosis of UTI.

In most populations, screening for asymptomatic bacteriuria is not indicated. Older adults with asymptomatic bacteriuria do not experience increases in mortality or development of subsequent UTI. It is only recommended to screen for asymptomatic bacteriuria in pregnant patients and patients who are going to be undergoing endoscopic urologic procedures associated with mucosal trauma (e.g. ureteroscopy). Diagnostic or other urologic procedures which do not breach the urinary tract mucosal lining (e.g. diagnostic cystoscopy, uncomplicated stent, or catheter removal) are low-risk for infection and do not require screening for asymptomatic bacteriuria.

Antibiotic treatment of asymptomatic bacteriuria is not recommended, except for the aforementioned patient populations. This "do not treat approach" is a paradigm shift over the last few decades. Antimicrobial therapy has not been found to have any benefit in the setting of asymptomatic bacteriuria and only increases the prevalence of antibiotic-resistant bacteria.

17.7 Special Circumstances

17.7.1 *Continuation of Case*

One year later, your patient presents to you with exciting news—she is 12 weeks pregnant. She is concerned about her history of recurrent urinary tract infections prior to pregnancy and her risk of having a UTI while pregnant. How do you counsel her about management of UTIs in pregnancy?

The incidence of UTIs is slightly higher in pregnant women compared to non-pregnant women, but there is a much greater risk of progression to pyelonephritis due to maternal anatomic and physiologic urinary tract changes. Moreover, bacteriuria in pregnancy (both symptomatic and asymptomatic) is associated with an increased risk of preterm labor, preeclampsia, and intrauterine growth restriction. Risk factors for bacteriuria in pregnancy include history of recurrent UTIs, diabetes, and abnormalities of the urinary tract. A screening urine culture should be collected at one of the initial visits early in pregnancy to assess for asymptomatic bacteriuria, which should be treated in pregnancy. The types of uropathogens in pregnant women are similar to the non-pregnant population, with *E. coli* being the most commonly isolated microbe.

Penicillin derivatives and cephalosporins are considered safe in pregnancy. Nitrofurantoin and TMP-SMX can be used as first-line agents in the second- and third-trimester of pregnancy, although there may be an increased risk of neonatal jaundice if used in the last week to month prior to delivery. Per the American College of Obstetricians and Gynecologists, these two agents may be also used in the first trimester if no other suitable alternative antibiotics are available. There is conflicting data on the effect of nitrofurantoin or TMP-SMX exposure in the first trimester on risk of fetal defects. Fluoroquinolones should be avoided in pregnancy due to their association with defects in fetal cartilage and bone in animal studies. However, data in human observational studies are mixed regarding the effect of fluoroquinolones on fetal defects and perinatal outcomes.

A follow-up urine culture should be collected within 1–2 weeks of treatment to ensure resolution of bacteriuria. Women with recurrent UTIs or who developed pyelonephritis during their pregnancy should be started on a prophylactic antibiotic until delivery.

17.8 Conclusion

Urinary tract infections (UTIs) are one of the most common bacterial infections in women and can present difficulties to the clinician when they become recurrent, complicated, or mistaken for asymptomatic bacteriuria. There are many available guidelines to aid in the care of these patients and many non-antibiotic alternatives to offer those with recurrent UTIs. Future research will continue to be geared toward novel therapies and dissemination of clinical guidelines to both patients and providers.

Suggested Reading

1. Rubin RH, Shapiro ED, Andriole VT, Davis RJ, Stamm WE. Evaluation of new anti-infective drugs for the treatment of urinary tract infection. Infectious Diseases Society of America and the Food and Drug Administration. Clin Infect Dis. 1992;15(Suppl 1):S216–27.
2. Bent S, Nallamothu BK, Simel DL, Fihn SD, Saint S. Does this woman have an acute uncomplicated urinary tract infection? JAMA. 2002;287(20):2701–10.
3. Gupta K, Hooton TM, Naber KG, Wullt B, Colgan R, Miller LG, et al. International clinical practice guidelines for the treatment of acute uncomplicated cystitis and pyelonephritis in women: a 2010 update by the Infectious Diseases Society of America and the European Society for Microbiology and Infectious Diseases. Clin Infect Dis. 2011;52(5):e103–20.
4. Foxman B. Epidemiology of urinary tract infections: incidence, morbidity, and economic costs. Dis Mon. 2003;49(2):53–70.
5. Raz R, Stamm WE. A controlled trial of intravaginal estriol in postmenopausal women with recurrent urinary tract infections. N Engl J Med. 1993;329(11):753–6.
6. Jepson RG, Williams G, Craig JC. Cranberries for preventing urinary tract infections. Cochrane Database Syst Rev. 2012;10:CD001321.
7. Peck J, Shepherd JP. Recurrent urinary tract infections: diagnosis, treatment, and prevention. Obstet Gynecol Clin N Am. 2021;48(3):501–13.
8. Stamatiou C, Petrakos G, Bovis C, Panagopoulos P, Economou A, Karkanis C. Efficacy of prophylaxis in women with sex induced cystitis. Clin Exp Obstet Gynecol. 2005;32(3):193–5.
9. Cai T, Nesi G, Mazzoli S, Meacci F, Lanzafame P, Caciagli P, et al. Asymptomatic bacteriuria treatment is associated with a higher prevalence of antibiotic resistant strains in women with urinary tract infections. Clin Infect Dis. 2015;61(11):1655–61.
10. ACOG. Committee opinion no. 717: sulfonamides, nitrofurantoin, and risk of birth defects. Obstet Gynecol. 2017;130(3):e150–2.

Chapter 18
A Primary Care Clinician's Focus on Sexually Transmitted Infections in the Female Gender

Anna Camille Moreno and Jeremy L. Kessler

18.1 Introduction

Sexually transmitted infections (STIs) are very common, and over half of individuals in the USA will have an STI in their lifetime. In fact, the CDC estimates that there are 20 million new STI cases each year among men and women living in the USA. According to the 2018 STD Surveillance Report, HPV is the most common STI (79 million cases), followed by genital herpes (24 million), trichomoniasis (3.7 million), and chlamydia (1.6 million). Gonorrhea, syphilis, hepatitis B, and HIV are less common, although rates of syphilis, gonorrhea, and chlamydia are rising up 71%, 63%, and 19%, respectively, from 2014 to 2018. The recently released 2020 STD Surveillance Report by the CDC cautioned that the COVID-19 pandemic caused some uncertainty in interpreting the surveillance data collected during 2020–2021. In this report, chlamydia infections were down by 13% from 2019, while gonorrhea cases were up 10% and primary and secondary syphilis were up 7% from 2019.

Sexually transmitted infections are most common among adolescents and young adults aged 15–24 but are increasing across many groups including racial and ethnic minority groups in addition to homosexual and bisexual men. According to the Surveillance Report, African American individuals were five to eight times greater in acquiring an STI than those of non-Hispanic white individuals. The STI rates for Native Americans, Alaskan Natives, Native Hawaiians, or other Pacific Islanders were three to five times higher than those of non-Hispanic whites. The STI rates

A. C. Moreno (✉)
University of Utah, Salt Lake City, UT, USA
e-mail: Camille.Moreno@hsc.utah.edu

J. L. Kessler
Ogden Regional Medical Center, Ogden, UT, USA

M. Mahmoudi (ed.), *Common Cases in Women's Primary Care Clinics*,
https://doi.org/10.1007/978-3-031-48569-5_18

were almost doubled for Hispanics or Latinos compared to non-Hispanic whites. In this chapter, we will focus on sexually transmitted infections in the female gender.

The CDC 2021 STI Treatment Guidelines include five major strategies:

1. Accurate risk assessment and education and counseling of persons at risk regarding ways to avoid STIs through changes in sexual behaviors and use of recommended prevention services
2. Pre-exposure vaccination for vaccine preventable STIs
3. Identification of persons with an asymptomatic infection and persons with symptoms associated with an STI
4. Effective diagnosis, treatment, counseling, and follow-up of persons who are infected with an STI
5. Evaluation, treatment, and counseling of sex partners of persons who are infected with an STI

This chapter seeks to provide detailed descriptions about STI screening/detection, risk assessment, evaluation/testing, treatment approach, prevention counseling, follow-up retesting, and treating partners.

18.2   Case 1

Ms. Thomas is a 24-year-old, healthy woman with an unremarkable medical history, presenting to a family medicine clinic for her annual exam. She is single and has never been pregnant. She identifies as a cis female. She takes birth control pills for contraception and does not take any other prescription medications. She takes an over-the-counter vitamin D3 supplement daily. She does not drink alcohol, smoke cigarettes, or use any recreational substances and/or intravenous drug use. She lives in an apartment by herself and works as a librarian. She reports that she has been sexually active with four male partners in the last year. She reports vaginal sex but denies oral and anal sex. She denies use of any protective STI barriers such as male condoms. She denies any prior history of sexually transmitted infections. Her last testing for gonorrhea and chlamydia was negative, at age 24. She also had a normal pap testing for cervical cancer screening at age 21. She has received the three HPV vaccine series. She denies any bothersome vulvovaginal symptoms and any associated sexual health concerns. She would like to know if she is at risk for acquiring STIs and if so, which ones she should be screened for today. She also inquires about how she can decrease her risk of STIs.

18.3 Discussion

Sexually transmitted infections are most common among adolescents and young adults aged 15–24. Rates of chlamydia, gonorrhea, and HPV infections are highest in females during their adolescent and young adult years. Those deemed at high risk for STIs are as follows:

- Individuals who initiate sex early
- Individuals living in detention or correctional facilities
- Individuals receiving services at STD clinics
- Individuals who are involved in commercial sex exploitation or those exchanging sex for drugs, money, food, or housing
- Individuals with disabilities
- Individuals with substance misuse
- Individuals with mental health disorders
- Pregnant females
- Females who have sex with females
- Individuals with HIV infection
- Immunocompromised individuals based on medication and disease

Moreover, those who are vulnerable to acquiring STIs specifically during adolescence include:

- Having multiple sexual partners
- Having sequential sex partnerships of limited duration or concurrent partnerships
- Failing to use barrier protection consistently and correctly
- Having lower socioeconomic status
- Facing multiple challenges or obstacles to health care access

1. Partners
- "Are you currently having sex of any kind?"
- "What is the gender(s) of your partner(s)?"

2. Practices
- "To understand any risks for sexually transmitted infections (STIs), I need to ask more specific questions about the kind of sex you have had recently."
- "What kind of sexual contact do you have or have you had?"
  - "Do you have vaginal sex, meaning 'penis in vagina' sex?"
  - "Do you have anal sex, meaning 'penis in rectum/anus' sex?"
  - "Do you have oral sex, meaning 'mouth on penis/vagina'?"

3. Protection from STIs
- "Do you and your partner(s) discuss prevention of STIs and human immunodeficiency virus (HIV)?"
- "Do you and your partner(s) discuss getting tested?"
- For condoms:
  - "What protection methods do you use? In what situations do you use condoms?"

4. Past history of STIs
- "Have you ever been tested for STIs and HIV?"
- "Have you ever been diagnosed with an STI in the past?"
- "Have any of your partners had an STI?"

Additional questions for identifying HIV and viral hepatitis risk:
- "Have you or any of your partner(s) ever injected drugs?"
- "Is there anything about your sexual health that you have questions about?"

5. Pregnancy intention
- "Do you think you would like to have (more) children in the future?"
- "How important is it to you to prevent pregnancy (until then)?"
- "Are you or your partner using contraception or practicing any form of birth control?"
- "Would you like to talk about ways to prevent pregnancy?"

Fig. 18.1 The five P's approach for health care providers obtaining sexual histories: partners, practices, protection from sexually transmitted infections, past history of sexually transmitted infections, and pregnancy intention

The American Academy of Pediatrics (AAP) recommends that providers should obtain thorough sexual histories from their patients and address their STI risk factors by providing prevention counseling. This is effectively performed by asking open-ended questions as depicted below in Fig. 18.1.

According to the CDC, prevention counseling is most effective if provided in a nonjudgmental and empathetic manner that is appropriate and responsive to the patient's culture, language, sex and gender identity, sexual orientation, age, and developmental level. Identifying high-risk behaviors such as oral, anal, vaginal sex; having multiple sex partners; having partners with STIs; or having substance misuse behaviors that increase one's risk for infections is highly encouraged.

In addition to obtaining a comprehensive sexual history from patients as well as performing a behavioral risk assessment, the following STI screening is recommended by the CDC for non-pregnant and pregnant females. The CDC and the United States Preventive Services Task Force (USPSTF) include the following screening recommendations and considerations by disease category, pregnant and non-pregnant status, and for females with HIV. A thorough and shared clinical discussion regarding these screening and retesting recommendations between the female and the provider is strongly encouraged. More frequent screening might be appropriate depending on individual risk behaviors, exposure, and the local epidemiology of the disease.

- **Chlamydia**
  Non-Pregnant Women

  - Sexually active women under 25 years of age.
  - Sexually active women 25 years of age and older if at increased risk. The risks are stated above.
  - Retest ~3 months after treatment.
  - Rectal chlamydia testing should be considered in females based on reported high-risk sexual behaviors and exposure as stated above.

Pregnant Women

- All pregnant women under 25 years of age.
- Pregnant women 25 years of age and older if at increased risk. The risks are stated above.
- Retest during the third trimester for women under the age of 25 or if at increased risk.
- Pregnant women with chlamydial infection should have a test of cure 4 weeks after treatment and be retested within 3 months.

Persons with HIV

- For sexually active individuals, screen at first HIV evaluation, and at least yearly thereafter.
- More frequent screening might be appropriate based on reported high-risk sexual behaviors as stated above.

- **Gonorrhea**
  Non-Pregnant Women

  - Sexually active women under 25 years of age.
  - Sexually active women 25 years of age and older if at increased risk. The risks are stated above.
  - Retest 3 months after treatment.
  - Pharyngeal and rectal gonorrhea testing should be considered in females based on reported high-risk sexual behaviors and exposure as stated above.

Pregnant Women

  - All pregnant women under 25 years of age.
  - Pregnant women 25 years of age and older if at increased risk. The risks are stated above.
  - Pregnant women with gonorrhea should be retested within 3 months.

Persons with HIV

  - For sexually active individuals, screen at first HIV evaluation, and at least yearly thereafter.
  - More frequent screening might be appropriate based on reported high-risk sexual behaviors as stated above.

- **Syphilis**
  Non-Pregnant Women

  - Screen asymptomatic women at increased risk. The risks are stated above.

Pregnant Women

  - All pregnant women at their first prenatal visit.
  - Retest at 28 weeks gestation and at delivery if at high risk (i.e., lives in a community with high syphilis rates or is at risk for syphilis acquisition during pregnancy).

Persons with HIV

  - For sexually active individuals, screen at first HIV evaluation, and at least yearly thereafter.
  - More frequent screening might be appropriate based on reported high-risk sexual behaviors as stated above and local epidemiology.

- **Herpes Simplex Virus**
  Non-Pregnant Women

  - HSV serologic testing (type-specific) should be considered for any woman presenting for STI screening.

Pregnant Women

- Routine HSV-2 serologic screening is not recommended among asymptomatic individuals.
- HSV serologic testing (type-specific) should be considered for pregnant women at risk for HSV infection.

Persons with HIV

- HSV serologic testing (type-specific) should be considered for persons presenting for STI screening.

- **Trichomonas**
  Non-Pregnant Women

- Screening should be considered for women receiving care in STD clinics and correctional facilities and for asymptomatic women at high risk for infection. The risks are stated above.

Persons with HIV

- For sexually active individuals, screen at first HIV evaluation, and at least yearly thereafter.

- **HIV**
  Non-Pregnant Women

- All women aged 13–64 years (could opt out).
- All women who seek STI screening.

Pregnant Women

- All pregnant women should be screened at first prenatal visit (could opt out).
- Retest during the third trimester if at increased risk. The risks are stated above and including having a new sex partner during pregnancy, living in areas with high HIV prevalence, or have partners with HIV.
- Rapid testing should be performed at delivery if not previously screened during pregnancy.

- **HPV, Cervical Cancer, Anal Cancer**
  Non-Pregnant Women

- Women 21–29 years of age every 3 years with pap cytology.
- Women 30–65 years of age every 3 years with pap cytology alone, or every 5 years with a combination of pap cytology and HPV testing.

Pregnant Women

- Should be screened at same intervals as non-pregnant women.

Persons with HIV

- Providers should refer for guidance to *Guidelines for the Prevention and Treatment of Opportunistic Infections in Adults and Adolescents with HIV.* This includes cervical cancer screening recommendations and management of results in persons with HIV.

- **Hepatitis B Screening**
  Non-Pregnant Women

  – Women at increased risk as stated above and including past or current injection drug use and an HBsAg-positive sex partner.

Pregnant Women

  – Test for HBsAg at first prenatal visit of each pregnancy regardless of prior testing.
  – Retest at delivery if at high risk. Risks are stated above.

Persons with HIV

  – Testing for HBsAg, anti-HBc, and anti-HBs.

- **Hepatitis C Screening**

  Non-Pregnant Women
  – All women over age 18 years should be screened for hepatitis C except in settings where the hepatitis C infection (HCV) positivity is <0.1%.

Pregnant Women

  – Should be screened for hepatitis C except in settings where HCV positivity is <0.1%.

Persons with HIV

  – For sexually active individuals, screen at first HIV evaluation.

18.3.1   *Understanding Sexually Transmitted Infections*

The term "sexually transmitted infection" (STI) differs from the term "sexually transmitted disease" (STD) in that STI refers to a pathogen that causes infection through sexual contact. STD, however, refers to the disease state that has developed from acquiring an infection. STIs are transmitted from one individual to another through vaginal, oral, and anal sex. However, they can also spread through intimate "skin-to-skin" contact such as heavy stroking or petting (hand job, fingering) and mutual masturbation.

Most STIs are asymptomatic or may cause only mild symptoms. If present, these symptoms may present like a vaginal infection that is accompanied by abnormal vaginal discharge, itching, burning, or odor. STIs can also cause symptoms related to urethritis including dysuria, urethral pruritus, and mucopurulent or purulent discharge. In addition, STIs can also cause cervicitis which refers to inflammation of the cervix and is frequently asymptomatic. However, some women may report an abnormal vaginal discharge and/or postcoital bleeding (vaginal bleeding after intercourse).

Untreated STIs can lead to serious reproductive health complications in women including pelvic inflammatory disease (PID) and continued sexual transmission. PID is an infection of a woman's reproductive organs often caused by infections such as chlamydia and gonorrhea. Unfortunately, 1 in 8 women with a history of PID experience infertility. Other sequelae of PID are uterine scarring, adhesions, ectopic pregnancy, and chronic pelvic pain.

STIs are preventable and treatable. If diagnosed and treated early, short-term and long-term complications such as PID could be prevented.

18.3.2 *Chlamydial Infections*

Introduction

Chlamydial infection is the most common bacterial infectious disease reported in the USA. It is one of the most common sexually transmitted bacterial infections worldwide. It is caused by an obligate, gram-negative intracellular bacterium, *Chlamydia trachomatis* (CT). CT can be found in the vagina, penis, anus, and oral mucosa. It is associated with 19 serologic variants (serovars), A, B/Ba, C, D/Da, E, F, G/Ga, H, I/Ia, J, K, L1, L2, L2a, and L3. In most cases at least >80% of the time, CT infection is asymptomatic. Most individuals with detected oropharyngeal CT infections do not present with oropharyngeal symptoms.

Diagnostic Considerations

Chlamydia trachomatis urogenital infections can be diagnosed by vaginal or cervical swabs or first-void urine. Nucleic acid amplification tests (NAATs), being the most sensitive tests for urogenital specimens, are the recommended screening tests for detecting CT. NAATs can be collected by a medical provider or the patient. In addition, NAATs are sensitive and specific in detecting rectal and oropharyngeal CT infections at the anatomic exposure sites among females engaging in receptive anal and/or oral intercourse. However, routine extragenital screening (oropharyngeal, rectal) is not recommended but must be considered for females based on reported high-risk sexual behaviors and exposure through shared clinical decision-making between the patient and medical provider.

Patient-collected vaginal swab specimens have been shown to be an acceptable and sensitive method to collect samples compared to conventional endocervical sampling by a medical provider. Some evidence suggests that liquid-based cytology specimens collected for pap smears might be acceptable specimens for NAAT, although test sensitivity might be lower than that associated with cervical or vaginal swab testing. NAAT-based point-of-care (POC) testing is newly available and appears to be promising.

Treatment Approach

Available evidence supports that doxycycline is efficacious in management for *Chlamydia trachomatis* infections of the urogenital, rectal, and oropharyngeal sites. However, azithromycin and levofloxacin are effective alternative options. To maximize medication adherence among those receiving multidose therapies, medication should be dispensed with all doses included. For individuals for whom adherence is a concern, on-site, directly observed azithromycin 1 g regimen should be available. Posttreatment evaluation and testing may be required because azithromycin 1 g regimen has demonstrated lower treatment efficacy among individuals with rectal infection.

- **Recommended regimen for chlamydial infection among adolescents and adults**
- **Doxycycline** 100 mg orally 2 times/day for 7 days
- **Alternative regimens**
- **Azithromycin** 1 g orally in a single dose or **levofloxacin** 500 mg orally once daily for 7 days
- **Recommended regimen for chlamydial infection during pregnancy**
- **Azithromycin** 1 g orally in a single dose
- **Alternative regimensAmoxicillin** 500 mg orally 3 times/day for 7 days

Management of Sex Partners and Other Considerations

To minimize disease transmission to sex partners, individuals treated for chlamydia should be instructed to abstain from sexual intercourse for 7 days after single dose therapy or until completion of a 7-day regimen and resolution of symptoms if present. To minimize risk for reinfection, patients should also be instructed to abstain from sexual intercourse until all their sex partners have completed the suggested treatment regimen. Individuals who receive a diagnosis of chlamydia should be tested for HIV, gonorrhea, and syphilis.

The most recent sex partners should be evaluated and treated if they had sexual contact with the infected partner during the 60 days (or greater) before the onset of the infected partner's symptoms or chlamydia diagnosis. Medical providers should provide patients with written educational materials and resources to give to their partners about chlamydia, specifically notification that partners have been exposed and the significance of treatment.

Follow-Up Testing

Most posttreatment infections do not result from failed treatment but rather from reinfection caused by failure of current sex partners to be treated or sexual activity with a new infected partner. Women treated for chlamydia should be retested approximately 3 months after completing therapy, regardless of whether their sex partner was treated or not. If retesting is not possible at 3 months, medical providers should retest whenever the next time the individual seeks for medical care.

18.3.3　Gonococcal Infections

Introduction

Gonococcal infection is the second most common reportable infectious disease in the USA. It is caused by a gram-negative bacterium, *Neisseria gonorrhoeae (N. gonorrhoeae)*. Urogenital tracts are the primary sites of *N. gonorrhoeae* although infections at extragenital sites, including the rectum and pharynx can also be detected. Most *N. gonorrhoeae* are asymptomatic, especially in females.

Diagnostic Considerations

N. gonorrhoeae genitourinary infections are detected using endocervical cultures, NAAT, and POC NAAT. Culture is also available for detecting rectal, oropharyngeal, and conjunctival gonococcal infection. NAAT sensitivity for detecting *N. gonorrhoeae* from urogenital and extra genital anatomic sites is superior to culture but varies by NAAT type. In females, optimal specimen types for gonorrhea screening using NAATs include vaginal swab specimens. Patient-collected specimens (urine, vaginal swabs, rectal swabs, oropharyngeal swabs) are reasonable alternatives to provider-collected swabs for gonorrhea screening by NAAT after clear patient instructions have been provided. In cases of suspected treatment failure or treatment resistance, medical providers should obtain both culture and antimicrobial susceptibility testing because NAATs cannot provide antimicrobial susceptibility results. Detection of *N. gonorrhoeae* using gram stains from endocervical, pharyngeal, and rectal specimens is not recommended due to poor sensitivity.

Treatment Approach

Clinical data supports that a single injection of ceftriaxone at higher than the strain minimum inhibitory concentration (MIC) for approximately 24 h is effective. However, gonococcal infections of the pharynx are more challenging to eradicate when compared to urogenital and rectal sites, so longer treatment times higher than the strains MIC are most likely needed to prevent development of mutant strains affecting the pharynx.

Dual therapy for gonococcal infection with ceftriaxone and azithromycin is no longer recommended. However, in cases in which chlamydial infections have not been excluded, patients should prophylactically receive chlamydial infection therapy.

Only ceftriaxone is recommended for gonorrhea treatment in the USA. Given the evolving nature of antimicrobial resistance of *N. gonorrhoeae* that have changed gonococcal treatment recommendations over time, medical providers must remain vigilant for treatment failures.

To maximize medication adherence among those receiving multidose therapies, medication should be dispensed with all doses included. For individuals for whom adherence is a concern, direct on-site administration should be provided.

- **Recommended regimen for uncomplicated gonococcal infection of the cervix, urethra, or rectum**

Ceftriaxone 500 mg IM in a single dose for persons weighing <150 kg. For persons weighing ≥150 kg, 1 g ceftriaxone should be administered.

If chlamydial infection has not been excluded, treat for chlamydia with doxycycline 100 mg orally 2 times/day for 7 days.

- **Alternative regimens**

If cephalosporin allergy:
Gentamicin 240 mg IM in a single dose
PLUS
Azithromycin 2 g orally in a single dose
If ceftriaxone administration is not available:
Cefixime 800 mg in a single dose

If chlamydial infection has not been excluded, treat for chlamydia with doxycycline 100 mg orally 2 times/day for 7 days.

- **Recommended regimen for uncomplicated gonococcal infection of the pharynx among adolescents and adults**

Ceftriaxone 500 mg IM in a single dose for persons weighing <150 kg. For persons weighing ≥150 kg, 1 g ceftriaxone should be administered.

Management of Sex Partners and Other Considerations

To minimize disease transmission to sex partners, individuals treated for gonorrhea should be instructed to abstain from sexual intercourse for 7 days after completing treatment regimen and until all sex partners have been treated. Individuals who receive a diagnosis of gonorrhea should be tested for HIV, chlamydia, and syphilis.

The most recent sex partners should be evaluated and treated if they had sexual contact with the infected partner during the 60 days (or greater) before the onset of the infected partner's symptoms or chlamydia diagnosis. Treatment of the sexual partner with cefixime 800 mg as a single dose is recommended, provided that concurrent chlamydial infection has been excluded. If chlamydia has not been excluded, then the partner may be treated with a single dose of oral cefixime 800 mg plus oral doxycycline 100 mg 2 times/day for 7 days. Medical providers should provide patients with written educational materials and resources to give to their partners about gonorrhea, specifically notification that partners have been exposed and the significance of treatment.

Follow-Up Testing

Most posttreatment infections do not result from failed treatment but rather from reinfection caused by failure of current sex partners to be treated or sexual activity with a new infected partner. Women treated for gonorrhea should be retested approximately 3 months after completing therapy, regardless of whether their sex partner was treated or not. If retesting is not possible at 3 months, medical providers should retest whenever the next time the individual seeks for medical care.

Any individual with pharyngeal gonorrhea should return 7–14 days after initial treatment for a test of cure by using either culture or NAAT; however, testing at 7 days might result in an increased likelihood of false-positive tests. If the NAAT is positive, confirmatory culture is advised. All positive cultures for the test of cure should undergo antimicrobial susceptibility testing. Symptoms that persist after treatment should be evaluated by culture for *N. gonorrhoeae* (with or without simultaneous NAAT) and antimicrobial susceptibility.

18.3.4　*Trichomonas Infections*

Introduction

Trichomonas infection is reported to be the most prevalent nonviral STI globally. Unlike other STIs, trichomonas is more common among women >24 years of age than in women <24 years. The infection, trichomoniasis, is caused by a protozoan parasite, *Trichomonas vaginalis (T. vaginalis)*. Its prevalence is highest among Black females (9.6%), followed by Hispanic women (1.4%) and non-Hispanic White women (0.8%). Most individuals who have trichomoniasis are asymptomatic or have minimal genital symptoms. In women, trichomoniasis presents with abnormal vaginal discharge that is typically described as malodorous, and yellow-green in color. A strawberry-appearing cervix may be detected on colposcopy.

Diagnostic Considerations

T. vaginalis infections are detected using NAATs from optimal specimen types including provider-collected endocervical swabs, provider-collected vaginal swabs, urine specimens, and liquid pap smear specimens. NAATs are more sensitive than traditional wet-mount microscopy and culture. However, they are inexpensive and can be performed at the point-of-care (POC). Vaginal specimens are the preferred specimen for obtaining cultures because urine specimens are less sensitive.

There are FDA-cleared rapid tests available at POC for detecting *T. vaginalis* with known improved sensitivities and specificities compared to traditional wet mount. Conventional and liquid-based pap smears are not considered diagnostic methods in detecting *T. vaginalis*. If *T. vaginalis* is found on a pap smear, performing a sensitive diagnostic test is recommended.

Treatment Approach

The nitroimidazoles are the only category of medications that have demonstrated the highest effectiveness against *T. vaginalis* infections. Clinical data supports that multi-dose metronidazole (500 mg orally 2 times/day for 7 days) reduced the number of women testing positive at 1-month after treatment initiation by half, compared with women who received the single dose (2 g orally).

Tinidazole, compared to metronidazole, has a longer half-life and thus could reach higher therapeutic levels in the serum and genitourinary tract. Evidence supports that tinidazole is equivalent or even superior to metronidazole in achieving *T. vaginalis* eradication but unfortunately, it is more expensive. Metronidazole gel, however, does not reach therapeutic levels in the urethra and genitourinary tract and thus is not recommended.

- **Recommended regimen for trichomoniasis among women**
  Metronidazole 500 mg 2 times/day for 7 days

- **Alternative regimen**
  Tinidazole 2 g orally in a single dose

Management of Sex Partners and Other Considerations

To minimize disease transmission to sex partners, individuals treated for trichomoniasis should be instructed to abstain from sexual intercourse until they and their sex partners have been treated. Individuals who receive a diagnosis of trichomoniasis should be tested for HIV, chlamydia, and syphilis.

Medical providers should provide patients with written educational materials and resources to give to their partners about trichomonas, specifically notification that partners have been exposed and the significance of treatment.

Follow-Up Testing

Most posttreatment infections do not result from failed treatment but rather from reinfection caused by failure of current sex partners to be treated or sexual activity with a new infected partner. Women treated for *T. vaginalis* should be retested approximately 3 months after completing therapy, regardless of whether their sex partner was treated or not. If retesting is not possible at 3 months, medical providers should retest whenever the next time the individual seeks for medical care.

18.3.5   Syphilitic Infections

Introduction

Syphilitic infection is known for its high variability in clinical presentation and is called "the great imitator." It is caused by a spirochete bacterium, *Treponema pallidum (T. pallidum)*. Syphilis infection presents clinically in different manifestations depending on the stage and timing of the disease. *Primary syphilis* typically presents with a single, painless, and ulcerated nodule (chancre) that occurs 3–90 days after exposure to the spirochete bacterium. It usually presents as a solitary nodule but can present atypically as multiple painful lesions usually on the sites of inoculation. It can be seen on the vagina, penis, perineum, anus, rectum, oral mucosa, nipples, or fingers and often accompanied by regional lymphadenopathy. *Secondary syphilis* consists of several mucocutaneous findings such as papulosquamous or macular rash on the trunk, scaly plaques on the palms and soles, alopecia, and condyloma lata that occur ~3 to 12 weeks from the disappearance of the chancre but can also present concomitantly. *Tertiary syphilis* can present with cardiac manifestations (aortic aneurysm, valvulopathy, aortic carditis), gummatous lesions, general paresis, and tabes dorsalis that occurs after 1 year to decades of latency. *Latent syphilis* lacks clinical manifestations but is characterized by positive serologic testing and can persist throughout life. At any syphilitic stage, the central nervous system, liver, kidney, and eye can also be affected and result in permanent loss of function of these organs. Mother-to-child transmission of *T. pallidum* can cause congenital infection and can cause antenatal and perinatal manifestations depending on the time of transmission. Most infants with congenital syphilis are infected in utero, but the newborn can also be infected by contact with an active genital lesion at the time of delivery.

Diagnostic Considerations

Treponema pallidum detection is based on the detection of spirochetes by direct examination with dark-field microscopy or direct immunofluorescence of mucocutaneous lesions of primary and secondary syphilis. Diagnosis is usually carried out by serological testing, categorized as *treponemal* and *nontreponemal*. The standard screening algorithm begins with a *nontreponemal* test [e.g., a rapid plasma reagin (RPR) or venereal disease research laboratory (VDRL) test] that detects serum antibodies to cardiolipin. These tests are positive after the development of the primary lesion, and search for antibodies produced against antigens released from the pathogenic tissues of *Treponema*. They are the only tests useful in the follow-up phase because they can highlight the activity of the infection and monitor the response to treatment. However, they are not very specific and therefore always need to be associated with a *treponemal* test. Reactivity is then confirmed with the use of highly sensitive and specific treponemal tests that detect serum antibodies to *T. pallidum*, such as *Treponema pallidum hemagglutination assay* (TPHA) and the *Treponema pallidum particle assay* (TPPA). *Treponemal* tests remain positive (reactive) even after treatment and so they are not useful in follow-up testing.

CSF tests including CSF cell count, protein, or reactive CSF-VDRL in the presence of reactive *treponemal* and *nontreponemal* results are warranted for individuals with clinical signs and symptoms of neurosyphilis. Individuals with ocular signs and symptoms and reactive serological testing will warrant a full ocular and cranial nerve examination.

Treatment Approach

Intramuscular (IM) penicillin G benzathine remains the first-line therapy administered in different dosages depending on the type of syphilis, stage, and clinical manifestations of the disease. For example, treatment for late latent syphilis (>1 years' duration), tertiary syphilis, and latent syphilis of unknown duration requires a longer duration of therapy. Resistance to penicillin has not been observed in the treatment of *T. pallidum*. Do not prescribe combination long- and short-acting benzathine-procaine penicillin (Bicillin C-R) since this is not approved for syphilis treatment.

Individuals should be informed about the Jarisch-Herxheimer reaction which is an acute febrile, self-limited reaction accompanied by headache and myalgia within the first 24 h after initiation of syphilis therapy. This is not an allergic reaction to penicillin but an immune-mediated reaction to treatment.

- **Recommended regimen for primary and secondary syphilis**
  benzathine penicillin G 2.4 million units IM in a single dose

  This is also the recommended regimen for syphilis during pregnancy. Pregnant women with primary or secondary syphilis who are allergic to penicillin should be desensitized and treated with penicillin G.

  This is also the recommended regimen among persons with HIV infection.

- **Recommended regimen for syphilis among infants and children**
  Benzathine penicillin G 50,000 units/kg body weight IM, up to the adult dose of 2.4 million units in a single dose

- **Recommended regimen for latent syphilis**

  - **Early latent syphilis: Benzathine penicillin G** 2.4 million units IM in a single dose
  - **Late latent syphilis: Benzathine penicillin G** 7.2 million units total, administered as 3 doses of 2.4 million units IM each at 1-week intervals

  This is also the recommended regimen among persons with HIV infection.

- **Recommended regimen for tertiary syphilis**
  Benzathine penicillin G 7.2 million units total, administered as 3 doses of 2.4 million units IM each at 1-week intervals

- **Recommended regimen for neurosyphilis, ocular syphilis, or otosyphilis**
  Aqueous crystalline penicillin G 18–24 million units per day, administered as three to four million units IV every 4 h or continuous infusion for 10–14 days
- **Alternative regimen for neurosyphilis, ocular syphilis, or otosyphilis**
  Procaine penicillin G 2.4 million units IM once daily PLUS
  Probenecid 500 mg orally 4 times/day, both for 10–14 days
- **Recommended regimens, confirmed or highly probable congenital syphilis**
- **Aqueous crystalline penicillin G** 100,000–150,000 units/kg/body weight/day, administered as 50,000 units/kg body weight/dose IV every 12 h during the first 7 days of life and every 8 h thereafter for a total of 10 days
  OR
  Procaine penicillin G 50,000 units/kg body weight/dose IM in a single daily dose for 10 days
- **Recommended regimens, possible congenital syphilis**
  Aqueous crystalline penicillin G 100,000–150,000 units/kg/body weight/ day, administered as 50,000 units/kg body weight/dose IV every 12 h during the first 7 days of life and every 8 h thereafter for a total of 10 days
  OR
  Procaine penicillin G 50,000 units/kg body weight/dose IM in a single daily dose for 10 days
  OR
  Benzathine penicillin G 50,000 units/kg body weight/dose IM in a single dose

Management of Sex Partners and Other Considerations

The sex partners of individuals with primary, secondary, or early latent syphilis should be notified of exposure, evaluated clinically and serologically, and treated. The following sex partners include *partners who have had sexual contact within*

3 months plus the duration of symptoms for persons who receive a diagnosis of primary syphilis, within 6 months plus duration of symptoms for those with secondary syphilis, and within 1 year for persons with early latent syphilis.

Persons who have had sexual contact with a person who receives a diagnosis of primary, secondary, or early latent syphilis <90 days before the diagnosis should be treated presumptively for early syphilis, even if serologic test results are negative.

Persons who have had sexual contact with a person who receives a diagnosis of primary, secondary, or early latent syphilis >90 days before the diagnosis should be treated presumptively for early syphilis if serologic test results are not immediately available and the opportunity for follow-up is uncertain. If serologic tests are negative, no treatment is needed. If serologic tests are positive, treatment should be based on clinical and serologic evaluation and syphilis stage.

In certain areas or among populations with high syphilis infection rates, health departments recommend notification and presumptive treatment of sex partners of persons with syphilis of unknown duration who have high nontreponemal serologic test titers (i.e., >1:32) because high titers might be indicative of early syphilis.

Long-term sex partners of persons who have latent syphilis should be evaluated clinically and serologically for syphilis and treated based on the evaluation's findings.

18.3.6 Herpes Simplex Virus

Introduction

Herpes simplex virus (HSV) is a lifelong viral infection categorized into two types, *HSV-1* and *HSV-2*. They have the potential to cause episodic flares consistent with painful, blister-like lesions that commonly develop on the orofacial and/or anogenital regions. However, HSV-2 rarely presents outside the anogenital region. Over the past two decades, HSV estimated seroprevalence has steadily declined, but specific populations remain disproportionately affected including Mexican Americans, non-Hispanic Blacks, and pregnant persons. Transmission of HSV during pregnancy often occurs during delivery when the infant comes into contact with genital lesions during delivery or when the pregnant person is experiencing prodromal symptoms. There have been rising cases of anogenital herpetic infections attributed to HSV-1, which has an increased prevalence among young women. Majority of people infected with HSV-2 who may have mild or unrecognized infections have the potential to shed the virus intermittently from the anogenital region. Thus, recurrence and subclinical shedding is more common in HSV-2 as compared to HSV-1. Furthermore, there is a large percentage of genital herpes infections transmitted by asymptomatic persons who are unaware that they have the infection.

Diagnostic Considerations

Serologic screening of HSV is complicated by the low predictive value of the available screening tests. It is imperative that healthcare providers know the high likelihood of false-positive results that occur when screening asymptomatic individuals. HSV is predominantly a clinical diagnosis and the disease can be self-limiting without the episodic recurrence of painful vesicular or ulcerative lesions that are classically seen. In fact, these classic lesions are absent at the time of clinical evaluation. The presence of HSV-1 antibodies often is acquired during childhood, which might be asymptomatic, but this does not distinguish anogenital from orolabial or cutaneous infection. In addition, regardless of the site of infection, these patients remain at risk for acquiring HSV-2 in the future. When genital lesions are present, clinical diagnosis of herpes can be confirmed by NAAT or culture from the fluid sampled of an unroofed lesion.

HSV NAAT assays detect HSV directly from the genital ulcers or other mucocutaneous lesions making this the most sensitive test. PCR is the test of choice for diagnosing HSV infections with central nervous system (CNS) involvement (meningitis, encephalitis, and neonatal herpes). HSV PCR is of low diagnostic value to diagnose genital herpes infection, with the exception of cases involving disseminated infection such as hepatitis. Viral culture is the only available virologic testing, providing low sensitivity, especially for recurrent lesions as viral load decreases rapidly as lesions begin to heal. Both PCR and viral cultures should be typed to determine whether HSV-1 or HSV-2 is causing the infection. Of note, failure to detect HSV by NAAT or culture, especially in the presence of older lesions or the absence of active lesions, does not reliably rule out an absence of HSV infection due to the intermittent nature of viral shedding. Even self-swabs in asymptomatic individuals provide low sensitivity and a negative result, which does not exclude the presence of HSV infection. Tzanck preparations are insensitive and nonspecific methods of diagnosing genital lesions and are not recommended. Direct immunofluorescence assay using fluorescein-labeled monoclonal antibodies is another modality available for detecting HSV antigen from genital specimens but this assay lacks sensitivity and is not recommended.

Antibodies that are type-specific and type-common develop during the first weeks following initial infection and persist indefinitely. Type-specific HSV serologic assays accuracy is based on the HSV-specific glycoprotein G2 (gG2) (HSV-2) and glycoprotein G1 (gG1) (HSV-1) and should be requested. False-negative results can occur more frequently in the early stages of infection; therefore, in instances of recent suspected HSV acquisition, repeat type-specific antibody testing 12 weeks after the presumed time of acquisition is recommended. The commercially available type-specific enzyme immunoassay (EIA) tests can have poor specificity; therefore, a confirmatory test with a Western blot as a second method should be performed before test interpretation to improve accuracy of HSV serologic testing. If confirmatory testing is unavailable, patients should be counseled about the existing limitations before obtaining serologic tests. Immunoglobulin M (IgM) testing for HSV-1 or HSV-2 has not proven to be useful and is not recommended due to not being type-specific with the potential to provide positive results during recurrent genital or oral episodes of herpes.

Type-specific HSV-2 serologic assays are useful in the following scenarios:

- Recurrent or atypical genital lesions with a negative HSV PCR or culture result.
- Clinical diagnosis of genital herpes without laboratory confirmation concurrently with a partner who suffers from genital herpes.
- Patients who are at higher risk for infection:

  - Those presenting for an STI evaluation,
  - Persons with ≥10 lifetime sex partners.
  - Persons with HIV infection.

    - HSV-2 genital infection increases the risk for acquiring HIV twofold to threefold—All persons with genital herpes should be tested for HIV.

Treatment Approach

Systemic antiviral medications partially control the symptoms of herpes for first-time and recurrent outbreaks. They are effective when used for daily suppressive therapy. However, antivirals neither eradicate the latent virus nor alter the risk, frequency, or severity of recurrences after the medication has been discontinued. Goals of treatment include prevention of symptomatic HSV recurrences and preventing transmission to sexual partners. Education and counseling of risk factors for reducing sexual and perinatal transmission are paramount in clinical management and prevention. FDA-approved antiviral medications such as *acyclovir*, *valacyclovir*, and *famciclovir* have proven efficacy against HSV infections. Topical therapy with these antiviral medications has proven to offer minimal clinical benefit and is not recommended. Management of HSV should address the chronic nature of the infection and not primarily on treating acute episodic outbreaks of the herpetic lesions. To date, there is no cure for the HSV infection.

Recommended regimen for first clinical episode of genital herpes:

Newly acquired HSV has the potential to develop into a complicated illness with severe ulcerations and neurologic involvement. Therefore, it is recommended that all patients with the first clinical outbreak of HSV should receive antiviral therapy. Treatment courses can be extended if the healing is incomplete after 10 days of therapy

Acyclovir: 400 mg orally 3 times/day for 7–10 days
or
Famciclovir: 250 mg orally 3 times/day for 7–10 days
or
Valacyclovir: 1 gram orally 2 times/day for 7–10 days

An overwhelmingly high percentage of patients with symptomatic first episode of HSV-2 infections subsequently experience recurrent episodes with the potential for intermittent asymptomatic shedding. Treatment can be administered either as suppressive therapy to reduce the frequency of recurrences or episodically at the first outbreak dosing to ameliorate or shorten the duration of lesions. The option for suppressive therapy also proves advantageous in decreasing the risk for transmitting the virus to susceptible partners.

Recommended regimens or suppression of recurrent HSV-2 Genital Herpes:

Suppressive therapy can reduce recurrences by 70–80%. The regimen selected should be individualized as it relates to frequency of outbreaks. Patients can use suppressive therapy for a period of time and cessation does not incur increased risk of adverse events or development of resistance. Suppressive therapy, consistent condom use, and avoidance of sexual activity during recurrences decrease the rate of HSV-2 transmission for discordant heterosexual couples in which a partner has a history of genital HSV-2 infection as well as for persons with a history of symptomatic genital herpes who have multiple partners.

HSV-1 genital herpes have less frequent recurrences following the first episode, when compared with genital HSV-2. Genital shedding in HSV-1 rapidly decreases during the first year of infection. There is limited data to support the use of suppressive therapy for preventing transmission of HSV-1 genital herpes infection and thus, suppressive therapy should be reserved for those with frequent recurrences through shared clinical decision-making between the patient and the provider.

Acyclovir: 400 mg orally 2 times/day
or
Valacyclovir: 500 mg orally once a day
or
Valacyclovir: 1 gram orally once a day
or
Famciclovir: 250 mg orally 2 times/day

Recommended regimens for episodic therapy for recurrent HSV-2 genital herpes:

Episodic treatment of recurrent HSV is most efficacious when therapy is initiated within 24 h of onset of lesions or during the symptomatic prodrome that precedes some outbreaks. Providing the patient with a prescription for the medication with instructions to initiate treatment immediately when symptoms begin has proved equally effective for episodic treatment of genital herpes.

Acyclovir: 800 mg orally 2 times/day for 5 days
or
Acyclovir: 800 mg orally 3 times/day for 2 days
o
Famciclovir: 1 g orally 2 times/day for 1 day
or
Famciclovir: 500 mg orally once, followed by 250 mg times/day for 2 days
or

Famciclovir: 125 mg orally 2 times/day for 5 days
or
Valacyclovir: 500 mg orally 2 times/day for 3 days
or
Valacyclovir: 1 g orally once a daily for 5 days

18.3.7   Severe Disease

Intravenous (IV) acyclovir therapy (5–10 mg/kg body weight IV every 8 h) should be provided for the following patients:

- Those who have severe HSV infection.
- Complications that necessitate hospitalization such as:

  - Disseminated infection
  - Pneumonitis
  - Hepatitis
  - CNS complications such as:

    - Meningitis
    - Encephalitis

HSV-2 meningitis is a rare complication of HSV-2 genital herpes infection affecting women predominantly than men. IV therapy should be the first line of therapy until clinical improvement is achieved. This is followed by an oral antiviral regimen to complete a total therapy of greater than 10 days to continuous treatment, with longer courses suggested for CNS complications.

HSV-2 meningitis is characterized clinically by the following signs:

- Headache
- Photophobia
- Fever
- Meningismus
- Cerebrospinal fluid (CSF)

  - Lymphocytic pleocytosis
  - Mildly elevated protein
  - Normal glucose

Treatment course for meningitis is recommended as follows:

- Acyclovir 5–10 mg/kg body weight IV every 8 h until clinical improvement is observed.
- Followed by high-dose oral antiviral therapy (valacyclovir 1 g 3 times/day) to complete a 10- to 14-day course of total therapy.

Patients with previous episodes of documented HSV-2 meningitis, treatment regimen with higher doses of oral valacyclovir can be equally efficacious during episodes of recurrent HSV-2 meningitis. HSV meningitis must be clinically distinguished from encephalitis, which requires a longer course (14–21 days) of IV therapy. Close attention to renal function is warranted.

18.3.8 Hepatitis

Hepatitis is a rare manifestation of disseminated HSV infection often seen in pregnant women who acquire HSV during pregnancy. In a pregnant woman with new onset fever and unexplained severe hepatitis, the clinician should have a high index of suspicion for HSV disseminated infection and have a low threshold to treat with empiric IV acyclovir pending confirmation diagnosis by HSV PCR from blood. HSV hepatitis can progress to fulminant liver failure with an accompanied mortality rate of up to 25%.

Management of Sex Partners and Other Considerations

In patients who have recently acquired HSV-2 and are asymptomatic, viral shedding is most frequent in the first year. Consistent and correct condom use has been shown to decrease, but not eliminate the risk for HSV-2 transmission from men to women, but are less effective for preventing transmission from women to men. There is decreased risk for HSV-2 acquisition among women with a male partner who has been circumcised. Pericoital intravaginal tenofovir 1% gel has been shown to decrease the risk for HSV-2 acquisition among heterosexual women. There is insufficient data to support the use of antiviral medications such as *acyclovir, valacyclovir*, or *famciclovir* in patients without HSV-2 as a form of prevention of acquisition of the virus.

Risk for transmission of HSV to the neonate is highest when genital herpes is acquired late in pregnancy near the time of delivery (30–50%). Women with the presence of prodrome/lesions at delivery should have a cesarean delivery to reduce the risk for neonatal HSV infection.

Recommended regimen for suppression of recurrent genital herpes among pregnant women to be started at 36 weeks' gestation:

Acyclovir: 400 mg orally 3 times/day
or
Valacyclovir: 500 mg orally 2 times/day

18.3.9   *Human Immunodeficiency Virus (HIV) and Acquired Immunodeficiency Syndrome (AIDS)*

Introduction

The human immunodeficiency virus (HIV) is a lifelong disease that attacks the body's immune system. If not treated, it can lead to *AIDS* (acquired immunodeficiency syndrome). There are no vaccines or medications available to cure HIV. Early in the disease course, HIV can present with brief, nonspecific influenza-like symptoms such as fever, fatigue, lymphadenopathy, pharyngitis, arthritis, or skin rash. Some are asymptomatic. Following an acute infection and if left untreated, this subsequently develops into a chronic illness that progressively depletes CD4+ T lymphocytes. Untreated HIV infection overtime will progress to a symptomatic and life-threatening immunodeficiency. Early diagnosis and effective antiviral therapy (ART) can suppress viral replication reducing morbidity, transmission, and early mortality. A history of another STI increases one's risk for HIV acquisition, especially among the following populations:

- Primary or secondary syphilis
- Men who have sex with men
- Rectal gonorrhea
- Rectal chlamydia

Diagnostic Considerations

There are strong recommendations to screen for HIV infection in the following populations:

- All pregnant patients—including those who present in labor or at delivery whose HIV status is unknown.
- Adolescents and adults aged 15–65 years.
- Younger adolescents and older adults who are at increased risk of infection.

Commercially available screening tests are highly accurate in diagnosing HIV, specifically testing for HIV infection with an antigen/antibody immunoassay that detects HIV-1 and HIV-2 antibodies and the HIV-1 p24 antigen. Reflex testing after a reactive assay to differentiate between HIV-1 and HIV-2 antibodies is recommended. An HIV-1 nucleic acid test is recommended to differentiate acute HIV-1 infection from a false-positive result for nonreactive or indeterminate results following an acute exposure. Available rapid antigen/antibody tests positive results should be confirmed. Repeat screening is reasonable for women known to be sexually active with someone who is known to be positive with HIV or women who engage in behaviors that may convey an increased risk of HIV infection. Such behaviors include IV drug use, commercial sex workers, and having multiple sex partners whose HIV status is unknown. Repeat screening is recommended for patients who receive medical care in a high-prevalence setting, live in a correctional facility, or homeless shelter. It is recommended to repeat prenatal screening for HIV during all pregnancies, repeated pregnancies, and in the third trimester of pregnancy in women with risk factors for HIV acquisition.

Treatment Approach

Prompt initiation of ART for all patients with HIV infection regardless of CD4+ T-cell count is recommended. Maintaining a viral load suppressed to <200 copies/mL with ART drastically reduces risk for sexual transmission of HIV and its progression to AIDS, AIDS-defining clinical events, and mortality. ART does not protect against other STIs that can be prevented by using condoms. Accompanied prophylaxis for opportunistic infections, immunizations, and cancer screening is recommended in this patient population. ART treatment of pregnant women living with HIV substantially decreases the risk of transmission to the fetus, newborn, or infant. The clinical treatment of HIV infection is constantly updated by subspecialists within the field. The Panel on Antiretroviral Guidelines for Adults and Adolescents of the US Department of Health and Human Services regularly updates guidelines for HIV treatment regimens. It is best to refer to their recommendations for the most up to date guideline approach to treatment.

Management of Sex Partners and Other Considerations

Patients and their partners face extensive challenges ranging from coping with HIV infection, reactions of others, maintenance of physical and emotional health, and transmission prevention while reducing the risk for acquiring additional STIs. Providing resources, access to health care and other support services such as behavioral, substance use, mental health, psychosocial services should be available to individuals upon diagnosis. Partner notification, early diagnosis and treatment of HIV among all potentially exposed sexual and injecting drug sharing partners are warranted in addition to offering HIV prevention services such as PrEP or PEP (if exposure was <72 h previous) and STI testing and treatment.

18.4 Hepatitis B Virus (HBV)

18.4.1 Introduction

The hepatitis B virus (HBV) is spread through contact with blood, semen, or other body fluids. The infection affects the liver and is vaccine preventable. Modes of transmission of HBV can be through sexual contact, IV drug use, perinatal, and household contacts of someone living with chronic HBV infection. New infections can be asymptomatic or present with symptoms including fatigue, GI disturbance, and jaundice, resulting in a short-term illness. Those with chronic infection subsequently develop cirrhosis, hepatocellular carcinoma, or liver failure. Increased risk for chronic infection includes factors related to age of onset of infection. Data shows that 90% of infants with hepatitis B go on to develop chronic infection, whereas 2–6% of adults who are infected with hepatitis B become chronically infected.

18.4.2   Diagnostic Considerations

According to the USPSTF recommendations, we must screen asymptomatic, non-pregnant adolescents and adults who are at increased risk for HBV infection, including those who were vaccinated before being screened. Screening tests include B surface antigen (HbsAg) testing with reflex confirmatory testing. If the test reveals a positive HBsAg result, this indicates a chronic or acute infection. However, sending a serologic panel allows for confirmatory diagnosis. Periodic screening is recommended for patients with results revealing a negative HBsAg. Use clinical judgment to determine screening frequency for those who have not received the HBV vaccine series and higher risk groups.

Important risk groups for HBV infection with a prevalence of $\geq 2\%$ that should be screened including the following:

- Born in any region with a high prevalence of HBV infection ($\geq 2\%$)

    - Asia
    - Africa
    - The Pacific Islands
    - South America

- If born in the USA, but not vaccinated as an infant and whose parents were born in regions with a very high prevalence of HBV infection ($\geq 8\%$)
- HIV-positive
- IV drug use
- Men who have sex with men
- Household contacts/sexual partners with HBV infection

18.4.3   Treatment Approach

Those who test positive for acute or chronic HBV infection should receive education about reducing the risk of transmission to others including preventative measures during childbirth, intercourse, needle sharing, and household contacts. There is no specific therapy available for patients diagnosed with acute HBV infection, as the treatment is supportive. However, vaccination is the most effective way to prevent HBV.

To verify the presence of chronic HBV infection, any patient testing positive for HBsAg should be retested. The absence of IgM anti-HBc or the persistence of HBsAg for ≥6 months would indicate that the patient is suffering from a chronic HBV infection. Between 20% and 40% of patients infected with chronic HBV will require treatment with antiviral medications approved by the US Food and Drug Administration (FDA) for treatment of chronic HBV infection. Patients with chronic HBV infection should be referred to a provider with experience managing such infections, given the fact that appropriate therapeutic agents approved by FDA for treatment of chronic HBV infection can achieve sustained suppression and remission of liver disease.

18.4.4 Management of Sex Partners and Other Considerations

Patients with HBV infection should be tested for HIV, syphilis, gonorrhea, and chlamydia. Any sexual partners, household members, and needle-sharing contacts that have not been vaccinated for HBV should be tested for susceptibility and receive the first dose of hepatitis B vaccine immediately following serologic testing. Those at risk should complete the dose and schedule vaccination series that is age-appropriate. Those at high risk of transmission secondary to sexual contact should be counseled to use condoms for protection from infectious body fluids such as semen and vaginal secretions. HBV could also be transmitted with blood contact; therefore, it is encouraged to cover cuts and skin lesions while refraining from the donation of the following:

- Blood
- Plasma
- Body organs
- Tissue
- Semen

Household contacts should refrain from sharing household articles such as toothbrushes, razors, or any article that could become contaminated with blood. To prevent further liver injury, patients diagnosed with HBsAg should avoid or limit alcohol consumption, refrain from starting any new medicines, including over-the-counter and herbal medicines, without discussion with their health care provider. Vaccination against Hepatitis A is also warranted.

18.5   Hepatitis C Virus (HCV)

18.5.1   Introduction

HCV is one of the leading causes of complications from chronic liver disease, is the most common chronic blood-borne pathogen in the USA, and is associated with more deaths than the top 60 other reportable infectious diseases combined, including HIV. IV drug use is the most important risk factor through sharing needles. Tattoos applied in non-regulated settings have been associated with HCV transmission. Transmission can also occur as a consequence of inadequate infection control in health care settings although rare nowadays. HCV prevalence has increased in women aged 15–44 years of age, with an increased detection rate in pregnant women, resulting in an increase in the proportion of infants born to mothers infected with HCV. Hepatitis C can be a short-term self-limiting illness consistent with jaundice, and/or flu-like symptoms. For more than half of those who become infected with the virus, it becomes a long-term, chronic infection resulting in serious health problems such as liver cirrhosis and hepatocellular carcinoma. Chronic hepatitis C can often be asymptomatic but when symptoms are present, patients may already have advanced liver disease. Currently, there is no available vaccine for long-term mitigation.

18.5.2   Diagnostic Considerations

The USPSTF recommends a one-time screening for all asymptomatic adults, including those who are pregnant, between the ages of 18–79 years, even without known liver disease. Anti-HCV antibody testing using a third-generation enzyme-linked immunosorbent assay, which has a 99% sensitivity and specificity, is the screening test of choice. Follow-up reflex HCV RNA polymerase chain reaction testing for positive results to confirm the active disease is recommended. HCV RNA can be detected in blood as early as 1–3 weeks following exposure. The average time from exposure to antibody to HCV (anti-HCV) seroconversion is approximately within 4–10 weeks. Once infected, 15–45% of patients can spontaneously clear the viral infection. The persistence of HCV RNA after 6 months indicates chronic HCV infection with detectable HCV antibodies in 97% of patients by 6 months following exposure. Chronic HCV infection develops among 75–85% of persons with HCV infection and 10–20% of patients with chronic infection will go on to develop liver disease related cirrhosis in 20–30 years, subsequently.

Consider periodically screening patients of any age, those between the ages of 18 and 79 years, who are younger than 18 years and older than 79 years, who are at high risk for infection, such as current or previous IV drug use. Due to the increasing prevalence of HCV in women aged 15–44 years and the infants born to mothers infected with HCV clinicians should consider screening pregnant patients younger than 18 years old. Patients with positive screening test results are followed up with a diagnostic evaluation. Pretreatment assessment with noninvasive evaluation of fibrosis/cirrhosis staging includes the following:

- Aspartate transaminase to platelet ratio index score
- FibroSure (combination of FibroTest and ActiTest)
- Fibrosis-4
- Direct serum markers
- Radiologic assessments—FibroScan—Transient elastography

Transient elastography plus an indirect serum marker are the optimal approach to testing. However, indirect serum markers that predict the presence/absence of significant fibrosis/cirrhosis do not accurately differentiate between the intermediate stages of fibrosis. More invasive testing, such as liver biopsy is recommended if two noninvasive tests are discordant.

18.5.3 Treatment Approach

Persons determined to have HCV infection with positive HCV RNA testing should be evaluated for treatment. Testing will remain positive for antibodies to HCV after spontaneous resolution or successful treatment. Therefore subsequent testing for HCV reinfection should be limited to HCV RNA. Patients who have spontaneously resolved HCV infection or have undergone successful medical treatment are not immune to reinfection. Antiviral treatment regimens for HCV infection are geared toward prevention of long-term complications of chronic HCV infection such as cirrhosis, liver failure, and hepatocellular carcinoma.

An 8–12 week course of the oral direct acting antiviral regimens has become the accepted gold standard of treatment for chronic HCV infection because they are more effective, better tolerated, and the treatment course is shorter. Antiviral therapy is not generally considered during pregnancy secondary to the lack of data available on the safety of newer oral direct acting antiviral regimens during pregnancy and breastfeeding. HCV infection is curable. Patients diagnosed with HCV infection should be linked to care and treatment with hepatitis specialists, as needed. The best way to prevent hepatitis C is by avoiding behaviors that can spread the disease, especially injecting drugs.

FDA-approved pangenotypic direct acting antiviral treatments that could be managed by primary care clinicians include glecaprevir/pibrentasvir (Mavyret), sofosbuvir/velpatasvir (Epclusa), and Sofosbuvir/velpatasvir/voxilaprevir (Vosevi). When patient presentation becomes more complex, referral to a hepatologist is recommended.

Glecaprevir/pibrentasvir (Mavyret: 100 mg/40 mg tablet)

- 3 tablets/day × 8 weeks
  - Simplified treatment regimen.

- Effective against all hepatitis C virus genotypes.
- Indicated for patients without cirrhosis and for those with compensated cirrhosis.
- Not recommended in Child-Pugh classification B cirrhosis and is contraindicated in Child-Pugh classification C cirrhosis.
- No restriction based on renal function.
- 8 weeks of treatment has exhibited a greater than 95% sustained viral response at 12 weeks posttreatment, regardless of the HCV genotype.

Sofosbuvir/velpatasvir (Epclusa: 400 mg/100 mg tablet)

- 1 tablet/day × 12 weeks

  - Simplified treatment regimen.
  - Genotype testing is required.
  - Genotype 3 requires Y93H resistance-associated substitution testing.
  - Patients without the Y93H variant—12 weeks of sofosbuvir/velpatasvir.
  - Presence of Y93H, treatment with glecaprevir/pibrentasvir or referral to a specialist is recommended.
  - Indicated for patients without cirrhosis and patients with compensated cirrhosis, including Child-Pugh classification B cirrhosis and Child-Pugh classification C cirrhosis (with ribavirin).
  - Approved for use in patients with advanced CKD with an eGFR of 30 mL per minute per m2 or less and patients on hemodialysis.
  - 12 weeks of treatment has exhibited a greater than 95% sustained viral response at 12 weeks posttreatment, regardless of the HCV genotype.

18.5.4   Management of Sex Partners and Other Considerations

Data supports that patients with HCV infection with one long-term monogamous partner do not need to change their sexual practices. It is encouraged that discussion about transmission risks and the need for testing be commonplace. Partners of those with diagnosed HCV and HIV should be tested for both infections. It is highly recommended that testing for HIV and HBV occur in all patients with diagnosed HCV infection.

18.6 Human Papillomavirus (HPV)

18.6.1 Introduction

HPV is a DNA virus that is spread by direct skin-to-skin contact, infects cutaneous and mucosal epithelial cells, and can be divided into low-risk and high-risk types based on their associated cancer risk. It is a sexually transmitted virus with more than 200 viral types, at least 40 of which infect the genital area, but the majority of which are self-limited and are asymptomatic. The Centers for Disease Control and Prevention reports that HPV is the most prevalent STI in the USA. The early HPV vaccine trial data report that the lifetime prevalence of the infection is 85% in women and 91% in men who have had at least one sexual partner. Risk factors that increase risk for persistent infection include multiple sex partners, initiation of sexual activity at an early age, not using barrier protection, other sexually transmitted infections such as HIV, an immunocompromised state, and alcohol/tobacco use. HPV types 16 and 18 have been deemed high risk, as they cause the majority of cervical, penile, vulvar, vaginal, anal, and oropharyngeal precancers/cancers. Low-risk types such as viral types 6 and 11 cause genital warts and recurrent respiratory papillomatosis. A decrease in HPV-attributable cancers has been seen since the introduction of the HPV vaccination.

18.6.2 Diagnostic Considerations

HPV screening focuses on the identification of precancerous lesions, allowing for early intervention and prevention of progression to carcinoma. Screening options include cytology-based testing (Pap smear), high-risk HPV testing, and cotesting (simultaneous cytology and high-risk HPV testing). Recommendations for cervical cancer screening can vary among medical societies and organizations, but this chapter focuses on the USPSTF recommendations.

Recommendations for screening as per the USPSTF guidelines are as follows:

- Women with increased risk factors such as HIV infection, a compromised immune system, in utero exposure to diethylstilbestrol, and previous treatment of a high-grade precancerous lesion or cervical cancer are not included in the following recommendation and should receive individualized follow-up.
- Women who have had a hysterectomy including the removal of the cervix, without the history of a high-grade precancerous lesion or cervical cancer, are not at risk for cervical cancer and should not be screened.
- Screen for cervical cancer every 3 years with cervical cytology alone in women aged 21–29 years.

- For women aged 30–65 years screening every 3 years with cervical cytology alone, every 5 years with high-risk human papillomavirus (hrHPV) testing alone, or every 5 years with hrHPV testing in combination with cytology (cotesting)
- Recommendations against screening for cervical cancer in women older than 65 years who have had adequate prior screening and are not otherwise at high risk for cervical cancer.
- Recommendations against screening for cervical cancer in women younger than 21 years.
- Recommendations against screening for cervical cancer in women who have had a hysterectomy with removal of the cervix and do not have a history of a high-grade precancerous lesion (i.e., cervical intraepithelial neoplasia [CIN] grade 2 or 3) or cervical cancer.
- The first 3 recommendations apply to individuals who have a cervix, regardless of their sexual history or HPV vaccination status. These recommendations do not apply to individuals who have been diagnosed with a high-grade precancerous cervical lesion or cervical cancer.
- These recommendations also do not apply to individuals with in utero exposure to diethylstilbestrol or those who have a compromised immune system (e.g., women living with HIV), cases of cervical cancer occur among women who have not been adequately screened.
- Strategies that aim to ensure that all women are appropriately screened and receive adequate follow-up are most likely to succeed in further reducing cervical cancer incidence and mortality in the USA.
- The USPSTF found convincing evidence that screening with cervical cytology alone, primary testing for high-risk HPV types (hrHPV testing) alone, or in combination at the same time (cotesting) can detect high-grade precancerous cervical lesions and cervical cancer.

18.6.3   Treatment Approach

Subclinical genital HPV infections are typically asymptomatic and resolve spontaneously. Specific antiviral therapy has not been recommended to eradicate such infections. Non-cancerous macroscopic genital warts can be treated with topical regimen as mentioned below or by local excision. The main focus of pathologic screening aims toward identification of high-grade precancerous cervical lesions. High-grade cervical lesions can be treated with excisional and ablative therapies. Early stages of cervical cancer can be approached with surgical interventions such as hysterectomy or chemotherapy. These more invasive procedures will require consultation and intervention with surgical subspecialists.

Recommended regimens for external anogenital warts:

- Medications that can be applied by the patient:

  - Imiquimod 3.75% or 5% cream

- Podofilox 0.5% solution or gel
- Sinecatechins 15% cream

- Provider administered:

  - Cryotherapy

    - Liquid nitrogen
    - Cryoprobe

  - Surgical excision

    - Tangential scissor excision
    - Tangential shave excision
    - Curettage
    - Lase
    - Electrosurgery

  - Trichloroacetic acid (TCA)
  - Bichloroacetic acid (BCA)

18.6.4 Management of Sex Partners and Other Considerations

Anogenital HPV infections are prevalent in those who are sexually active and the majority of people will suffer infections at some time during their lifetime. Partners tend to share the virus, and it is not possible to determine where the infection originated. Persistent HPV infections can lead to genital warts, precancers, and even progress to cancers of the cervix, anus, penis, vulva, vagina, head/neck. Discussion of tobacco/alcohol use in addition to cessation counseling is paramount due to its contribution to the progression of precancer and cancer. HPV infection does not complicate conception of carrying a fetus to term, but in rare instances, a pregnant woman can transmit HPV to an infant during delivery. Certain surgical procedures required to treat HPV related precancers or cancers can affect a woman's ability to get pregnant or carry a pregnancy to term.

18.7 Mycoplasma Genitalium

18.7.1 Introduction

Mycoplasma genitalium is a sexually transmitted bacteria that has an affinity for the mucosal epithelium of the urogenital tracts. It has been estimated that 15–25% of nongonococcal urethritis is caused by Mycoplasma genitalium and is a common cause of recurrent urethritis in the USA. Mycoplasma genitalium among women are frequently asymptomatic, but can cause symptomatic urethritis, cervicitis, PID, pre-term delivery, spontaneous abortion, and infertility. Mycoplasma genitalium can be detected among 10–30% of women with clinical cervicitis and ranges from 4% to 22% among women with PID.

18.7.2   Diagnostic Considerations

Mycoplasma genitalium is an extremely slow-growing organism, and cultures can take up to 6 months to provide results. Nucleic acid amplification test, or NAAT for Mycoplasma genitalium is FDA approved for testing of urine, urethral, penile meatal, endocervical, and vaginal swab samples and has a specificity of 97% or higher for all specimen types. Vaginal swab is the preferred specimen type because of higher sensitivity. Women with recurrent cervicitis or PID should be tested for Mycoplasma genitalium accompanied with resistance testing for macrolide (azithro-mycin) or quinolone (moxifloxacin) resistance markers, if available. Routine screening for asymptomatic Mycoplasma genitalium infection has not been recommended.

18.7.3   Treatment Approach

Mycoplasma genitalium has been complicated by high rates of macrolide resistance. A two-tiered treatment regimen has been recommended for treatment, ideally using resistance-guided therapy.

Recommended treatment regimen of Mycoplasma genitalium if resistance testing is available:

If macrolide sensitive:

- Doxycycline 100 mg PO BID × 7 day course, followed by
- Azithromycin 1 gram PO × 1 day, followed by
- Azithromycin 500 mg PO QD × 3 additional days (total of 2.5 grams)

Recommended treatment regimen of Mycoplasma genitalium if resistance testing is not available and Mycoplasma genitalium has been detected by FDA-approved NAAT:

- Doxycycline 100 mg PO BID × 7 day course, followed by
- Moxifloxacin 400 mg PO QD × 7 days

In settings without access to resistance testing and when moxifloxacin cannot be used, an alternative regimen can be:

- Doxycycline 100 mg PO BID × 7 day course, followed by
- Azithromycin 1 gram PO × 1 day, followed by

- Azithromycin 500 mg PO QD × 3 additional days (total of 2.5 grams)
- Test of cure 21 days after completion of therapy. This regimen should be used only when a test of cure is possible, and no other alternatives exist.

Initial empiric therapy for PID includes:

- Doxycycline 100 mg PO BID × 14 days should be provided at the time of presentation for care.
- If Mycoplasma genitalium is detected.
- Moxifloxacin 400 mg PO QD × 14 days has been effective in eradicating the organism.

18.7.4 Management of Sex Partners and Other Considerations

There is high co-infection rate among sexual partners and those with symptomatic Mycoplasma genitalium infection. If testing the partner is not feasible, it is recommended to treat the partner with the same antimicrobial regimen that was provided to the patient.

18.8 Ectoparasitic Infections

18.8.1 Pediculosis Pubis (Pubic Lice)

Introduction

Pediculosis pubis or pubic lice is caused by the parasite *Phthirus pubis,* which can be transmitted by skin-to-skin contact and sexual contact. Patients seek medical attention secondary to the visualization of lice or nits in their pubic hair and/or from pruritus in the anogenital region. The life cycle of this ectoparasite has three phases. Nits are eggs, oval, yellow/white, hard to see, are found firmly attached to the hair shaft, and take about 6–10 days to hatch. The nymph is an immature louse, small, and once they hatch take about 2–3 weeks to mature into adults that are capable of reproducing. Nymphs require blood meals during three separate molts in the maturation process to achieve the adult phase. The adult pubic louse has six legs, with two large front legs that are pincher/claw-like, with phenotypic features resembling a crab. The louse can live for 24–48 h off the body of its human hosts and be transmitted via fomites in bedding or clothing, which plays a minor role in their transmission. The louse is not known to transmit any diseases, but the intense pruritus in the anogenital region leads to scratching, which can cause breakdown in the skin integrity allowing for secondary bacterial infection of the skin.

Diagnostic Considerations

The parasite is diagnosed visually and clinically.

Treatment Approach

Treatment for non-pregnant/non-breastfeeding patients consists of the following:

- Permethrin 1% cream:

  - Applied to affected areas and washed off after 10 min

or

- Pyrethrins with piperonyl butoxide

  - Applied to affected areas and washed off after 10 min

or

- Malathion 0.5% lotion

  - Applied to affected areas and washed off after 8–12 h

or

- Ivermectin

  - 250 mcg/kg/dose PO × 1
  - Repeat in 2 weeks

  Treatment for pregnant/breastfeeding patients consists of the following:

- Permethrin 1% cream:

  - Applied to affected areas and washed off after 10 min

  or

- Pyrethrins with piperonyl butoxide

  - Applied to affected areas and washed off after 10 min

Management of Sex Partners and Other Considerations

Recommendations include decontaminating bedding and clothing by machine washing on hot water cycle and drying using a high heat cycle. Clothing and items that are not washable can be dry-cleaned or they can be sealed in a plastic bag and stored for a 2 week period. Remove clothing or bedding from body contact for a minimum of 72 h. There is no need to fumigate the living areas. Sexual partners from the past 30 days must be treated.

18.9 Scabies

18.9.1 Introduction

Human scabies is caused by the human itch mite *Sarcoptes scabiei var. hominis.* Scabies infestation is spread by direct, prolonged, skin-to-skin contact such as sexual intercourse. Outbreaks are common in congesting living quarters such as nursing homes, extended-care facilities, dormitory sleeping arrangements such as hostels/military barracks and prisons. The mite is microscopic, burrows into the epidermis but never below the stratum corneum, where it lives/lays its eggs causing intense itching and a pimple-like skin rash. The burrows can appear as tiny raised serpentine lines and can be a centimeter or more in length. Areas commonly affected are the hands/wrist, interdigitary webbed spaces of the fingers/toes, axilla, waistline, anogenital region, elbows, and knees. *Sarcoptes scabiei* undergoes four stages in its life cycle including egg, larva, nymph, and adult. This process can be greater than 2 months. Initial symptoms usually do not appear for up to 2 months; however, an infested person still can spread scabies during this time. In subsequent infestations, symptoms appear much sooner, ~1 to 4 days following exposure. Those infected with scabies may continue to transmit the mite until successfully treated and the mites/eggs have been eradicated.

Crusted or Norwegian scabies are an aggressive infestation noted in the immunosuppressed, debilitated, or malnourished patient population, including those receiving potent glucocorticoids, organ transplant recipients, those infected with HIV infection or human T-lymphotropic virus-1 infection, and those suffering from hematologic malignancies. Patients present with thick crusts of skin that contain large numbers of scabies mites and eggs that are far more numerous making them extremely contagious to others.

18.9.2 Diagnostic Considerations

Scabies infestation is usually a clinical diagnosis given the customary appearance and distribution of the rash and the presence of burrows. The diagnosis of scabies can be confirmed by identifying the mite, mite eggs, or fecal matter under a microscope. However, this method has low sensitivity because of operator dependence and can be time-consuming. Noninvasive techniques such as videodermatoscopy have high sensitivity and specificity when performed by experienced operators. Low-technology strategies include the burrow ink test and the adhesive tape test.

18.9.3 Treatment Approach

Typical scabies in non-pregnant, non-breastfeeding patients:

- Permethrin 5% cream:
  - Applied to all areas of the body from the neck down and washed off after 8–14 h

or

- Ivermectin
  - 200 mcg/kg/dose PO × 1
  - Repeat in 2 weeks

or

- Ivermectin 1% lotion
  - Applied to all areas of the body from the neck down and washed off after 8–14 h
  - Repeat in 1 week if symptoms persist

Typical scabies in pregnant/breastfeeding patients:

- Permethrin 5% cream:
  - Applied to all areas of the body from the neck down and washed off after 8–14 h

  or

- Ivermectin
  - 200 mcg/kg/dose PO × 1
  - Repeat in 2 weeks

Crusted (Norwegian) Scabies in non-pregnant, non-breastfeeding patients:

- Permethrin 5% cream daily + ivermectin 200 mcg/kg/dose PO on days 1, 2, 8, 9, and 15

  or

- 25% topical benzyl benzoate daily + ivermectin 200 mcg/kg/dose PO on days 1, 2, 8, 9, and 15

Severe cases potentially could require additional Ivermectin treatment on days 22 and 29.

Crusted (Norwegian) Scabies in pregnant/breastfeeding patients:

- Permethrin 5% cream daily + ivermectin 200 mcg/kg/dose PO on days 1, 2, 8, 9, and 15 or

- 25% topical benzyl benzoate daily + ivermectin 200 mcg/kg/dose PO on days 1, 2, 8, 9, and 15.

Severe cases potentially could require additional ivermectin treatment on days 22 and 29.

18.9.4 Management of Sex Partners and Other Considerations

Recommendations include decontaminating bedding and clothing by machine washing on hot water cycle and drying using a high heat cycle. Clothing and items that are not washable can be dry-cleaned or they can be sealed in a plastic bag and stored for a 2 week period. Remove clothing or bedding from body contact for a minimum of 72 h. There is no need to fumigate the living areas. Sexual partners from the past 30 days must be treated. Advise patients to keep their fingernails clean and trimmed in order to prevent breakdown in the skin integrity as a result of scratching.

Ms. Thomas, who you counseled above on her risks of getting an STI(s) and STI screening, asks you specifically about how she can protect herself from getting a sexually transmitted infection and passing it on to others. She reports that she has been sexually active with four male partners in the last year. She reports vaginal sex but denies oral and anal sex. She denies use of any protective STI barriers such as male condoms. She denies any prior history of sexually transmitted infections.

18.10 STI Prevention Counseling

The USPSTF recommends provision of behavioral counseling for all sexually active adolescents, adults, and those who are at increased risk of sexually transmitted infections (STIs). Furthermore, the USPSTF recommends with moderate certainty that behavioral counseling interventions reduce the likelihood of STI transmission among sexually active adolescents and adults at high risk of STIs.

The USPSTF recommends implementation of this recommendation by doing the following. This is as stated in their publication in August 2020.

1. Assessing whether adolescents are sexually active and, for adults, assess risk for STIs. Factors that put a person at increased risk include:

   (a) Being diagnosed with an STI within the past year
   (b) Not consistently using condoms
   (c) Having multiple sex partners or having a partner(s) at high risk for STIs
   (d) Belonging to a population that has a high STI prevalence (such as persons seeking STI testing or attending an STI clinic, sexual and gender minorities,

persons living with HIV, persons with injection drug use, persons who exchange sex for money or drugs, persons who have recently been in a correctional facility, and some racial/ethnic minority groups)

2. Providing behavioral counseling to sexually active adolescents and to adults at increased risk:

  (a) Deliver counseling in person, refer patients to outside counseling services, or inform patients about media-based interventions
  (b) Interventions that include group counseling, involve more than 120 min of counseling, and are delivered over several sessions have the strongest effect in preventing STIs

    (i) Counseling interventions shorter than 30 min delivered in a single session may also be effective

  (c) Provide information on common STIs and STI transmission; aim to increase motivation or commitment to safer sex practices; and provide training in condom use, communication about safer sex, problem solving, and other pertinent skills.

18.11 STI Prevention Tips

STIs are preventable. Knowing your STI health history is a critical step to stopping STI transmission. Counseling women on the following tips will reduce their risk of getting an STI.

- Know your sexual partners and reduce the number of sex partners. The more partners you have, the higher the risk of acquiring an STI. STI testing of partners is highly encouraged.

  - Mutual monogamy with an uninfected sex partner is encouraged.

- Abstaining from intercourse (vaginal, anal, oral) is the most reliable way of avoiding infection.
- Using male and female synthetic latex and non-latex (for latex allergic) condoms correctly and consistently every time vaginal, anal, and oral sex. Natural membrane condoms are not reliable for STI prevention.
- Getting vaccinated to help protect against HPV and hepatitis B infections.

  - Routine HPV vaccination can start as early as age 9 and recommended through age 26. For adults ages 27–45 years, clinicians can consider discussing HPV vaccination with people who are most likely to benefit.
  - Routine hepatitis B vaccination is recommended for all infants, children, and adolescents younger than 19 years who have not been vaccinated, all adults age 19–59 years, and adults age 60 years or older with risk factors for acquir-

ing hepatitis B infection. Adults 60 years or older who have no risk factors for hepatitis B may also receive the vaccine if they choose to.

Ms. Thomas was grateful for the comprehensive counseling you have given her about common STIs and STI transmission. She is committed to safer sex practices and is motivated to increase educational awareness about STI-related stigma, fear, and discrimination.

18.12 Conclusion

Sexually transmitted infections are on the rise and continue to be a significant public health concern. This prompts a call for action among clinicians to educate themselves on up-to-date evidence-based information on STI screening/detection, risk assessment, evaluation/testing, management, prevention counseling, follow-up retesting, and treating partners. By doing this, the medical community can decrease the overall health burden attributed to the serious health consequences of untreated and undiagnosed STIs including pelvic inflammatory disease (PID) and continued sexual transmission.

STIs are preventable and treatable. If diagnosed and treated early, short-term and long-term complications could also be prevented.

Suggested Reading

1. Centers for Disease Control and Prevention. Sexually transmitted disease surveillance, 2020. Centers for Disease Control and Prevention. 2022, August 22. Retrieved January 2, 2023, from https://www.cdc.gov/std/statistics/2020/default.htm
2. Centers for Disease Control and Prevention. Sexually transmitted disease surveillance 2018. Atlanta: U.S. Department of Health and Human Services; 2019. https://doi.org/10.15620/cdc.79370.
3. Workowski KA, Bachmann LH, Chan PA, et al. Sexually transmitted infections treatment, 2021. MMWR Recomm Rep. 2021;70(RR-4):3–127.
4. U.S. Preventive Services Task Force. Screening for chlamydia and gonorrhea: U.S. preventive services task force recommendation statement. JAMA. 2021;326(10):949–56.
5. Panel on Opportunistic Infections in Adults and Adolescents with HIV. Guidelines for the prevention and treatment of opportunistic infections in adults and adolescents with HIV: recommendations from the Centers for Disease Control and Prevention, the National Institutes of Health, and the HIV Medicine Association of the Infections Diseases Society of America. Available at https://clinicalinfo.hiv.gov/sites/default/files/guidelines/documents/Adult_OI.pdf
6. Rodrigues R, Sousa C, Vale N. *Chlamydia trachomatis* as a current health problem: challenges and opportunities. Diagnostics (Basel). 2022;12(8):1795. https://doi.org/10.3390/diagnostics12081795. PMID: 35892506; PMCID: PMC9331119
7. Knox J, Tabrizi SN, Miller P, et. al. Evaluation of self-collected samples in contrast to practitioner-collected samples for detection of chlamydia trachomatis, Neisseria gonorrhoeae, and trichomonas vaginalis by polymerase chain reaction among women living in remote areas. Sex Transm Dis 29(11):p 647–654 2002.

8. Sunkavalli A, McClure R, Genco C. Molecular regulatory mechanisms drive emergent Pathogenetic properties of *Neisseria gonorrhoeae*. Microorganisms. 2022;10(5):922. https://doi.org/10.3390/microorganisms10050922. PMID: 35630366; PMCID: PMC9147433

9. Mercuri SR, Moliterni E, Cerullo A, Di Nicola MR, Rizzo N, Bianchi VG, Paolino G. Syphilis: a mini review of the history, epidemiology and focus on microbiota. New Microbiol. 2022;45(1):28–34. Epub 2021 Dec 11. PMID: 35403844

10. US Preventive Services Task Force, Krist AH, Davidson KW, Mangione CM, Barry MJ, Cabana M, Caughey AB, Donahue K, Doubeni CA, Epling JW Jr, Kubik M, Ogedegbe G, Pbert L, Silverstein M, Simon MA, Tseng CW, Wong JB. Behavioral counseling interventions to prevent sexually transmitted infections: US preventive services task force recommendation statement. JAMA. 2020;324(7):674–81. https://doi.org/10.1001/jama.2020.13095. PMID: 32809008

11. McQuillan G, Kruszon-Moran D, Flagg EW, Paulose-Ram R. Prevalence of herpes simplex virus type 1 and type 2 in persons aged 14-49: United States, 2015-2016. NCHS Data Brief. 2018;304:1–8.

12. US Preventive Services Task Force, Mangione CM, Barry MJ, Nicholson WK, Cabana M, Chelmow D, Coker TR, Davis EM, Donahue KE, Jaén CR, Kubik M, Li L, Ogedegbe G, Pbert L, Ruiz JM, Stevermer J, Wong JB. Serologic screening for genital herpes infection: US preventive services task force reaffirmation recommendation statement. JAMA. 2023;329(6):502–7. https://doi.org/10.1001/jama.2023.0057. PMID: 36786784

13. US Preventive Services Task Force, Krist AH, Davidson KW, Mangione CM, Barry MJ, Cabana M, Caughey AB, Donahue K, Doubeni CA, Epling JW Jr, Kubik M, Ogedegbe G, Owens DK, Pbert L, Silverstein M, Simon MA, Tseng CW, Wong JB. Screening for hepatitis B virus infection in adolescents and adults: US preventive services task force recommendation statement. JAMA. 2020;324(23):2415–22. https://doi.org/10.1001/jama.2020.22980. PMID: 33320230

14. Scott H, Volberding PA. HIV screening and preexposure prophylaxis guidelines: following the evidence. JAMA. 2019;321(22):2172–4. https://doi.org/10.1001/jama.2019.2590. PMID: 31184721

15. Maness DL, Riley E, Studebaker G. Hepatitis C: diagnosis and management. Am Fam Physician. 2021;104(6):626–35. PMID: 34913652

16. US Preventive Services Task Force, Curry SJ, Krist AH, Owens DK, Barry MJ, Caughey AB, Davidson KW, Doubeni CA, Epling JW Jr, Kemper AR, Kubik M, Landefeld CS, Mangione CM, Phipps MG, Silverstein M, Simon MA, Tseng CW, Wong JB. Screening for cervical cancer: US preventive services task force recommendation statement. JAMA. 2018;320(7):674–86. https://doi.org/10.1001/jama.2018.10897. PMID: 30140884

17. Quinlan JD. Human papillomavirus: screening, testing, and prevention. Am Fam Physician. 2021;104(2):152–9. PMID: 34383440

18. Clebak KT, Sell JK, Koontz A. Aptima assay for detection of mycoplasma genitalium infection. Am Fam Physician. 2021;104(5):517–8. PMID: 34783498

19. US Preventive Services Task Force, Owens DK, Davidson KW, Krist AH, Barry MJ, Cabana M, Caughey AB, Donahue K, Doubeni CA, Epling JW Jr, Kubik M, Ogedegbe G, Pbert L, Silverstein M, Simon MA, Tseng CW, Wong JB. Screening for hepatitis C virus infection in adolescents and adults: US preventive services task force recommendation statement. JAMA. 2020;323(10):970–5. https://doi.org/10.1001/jama.2020.1123. PMID: 32119076

20. Centers for Disease Control and Prevention. Sexually transmitted disease surveillance, 2020. Centers for Disease Control and Prevention. 2023, March 9. Retrieved January 2, 2023, from https://www.cdc.gov/hepatitis/hbv/index.html.

21. Centers for Disease Control and Prevention. Sexually transmitted disease surveillance, 2020. Centers for Disease Control and Prevention. 2023, June 15. Retrieved January 2, 2023, from https://www.cdc.gov/parasites/lice/pubic/index.html.

22. Centers for Disease Control and Prevention. Sexually transmitted disease surveillance, 2020. Centers for Disease Control and Prevention. 2023, June 6. Retrieved January 2, 2023, from https://www.cdc.gov/parasites/scabies/index.html.

Part IV
Heath Maintenance

Chapter 19
Mammography/Cervical Cancer Screening

Ramya Parameswaran and Massoud Mahmoudi

19.1 Case

Sally is a 35 yo woman with no significant past medical history who presents to establish care. She has not seen a primary care doctor in 10 years and wonders about cancer screenings as her mother was diagnosed with breast cancer at the age of 47.

19.2 Breast Cancer Screening

19.2.1 Introduction

In 2020, there was an estimated 3.8 million women living with breast cancer. Approximately 13% of women in the USA will be diagnosed with breast cancer during their lifetime and the death rate for these cancers is 19.6 for every 100,000 women every year. Breast cancer mortality rates have decreased substantially over the past half a century due to improvements in treatment options as well as available modalities for and frequency of screening, thus allowing for detection at earlier stages. Current 5-year survival rates are 90%, compared to 75% in the mid-1970s.

R. Parameswaran (✉)
Department of Internal Medicine Residency Program, University of California, San Francisco, San Francisco, CA, USA
e-mail: ramya.parameswaran@ucsf.edu

M. Mahmoudi
Department of Medicine, University of California, San Francisco, San Francisco, CA, USA

© The Author(s), under exclusive license to Springer Nature Switzerland AG 2024
M. Mahmoudi (ed.), *Common Cases in Women's Primary Care Clinics*,
https://doi.org/10.1007/978-3-031-48569-5_19

Screening should be a shared decision between the physician and the patient, and whether to order screening tests for a patient should be determined by a combination of risk factor assessment, age, and a thorough discussion of both the risks (false positives, cost, anxiety, and overdiagnosis) and benefits (early detection and decreased mortality) of performing screening tests. Screening modalities include breast self-awareness, clinical breast examination, breast MRI, genetic testing, and mammography, and recommendations from various medical organizations regarding which of these to use and in which patients will be discussed in detail below. It is imperative that primary care doctors are equipped to use a shared decision framework to assist patients in making personal screening choices from within a range of reasonable options that depend on their risk factors, age, and discussion of potential benefits and harms. This chapter is aimed at providing guidance for primary care physicians as they broach these topics with their patients.

19.2.2   *Risk Factors for Breast Cancer*

Case Continued

Upon gathering more history, we find out that Sally has never had children and achieved menarche at the age of 13. She has no personal history of cancer, breast disorders, or radiation to the chest. She is of Ashkenazi Jewish heritage and, other than her mother, is not aware of any other relatives with cancer diagnoses. Her BMI is within normal range and she does not smoke or drink alcohol. Sally wonders what her own risk of developing breast cancer will be.

In the primary care office, it is important to assess for specific risk factors for breast cancer. While the main risk factors for breast cancer include advanced age and sex, eliciting more detailed medical, family, and social history from our patients can help us more thoroughly risk stratify patients. Specifically, this information can help us determine whether an individual is deemed to be high risk or low risk for developing breast cancer, and counsel our patients on lifestyle changes for modifiable risk factors and consideration of genetic testing for non-modifiable risk factors. Importantly, these factors can change how often, when, and via what modalities we screen patients for breast cancer. It can be helpful to think about risk factors for breast cancer in the following five categories: reproductive, therapies, familial, breast disorders, and others (Table 19.1).

Reproductive Risk Factors: Studies have consistently demonstrated that nulliparity and longer intervals between menarche and age of first pregnancy are associated with increased risk of hormone receptor positive breast cancer, specifically estrogen receptor (ER) and progesterone receptor (PR) positive cancers. Specifically, in a systematic review of the literature, 19 of 22 case control and cohort studies showed an inverse association between parity and hormone positive breast cancers and in one study, this association was specifically seen in women who were diagnosed with breast cancer at age 40 or greater. Other studies have reported links between

Table 19.1 Breast cancer risk factors

Reproductive	Therapies	Familial	Breast disorders	Others
Nulliparity	Menopausal combined hormone replacement therapy	Germline mutation-associated cancers (prostate, pancreas)	Atypical ductal hyperplasia	Dense breasts
Longer intervals between menarche and first birth	Ionizing radiation to chest	Family history of breast cancer	Atypical lobular hyperplasia	Increasing age
Older age at first birth		Family history of ovarian cancer	Lobular carcinoma in situ	Higher BMI
Older age at menopause		Ashkenazi Jewish heritage		Smoking
Younger age at menarche				Increased alcohol consumption
No breastfeeding				Female sex

older age at first pregnancy, older age at menopause, and younger at menarche and increased breast cancer risk. However, these studies have been less consistent overall.

Increased parity and breastfeeding, however, confer a decreased risk for developing hormone receptor positive breast cancer, and in the case of breastfeeding, also a reduced risk of triple negative breast cancer as well.

Therapies: The two main therapies that are associated with increased risk for breast cancer are combination hormone replacement therapy (HRT) in post-menopausal women and prior therapeutic chest radiation. Regarding HRT, Chlebowski et al. performed the Women's Health Initiative randomized control trial (RCT) in 2015 in which 16,608 post-menopausal women with a uterus were randomized to estrogen-progestin HRT versus placebo with a median duration of 5.6 years. Hazard ratios for the effect of combined HRT on breast cancer were 0.71 for the first 2 years of the study and increased to 1.24 by the end of the study. This study also assessed breast cancer risk in women who previously had a hysterectomy and were treated with estrogen alone versus placebo with a median duration of 7.2 years. In this population, the hazard ratio for invasive breast cancer was 0.79 throughout the intervention. Thus, combined HRT confers an increased risk of invasive breast cancer in post-menopausal women.

Regarding therapeutic chest radiation, in a systematic review of literature from 1993 to 2008, it was determined that cumulative incidence of breast cancer by 40–45 years of age in patients who received chest radiation for treatment of Hodgkin's lymphoma between the ages of 10 and 30 years was 13–20% with standardized incidence ratios in the 13–55 range. Risk for breast cancer was shown to increase linearly with chest radiation dose. Patients who received radiation between the ages of 10 and 14 were at greatest risk in these studies. Thus, obtaining a thorough medication, prior cancer, and radiation exposure history is vitally important to understanding a patient's risk of breast cancer.

Familial: Hereditary breast cancer syndromes can be suspected in patients who currently have or previously had ovarian cancer or have a personal or family history of ovarian or breast cancer. Germline mutations in the BRCA1 and BRCA2 genes account for most cases of hereditary breast cancer syndrome and these mutations are found in 4.5% of breast cancer cases. The BRCA genes are tumor suppressor genes that encode for proteins that are vital to DNA repair and patients with hereditary breast cancer inherit one defective allele from one parent. In the two-hit hypothesis, if the second normal allele becomes nonfunctional as a result of a somatic mutation, cancer develops. In a systematic review of 1641 patients carrying BRCA mutations from multiple countries, the mean cumulative risk of breast cancer was 57% for BRCA1 and 49% for BRCA2. BRCA1 mutations are more commonly associated with triple negative breast cancers and BRCA2 mutations are more commonly associated with ER/PR positive cancers. Ashkenazi Jewish populations have also been found to have increased risk of developing breast cancer, often due to BRCA associated hereditary cancer syndromes. Genetic mutations in other genes, such as ATM, CDH1, CHEK2, PALB2, PTEN, STK11, and p53, are also associated with increased breast cancer risk, and some are associated with other hereditary cancer syndromes like Lynch and Cowden syndrome. Given this, it is important to obtain information about ethnic background and a thorough personal and family history of cancer, including first- and second-degree relatives from both paternal and maternal lineages, a description of the type of primary cancer, and age of diagnosis. Detailed criteria that primary care doctors can use to determine which patients need genetic testing and counseling is addressed below.

Pre-existing Breast Disorders: Benign breast lesions are often diagnosed upon evaluation of a breast mass or abnormal mammogram. Atypical ductal hyperplasia, atypical lobular hyperplasia, and lobular carcinoma *in situ* are associated with a fourfold risk of developing breast cancer in the affected and contralateral breasts, with a cumulative incidence of 30% at 25 years of follow-up.

Others: This category includes both modifiable and non-modifiable risk factors. Modifiable risk factors include at-risk alcohol use or alcohol use disorder, smoking, and higher BMI. Patients with any of these risk factors should be counseled on their association with breast cancer incidence. Female sex and dense breast tissue also confer risk for breast cancer. Ninety-nine percent of people with breast cancer are women. Women with dense breasts diagnosed by mammography have a slightly increased risk of developing breast cancer, and mammograms often have difficulty detecting cancer in women in dense breasts. There is currently no data that demonstrates reduction in breast cancer mortality via the use of supplemental screening modalities like ultrasonography, MRI, or tomosynthesis in patients without other significant risk factors. Thus, screening guidelines are the same for average risk women with and without dense breasts.

19.2.3 Risk Assessment Tools

Several risk assessment tools have been developed to identify patients who are high risk for developing breast cancer and thus may require genetic testing, more intensive screening measures, and risk reduction therapies or surgeries. Some of these models include the Gail model, the BRCAPRO, and the IBIS calculators. These calculators use factors such as age, personal history of cancer or other benign breast disorders, family history of cancer, BMI, race/ethnicity, age of menarche, and age of first pregnancy, in order to estimate a personal lifetime risk of developing breast cancer. No single model has been agreed upon as the standard in the field. The Gail model, for example, is widely used but is not as accurate in patients younger than 35, with a paternal family history of breast cancer, with a family history of non-breast cancers that are associated with genetic cancer syndromes, or high-risk biopsy lesions other than atypical hyperplasia. The American Cancer Society (ACS), National Comprehensive Cancer Network (NCCN), and American College of Radiology would designate any patient with a lifetime risk of 20% or greater to be high risk, as well as women 35 years of age or older with a 5 year risk of invasive breast cancer of 1.7% or greater high risk as well. Patients with BRCA or other genetic mutations associated with hereditary cancer syndromes are automatically considered to be high risk.

19.2.4 Screening Modalities

Case Continued

Given her Ashkenazi Jewish heritage and first degree relative with breast cancer, Sally is determined to have a high risk for developing breast cancer and is recommended for a screening mammogram and breast MRI yearly, along with genetic counseling and clinical breast exams every 6 months.

Average Risk Patients

Breast Self-Awareness: Breast self-awareness is defined by the American College of Obstetrics and Gynecology (ACOG) as a patient's awareness of the normal appearance and feel of their breasts. Unlike the breast self-examination, which was previously recommended for women to perform systematically and on a regular basis, this methodology encourages patients to be attuned to any changes in their breasts. Thus, it is important for primary care doctors to educate patients about the specific changes to take notice of including pain, new masses, new onset nipple discharge, or redness in the breast skin. Self-examination is no longer recommended due to risk of harm from false positive results and lack of benefit. However, self-awareness is imperative as almost 50% of breast cancer diagnoses in women 50 years and older and 71% in women younger than 50 years are made after detection by patients themselves.

Clinical Breast Exam: The clinical breast exam is performed in the primary care office first with visual inspection with arms at the patient's side and arms above the head. Palpation is then performed in all sections of breast tissue, including the areola, nipple, and under the breast, in addition to the axilla. It is important to document the shape, texture, nipple–areolar complex color and skin texture, skin color and appearance, and symmetry.

Screening Mammogram: The screening mammogram is a low dose X-ray of the breast that allows for detection of high density tissue in both a top and side view of the breast. Radiology examines the images to determine whether they can visualize any abnormal masses as well as microcalcifications that can represent cancer. When abnormal findings appear on screening mammograms, diagnostic mammogram, breast MRI, or biopsy may be recommended to further evaluate.

High-Risk Patients

Breast MRI: The breast MRI with contrast is a more sensitive method to screen for breast cancer. Thus, a combination of breast MRI and traditional mammography (alternating every 6 months) can be a useful tool for screening high risk patients.

Genetic Screening: Both BRCA mutation testing and multigene panels are used in patients with family history that is suspicious for a hereditary cancer syndrome. These patients should be referred first to a genetic counselor, who can perform a detailed pedigree analysis, a thorough risk assessment to determine eligibility for genetic testing and identification of appropriate family members to test, and an informed consent process in which the risks, benefits, and limitations of genetic testing can be explained.

Special Considerations

Transgender Men: Screening for transgender men depends on the presence of breast tissue. Patients who continue to have breast tissue after their transition should receive the same screening as the cis female population. It is important to review operative reports if your patient had gender affirming surgery to understand if they had a mastectomy or breast reduction. Family history of breast and ovarian cancer should be assessed prior to surgery to determine whether further genetic testing is needed in these individuals.

Transgender Women: Overall, it is thought that transgender women have a lower risk of breast cancer due to decreased length of lifetime exposure to estrogen. A Dutch retrospective study showed that the incidence of breast cancer in transgender women was 4.1 in 100,000, compared with 155 in 100,000 in the cis female population. General consensus is to start screening this population at the age of 50 years old and a minimum of 5 years after feminizing hormone use.

Importantly, our transgender patients often face discrimination when interacting with the healthcare system. Thus, it is important to ask all patients about their gender identity and pronouns prior to starting an interaction. Training other staff and providing access to gender neutral bathrooms can make this patient population feel safer as well. Lastly, acknowledging that it can be emotionally and physically traumatizing to undergo cancer screenings for anatomical structures that the patient may not identify with can create a safe space for shared decision-making.

19.2.5 Screening Recommendations

Average Risk Patients

In average risk patients, the screening recommendations from four clinical organizations are listed in Table 19.2. Breast self-awareness is a concept supported by the ACS and USPSTF. The clinical breast exam is no longer recommended by the USPSTF and ACS. It is encouraged as a shared decision with patients by ACOG and

Table 19.2 Recommended breast cancer screening modalities and frequency

Screening modality	American College of Obstetricians and Gynecologists (ACOG)	US Preventative Services Task Force (USPSTF)	American Cancer Society (ACS)	National Comprehensive Cancer Network (NCCN)
Breast self-awareness	No clear answer	Supportive	Supportive	No clear answer
Clinical breast exam	May offer every 1–3 years for women 25–39 yo and annually for women 40 + yo	Insufficient evidence	Not recommended	Every 1–3 years in women 25–39 yo; annual for 40 years and older
Screening mammogram initiation age	Offer at 40 yo; recommend strongly by no later than 50 yo if not initiated yet	Recommend at 50 yo; shared decision-making regarding starting between 40 and 49 yo	Offer 40–45 yo; recommend at 45 yo	40 yo
Screening mammogram interval	Annual or once every 2 years	Once every 2 years	Annual for women 40–54 yo; once every 2 years or annual for 55 yo and older	Annual
Screening mammogram discontinuation age	Until 75 yo; beyond 75 yo should be a shared decision	Insufficient evidence to screen women 75 yo and older	When life expectancy is less than 10 years	When severe comorbidities limit life expectancy to 10 years or less

NCCN every 1–3 years under the age of 40 and annually in patients who are 40 years and older. Screening mammograms are recommended by all groups, some recommending a start age of 40 yo, others recommending 50 yo as the start age with shared decision-making for screening earlier. Frequency of screening is between 1 and 2 years and screening stops at the age of 75 or when life expectancy is less than 10 years.

High-Risk Patients

In patients who are determined to be high risk via the risk assessment tools described earlier in this chapter (20% or greater lifetime risk of developing breast cancer) or any patient found to have a hereditary cancer syndrome or history of radiation therapy in the chest, more intensive screening is recommended. In patients between the ages of 25 and 29 years old, clinical breast examination every 6–12 months and annual breast MRI with contrast are recommended. MRI is recommended over mammography in this age group as it has been shown to decrease breast cancer risk from radiation exposure in European patients with BRCA mutations; these studies have not been replicated in other populations. For patients age 30 years or older, annual breast MRI with contrast and mammography (alternating each every 6 months), with clinical breast examination every 6 months is recommended.

For patients with strong family history of ovarian or breast cancers, specifically meeting the following criteria, genetic testing for both BRCA mutations and other mutations via a multigene panel is important:

Women affected by one or more of the following:

- Epithelial ovarian, tubal, or peritoneal cancer
- Breast cancer at 45 years old or less
- Breast cancer and have a close relative (first degree relative, second-degree relative, or third degree relative) with breast cancer at age 50 years or less or close relative with epithelial ovarian, tubal, or peritoneal cancer at any age
- Breast cancer at age 50 years or less with limited or unknown family history
- Breast cancer and have two or more close relatives with pancreas cancer or Gleason 7 or higher prostate cancer
- 2 breast cancer primaries, with first diagnosed before 50 years old
- Triple negative breast cancer at age 60 years old or less
- Breast cancer and Ashkenazi Jewish heritage at any age
- Pancreas cancer and two or more close relatives with breast, ovarian, tubal, peritoneal, pancreas, or Gleason 7 or higher prostate cancer

or women without cancer, but with one or more of the following:

- First degree or several close relatives that meet one or more of the criteria above
- Close relative with a known BRCA1 or BRCA2 mutation
- Close relative with male breast cancer

19.2.6 Benefits and Harms of Screening

Benefits of screening patients for breast cancer include increases in life expectancy due to decreases in breast cancer mortality and earlier detection of breast cancer. Adverse consequences include false positive test results, especially in those who use combination hormone therapy and have dense breasts in the age group of 40–49 years, anxiety, discomfort during procedures that result from false positives, overdiagnosis and overtreatment of cancers that may have remained indolent. Lastly, mammography induced radiation can in rare cancers cause cancer (2 in 100,000 women aged 50–59 years). However, the benefits outweigh the radiation risks.

19.3 Cervical Cancer

19.3.1 Introduction

In 2020, there was an estimated 296,000 women living with cervical cancer. Approximately 0.7% of women in the USA will be diagnosed with cervical cancer during their lifetime and the death rate for these cancers is 2.2 for every 100,000 women every year. Cervical cancer mortality rates have decreased over time with the HPV vaccine and our ability to perform routine screening with PAP smears and HPV co-testing in the primary care clinic. In this section of the chapter, we will discuss risk factors for cervical cancer, screening methodologies and guidelines for different age groups, and risks and benefits of screening.

19.3.2 Risk Factors for Cervical Cancer

Modifiable Risk Factors: Multiple sexual partners and having a sexual partner with HPV (asymptomatic or in the form of genital warts) could increase our patients' risks of cervical cancer. Counseling on using protection and education on genital lesions can be helpful in the primary care office for risk reduction. Smoking and immunosuppression via HIV are also risk factors for cervical cancer. Motivational interviewing to counsel patients on tobacco cessation can reduce risk and encouraging adherence to intensive screening and HIV treatments can reduce risk as well. Obtaining a thorough sexual and social history is important for understanding your patient's overall risk.

Non-modifiable Risk Factors: Diethylstilbestrol exposure in utero is a risk factor for both cervical and vaginal cancers. Women used this drug to prevent miscarriages in the 1930s–1970s. Ninety-nine percent of patients exposed to this drug in utero do not develop cancer; however, this risk of developing clear cell carcinoma of the vagina or cervix is greater than the general population. These patients require more intensive screening, and so obtaining a thorough history in the primary care office is important for determining each patient's screening regimen.

19.3.3 Screening Methodologies

PAP (Papanicolaou) Smear. A PAP smear is a procedure in which a small brush is used to collect cervical cells. These cells can be tested for human papilloma virus (HPV) and can be analyzed under a microscope to look for changes that could be consistent with cancer. The HPV types that are tested for are high-risk subtypes that are known to cause oncogenic transformation in cervical epithelial cells.

Special Considerations

Transgender Men: Self-collection of HPV specimens, while not FDA approved, may be appropriate for individuals for whom speculum insertion may be physically challenging and emotionally traumatic and thus a barrier to accessing care. Atrophy due to testosterone treatment can make the testing challenging as well and increase the rates of unsatisfactory pap tests. In a study comparing self-collected tests in transgender men to health care professional collected tests, there was a 71.4% concordance in results of samples.

Transgender Women: Neovaginas constructed via gender affirming surgery do not require routine cytologic testing.

19.3.4 Screening Recommendations

Average Risk Patients: In average risk patients, screening is recommended by ACOG, American Society for Colposcopy and Cervical Pathology (ASCCP), and Society for Gynecologic Oncologists (SGO) starting at age 21 (Table 19.3). ACS released updated guidelines in 2020 raising screening age initiation to 25 years old given the

Table 19.3 Screening guidelines in average risk patients

Population	Recommendation
<21 years old	No screening
21–29 years old	Cytology alone every 3 years
30–65 years old	Cytology every 3 years or high-risk HPV testing every 5 years or high-risk HPV testing and cytology every 5 years
>65 years old	No screening if adequate negative prior screening results
Hysterectomy with removal of cervix	No screening if no history of high grade cervical precancerous lesions or cervical cancer

availability of the HPV vaccine. However, while HPV vaccination rates are improving nationwide, racial and socioeconomic disparities still exist making both vaccinations and screening rates below target levels more broadly. An increase in screening age to 25 years old could exacerbate these existing health care inequities. Data from several RCTs, cohort studies, and modeling studies have demonstrated that HPV based cervical cancer screening has superior sensitivity and longer term negative predictive value than cytology alone. Thus, current guidelines state that patients between the ages of 30 and 65 should receive high risk (hr) HPV testing alone every 5 years, cytology alone every 3 years, or co-testing every 5 years. Given the natural history of the disease, it is not recommended for patients under the age of 29 to receive high-risk HPV co-testing, as it can result in more harm than benefit. Regarding when to stop testing, two consecutive negative HPV tests or co-tests or three consecutive negative cytology tests within the past 10 years after the age of 65 years old are adequate to end testing. Additionally, if a patient has a life expectancy limiting diagnosis before the age of 65 years old, it is also appropriate to cease testing.

High-Risk Patients: In high-risk patients, namely those who have previously received a diagnosis of a high grade precancerous cervical lesion, were exposed to diethylstilbestrol in utero, or those with HIV, more intensive screening is recommended. In patients with HIV, annual screening with cytology and high-risk HPV co-testing is recommended by the CDC and after 3 years of consecutive normal cytology results and negative HPV testing, the screening interval can be spaced to every 3 years. Annual cytology and co-testing are recommended in those individuals in the other aforementioned high-risk categories.

19.3.5 Benefits and Harms of Screening

The main benefits of cervical cancer screening include decreased mortality from cervical cancer and early detection and thus early intervention. An optimal screening regimen for cervical cancer will maximize these benefits while reducing harm. Some of the harms related to screening and diagnostic procedures include psychological distress and anxiety, bleeding and cramping from repeated pelvic examinations, pain and infection from coloscopy, preterm deliveries, and overall overdiagnosis and overtreatment. It is important to both adhere to the guidelines and engage in shared decision-making with our primary care patients regarding frequency, initiation, and cessation of screening.

19.3.6 Summary

Regular breast and cervical cancer screening are incredibly important for reducing mortality from and increasing the chances of early detection of these cancers. A thorough history can help with risk stratification of these patients. Adhering to guidelines in combination with shared decision-making with our patients allows us to weight risks and benefits of screening tests and recommend appropriate screening regimens for both cancers.

Suggested Reading

1. Surveillance, Epidemiology, and End Results (SEER) program. https://seer.cancer.gov/statfacts/html/breast.html. Cancer Stat Facts: Female Breast Cancer. 1975–2020.
2. Breast cancer risk assessment and screening in average-risk women: ACOG practice bulletin, number 179. Obstet Gynecol. 2017;130(1):e98–e109.
3. Dyrstad SW, Yan Y, Fowler AM, Colditz GA. Breast cancer risk associated with benign breast disease: systematic review and meta-analysis. Breast Cancer Res Treat. 2015;149:569–75.
4. Page DL, Kidd TE Jr, Dupont WD, Simpson JF, Rogers LW. Lobular neoplasia of the breast: higher risk for subsequent invasive cancer predicted by more extensive disease. Hum Pathol. 1991;22:1232–9.
5. Warner ET, Colditz GA, Palmer JR, Partridge AH, Rosner BA, Tamimi RM. Reproductive factors and risk of premenopausal breast cancer by age at diagnosis: are there differences before and after age 40? Breast Cancer Res Treat. 2013;142(1):165–75.
6. Anderson KN, Schwab RB, Martinez ME. Reproductive risk factors and breast cancer subtypes: a review of the literature. Breast Cancer Res Treat. 2014;144(1):1–10.
7. Chlebowski RT, Rohan TE, Manson JE, Aragaki AK, Kaunitz A, Stefanick ML, Simon MS, Johnson KC, Wactawski-Wende J, O'Sullivan MJ, Adams-Campbell LL, Nassir R, Lessin LS, Prentice RL. Breast cancer after use of estrogen plus progestin and estrogen alone: analyses of data from 2 women's health initiative randomized clinical trials. JAMA Oncol. 2015;1(3):296–305.
8. Henderson TO, Amsterdam A, Bhatia S, Hudson MM, Meadows AT, Neglia JP, Diller LR, Constine LS, Smith RA, Mahoney MC, Morris EA, Montgomery LL, Landier W, Smith SM, Robison LL, Oeffinger KC. Systematic review: surveillance for breast cancer in women treated with chest radiation for childhood, adolescent, or young adult cancer. Ann Intern Med. 2010;152(7):444–55. W144-154
9. Hartmann LC, Degnim AC, Santen RJ, Dupont WD, Ghosh K. Atypical hyperplasia of the breast – risk assessment and management options. NEJM. 2015;372(1):78–89.
10. Roa BB, Boyd AA, Volcik K, Richards CS. Ashkenazi Jewish population frequencies for common mutations in BRCA1 and BRCA2. Nat Genet. 1996;14:185–7.
11. Hereditary Breast and Ovarian Cancer Syndrome. ACOG Practice Bulletin, Number 103 (Revised: 182). Obstet Gynecol. 2017; Obstet Gynecol. 2009;113(4):957–66.
12. Health Care for Transgender and Gender Diverse Individuals. ACOG Pract Bull. 202;1823.
13. Surveillance, Epidemiology, and End Results (SEER) program. https://seer.cancer.gov/statfacts/html/breast.html. Cancer Stat Facts: Cervical Cancer. 1975–2020.
14. Screening for Cervical Cancer: ACOG Practice Bulletin, Number 131. Obstet Gynecol. 2012;120(5):1222–38.
15. Fontham ETH, Wolf AMD, Church TR, Etzioni R, Flowers CR, Herzig A, Guerra CE, Oeffinger KC, Shih YT, Walter LC, Kim JJ, Andrews KS, DeSantis CE, Fedewa SA, Manassaram-Baptiste D, Saslow D, Wender RC, Smith R. Cervical cancer screening for individuals at average risk: 2020 guideline update from the American Cancer Society. CA Cancer J Clin. 2020;70(5):321–46.

Index

© The Editor(s) (if applicable) and The Author(s), under exclusive license to
Springer Nature Switzerland AG 2024
M. Mahmoudi (ed.), *Common Cases in Women's Primary Care Clinics*,
https://doi.org/10.1007/978-3-031-48569-5